"WOW I started reading Sebern's book and 30-something pages in there are so many things that I've related to in a way that is almost beyond words. Like I keep starting to cry and not even fully knowing the reason - just feeling like she is articulating something so deep and fundamental that I've never experienced being reflected externally. And I too have had recurring dreams about kittens left in my care dying or nearly dying - it's eerie! Thank you for sharing it with me - you're doing a real service getting it out into the world and please thank her for me"

— J.W. JOURNALIST

"Some thoughts/feelings on experiencing your book: I couldn't read it and I couldn't not. Anger, fury, shame, fascination - all erupted without rhythm or mercy. How dare she speak all of this! These truths are to be hidden, banished, not allowed. I wanted to banish the scapegoat, silence her, hurl stones at her like those men in the Bible when Christ, drawing in the dust, dared them to begin. This is like Christ whom we would crucify again if we cannot look in the mirror. And through it all, the shards of memory too sharp to hold, a flame flickered. It was not steady but luminous and it kept drawing me in - it lured me in with a powerful magnetic force. I kept reading more and more and again and again. I couldn't turn away. I read until I cried and quietly wept for the child parts in me so brutally violated and abandoned, shamed, scattered and literally left voiceless. And I read yet again. I am now discovering new depths of compassion and this too is a painful journey. For the rest of my life I will be exploring this book in me, this book in every person I work with, from a vantage point beyond the hell and suffering."

— HELENA BESTER, TRAUMA THERAPIST

In *The Hidden Book of First Things*, Sebern Fisher does something rare and courageous - she turns the clinician's gaze inward, weaving her lived experience of a fragmented self together with the hard-won wisdom of a master therapist. The result is a book that illuminates, from the inside, what so many clients struggle to put into words and offers practitioners a depth of understanding that no textbook can provide. This is essential reading for those who have walked this terrain themselves, and for every clinician who sits with them.

— Ed Hamlin, PhD., Clinical Director,
Institute for Applied Neuroscience

Sebern's masterful use of metaphor took me to that place where there are no words, only feelings. Feelings of being deeply held and understood. A feeling of peace because there is a reason for the "me"□ that didn't exist for decades, the "me"□ that exists now, and the "me" that is a work in progress. A feeling that I am worthy and deserving of the many treatments I've needed. The shame of needing so many treatments drifted away.

I don't know how women with severe trauma histories get through life without neurofeedback.

— Debbie Asplen Ingraham

The Hidden Book of First Things

The Hidden Book of First Things

Sebern F. Fisher

Sebern F. Fisher
The Hidden Book of First Things

Printed in the United States of America.

Published by Spines
ISBN: 979-8-90419-375-1

Spines

For my mother

Contents

Preface

As you will come to see, this memoir is not about me. It is a memoir of becoming me. It is a memoir of the aftermath that almost everyone who has a history of severe childhood trauma suffers. It is a memoir of how a child's mind develops when they lose their mother. It is a memoir of a profound therapeutic relationship, and some may think of it as a radical 'treatment.' It is a memoir of my brain, its alignment with the absence of my parents, and its adaptations to events I discovered while writing the journal on which this book depends. Because it is taken from journals I kept over the years, this book unfolds in a facsimile of 'real time.' You will learn what happened as I do.

It is a memoir about memory, in the mind, the brain, and the body. It is about the experience of 'body memories' and the therapists who took me through them as they arose and arose again. It is a memoir about identity and a memoir about race. It is the story of turning slowly, almost blindly, toward what happened to me, what didn't happen and what happened within me as a result. My interior world echoed. It had no landscape. There was no horizon.

There is an inescapable paradox in writing about the absence of self and other, particularly as I am doing so, from within it. As you read, you may find yourself feeling lost, without bearings. If you can, join me there. Go with it. I am writing, I had to write of it, from it, not about it. I am writing from the inchoate 'presence of absence' experienced in some way by every child whose mother has turned away. This is the core of early childhood trauma, not the events, the absence.

I think if I understood what others mean when they say recovery, this would be a book about recovery. But recovery is about disease. There is a state of wellness before the onset of illness that you return to when you recover. I could never find that state of wellness or wholeness. There was no 'before.' There is no disease. And yet, I did recover. It was not will or understanding. It was, in a way that was not even personal, but the triumph of life force when it is recognized, nurtured, and challenged, when it is demanded of. Everyone traumatized as a young child has no choice but to identify with what happened. It is impossible not to; it is you. 'Healing' from an identity may not be possible, but healing a brain injury is. It is the imperative of the brain, as much as it is the imperative of bone or skin. As a colleague of mine said, "The brain privileges its own regulation. It has to." This is a memoir of healing my brain and, directly as a result, discovering a mind.

The book begins in stanzas. You can read it as a tone poem. This is a memoir of interior life that is never, if it stays true, a story. I came into psychotherapy mummified by the stories I had, and often told, of significant mental illness. At some point, I wrote, "The story was the container. It had protected me from seeing what the story was about."

Arles, the therapist you will meet, recognized that I did not understand the tragedy of the story I told, and, more importantly, he saw how little of 'me' there was in telling it. He insisted on my presence in the room and on my recognizing his; neither came readily. Establishing 'self' and 'other' had to be the first order in therapy. What is therapy without the self and the other, without him and me? He saw me through episodes of flashback that overtook me, and he cared for me in their aftermath. He taught me the rules of relationships that I had missed. But it was a steep learning curve for me and often frustrating for him. It is important to say that neither he nor I is recommending the psychotherapy that I am writing about. Like any other deep relationship, its conditions arise from within it. It does underscore, however, the need to establish attachment where it has failed, and the great difficulty in doing so.

In the course of the memoir, I learn that the traumatized brain, my brain, is significantly different from one that is not. One of those ways is the failure of the Default Mode Network, the network that underwrites Self and Other in the brain. I didn't have a Self to bring to Arles, and I couldn't recognize the reality of a Self in him. His insistence that I do so, though, was crucial to its development. He became the being around which I began to scaffold my own. He was the spinal column. He gave me the template of Self and Other. But he could not give me the brain for it.

I met Ruth Lanius, the eminent trauma researcher, in a workshop Bessel van der Kolk asked me to give on neurofeedback for his staff at the Trauma Center. I taught Ruth about neurofeedback, and she taught me about the Default Mode Network. Generally speaking, this network develops naturally when children are cared for 'well enough.' Arles and I were trying to establish a brain network with psychotherapy. I don't think it can be done. My brain was wild with absence and fear. The eruptions in me began with those in my brain, which I could not control. Neurofeedback quieted them and prompted the activation of the Default Mode Network in my brain. Without neurofeedback, I would have lived within the adaptations I had already made to no core self, to ambient terror, to the thrall of absence. Most do. I would have understood it better, but I would have, like most trauma survivors, lived with it. It was pure chance that I came across my brain and how to help it—I found one when I found the other—and I don't want it to be pure chance for you. I am in a privileged position to have trained my brain, and it comes with this responsibility: to tell you about it.

Throughout my course of treatment as a trauma patient, I was a therapist treating trauma patients. When I felt the changes that neurofeedback brought in me, I needed to learn it. When I did, I offered neurofeedback to my patients, some of whom you will meet. I continued in therapy, and I continued to train my brain. I wrote a professional book about neurofeedback and psychotherapy, *Neurofeedback in the Treatment of Developmental Trauma: Calming the Fear-*

Driven Brain, published in 2014. This book you are about to begin will bring you into the brain as it changes the mind. This is, perhaps most importantly, a neurofeedback memoir. I will ask of you what I ask of my patients, that once neurofeedback begins, you relate everything—everything—to the brain that is changing. Neurofeedback is always the first thing to be ruled out. In this memoir, it can never be.

The text will not identify the early changes I experienced with training my brain because I didn't recognize them. Look for them. Had I understood it, the first change would have helped me appreciate the instability of my brain. It happens in front of Ted's Boot Shop. I feared that I might plummet through the plate-glass window. When I wrote about this in my journal, I had no recall of the session I'd had with Arles just before it. I still don't. This, too, the explosion of terror and amnesia for it, most likely related to the new demand I was putting on my brain, but neither Arles nor I recognized it.

As my brain regulates itself, everything begins to quiet. I begin to recognize myself and to recognize Arles. I become more able to comment on the effects training is having. An encounter with one's own brain is profound, particularly so when you can nudge it into its own functionality, or momentarily, with the wrong protocol, into its own dysfunction. Training could change a snarl to a smile, a state of terror to a sense of ease.

I did have setbacks with this brain, and these are often what I write about. I used the journal to write about the interior of the state I was in, just to bear it, and these states arose fiercely and almost exclusively when Arles went away on a trip or was absent with me in the room. Neither of these happened more than would happen in any therapeutic relationship. In terms of absence in the room, I think much less. His presence was foundational. It could seem so, however, reading this memoir, because that is when I needed the most to write. His absence was not bearable. This changes too, and you will be there with me as it happens.

Neurofeedback opened the door to my brain and paved the way for other therapies. I tried hyperbaric oxygen (HBOT), hemoencephalography (HEG), the Listening Program, the Symmetron, Nexalin, acupressure, the Rosen Method and trauma-informed physical therapy. So many of these histories are written in the body. I'll tell you about these, too. They all helped. And throughout this time, I was becoming a meditator, but as those who are also meditators know, meditation is not a treatment. Before neurofeedback, I could only inhabit the form of meditation, but as I gained a mind, I was also gaining the practice to work with it, to settle it.

This book is in your hands now. If you are a trauma therapist, I hope it helps you to better understand and treat your most complicated patients. Although this may not be the psychotherapy you want to offer or should, it does lay open what people with histories like these, many far worse than mine, need. Attune to motherlessness in your patient and know that you just cannot address it without regulating the motherless brain. It's not your failure or your patient's failure; it's the brain, and you will want to learn how to help it regulate. If you are a trauma patient, I offer you my interior experience and hope it might help you put words to the unspeakable, to seek out a therapist who understands what you are saying and one who will help you train your brain. If you are reading this book because you are trying to understand the complex and difficult experience of a traumatized relative or friend, bless you. I think it will help. Meditation halls in the US are filled with people trying to address terrible trauma early in their lives. If you are reading this as a meditator or a meditation teacher, I hope it helps you to appreciate the brain and its reluctant but persistent adaptations to its earliest experiences. Trauma is neurological before it is psychological. It was my brain that threw me off the cushion, and you will see that change as well.

Standard trauma treatments are failing traumatized patients; these patients are not failing their treatment. They are not "treatment resistant." They suffer from these failures. They suffer believing it signals something inherently broken in them, and they are further degraded by it. They are failing trauma therapists, too. Therapists suffer in a different way. They are taught that therapy, if they do it right, will help their traumatized patients, and when it doesn't, they can resent the patient, get angry at themselves, and become disheartened with their profession. All too many learn to turn these, the most injured, patients away.

I wrote this memoir to describe the aftermath of absence and abuse from the interior of it and to lay bare its complexity. I wrote it to better understand my brain and my mind that arose through it. I wrote to provide a narrative for the brain that cannot speak, so that you might hear its plea. I wrote so you would know that you can help this brain, injured so profoundly by what happens and what doesn't happen early in its own history and that when you do, you, or your patient, your friend or your student will get better.

The therapy I had with Arles is not replicable, but the understanding that developed within it, I hope, informs every therapy. The core dilemma is attachment failure. The core dilemma is the absence of a key brain network. Neurofeedback is replicable, and every person who has endured these childhoods should have access to it.

By the time you finish this book, you will understand why I begin by saying this memoir is not about me. With Arles and neurofeedback, I established a 'me' and then astonishing things happened.

One last important note. Although neurofeedback is essential in the treatment of trauma, as you will see, it is not specifically a treatment for trauma. Human consciousness is encoded in the brain's frequencies. Appealing to these frequencies can change the nature of that consciousness and how it expresses itself in mind and body. Join me here and watch this happen.

Part One

Chapter 1

Hall of Mirrors

This past weekend, I touched down in a state of madness. I went to Cape Cod.

My mother lives in a small white house on a pretty tree-lined street in Yarmouth Port, with blue hydrangeas. Inside, handrails are missing, and the floor moves. Everything that was true the last time we talked is no longer. She constructs my collapse as her tragedy. I am not there, in her mind. Hurt and angry, she tells me that it is all in the past, it's over. I wonder now what else I could have done to right myself. My mother beckons me and turns away.

When I was eight, and my sister Kevy was five, she insisted on coming with me into the Fun House at Playland. My mother gave up more than she agreed, sat down on a bench, and lit a cigarette. When we arrived in the Hall of Mirrors, Kevy froze in place and started to scream. I huddled over her and pushed her against a stream of kids to get out the way we'd come in. Something stopped us. I started to lose track of which way was which. Her panic ricocheted. Other kids turned and stared at us, the only focal point. A door opened in the wall. A man grabbed Kevy's arm, pulled her out and closed the panel. I caught a glimpse of plywood and a bare wooden beam, and then I was back in the Hall of Mirrors.

I slip in and out of a malaise as heavy as the August air. It is wordless. I have chronic inflammatory disease: my lower back, my neck, my shoulders, my left arm, and the juncture between the first and second finger. Migraine. The broken neck, the concussions, the loss of teeth, the psychosis. I needed all of it.

I don't think about recovery anymore. There is no 'before.'

MEETING THE BUDDHA 1990

"Oh, you are Madame Fisher! What a problem!"

The owner of the little hotel greeted me. She looked around her behind the counter and came up with the telex from my mother's office. "We have no room for you... But fortunately, a man checked out a day early! Now we have a room!"

I stowed my stuff with her, and after getting my ticket at the Gare d'Austerlitz, I walked back through the Jardin du Plants, exhausted. I tried to practice mindfulness at the edge of the rose garden, beneath the sky that alternated between hopeful and hopeless.

I must stop now to prepare for tea meditation. I have made it here. Thich Nhat Hanh, Thầy to everyone here, will give an orientation talk tonight in the Lower Hamlet. It's cold and raining. I didn't bring a sweater. Today I spent 3 hours in semi-sleep in my bedroom in the old farmhouse, "The Middle Hamlet." When I registered, I heard others refusing this placement, but I don't understand why. I have it to myself.

I want to remember the plump French woman on the train, my mother's age, in her oversized gray cardigan, who offered me her magazine. I could only read the horoscope. I was shy, embarrassed that I didn't know the language. She understood then that I spoke no French. She tried speaking softly and slowly, using gestures. I only understood her kindness. (Mlle Calais took me aside after our last class at the end of my sophomore year in high school. She whispered, like a conspirator, asking what language I was taking next year. I hadn't decided between Latin and French. She made me an offer: "If you take Latin, I will give you a 'B' for the year. If you take French, a 'C'.") This is a retreat for psychotherapists and Vietnam vets in the home of a Vietnamese diaspora and Thich Nhat Hanh's retreat center, Plum Village. That war, as it was waged in me, at Columbia and on the streets of New York, is fresh and raw. I watch the men who I think are vets. Vietnamese is the first language here. The rain beat relentlessly on the metal roof.

"We fall back into the past, we leap ahead into the future, and in that we lose our entire lives."

When Thầy finished speaking, I was crying and smiling at the same moment. He tells us to rest.

I come to measure the speed of my mind in judgments per second. I envy the 'in group' for their specialness, for their comfort with each other and with being here; for leaving me out, the fat child.

MAITRI MEDITATION

Monday: Loving kindness and deep, clear sadness seem inextricable. Sadness does not feel at all like suffering.

Tuesday: Constant pushing to keep my heart open; not to be ashamed of the migraine; not to be ashamed of asking for help. I talked with Evie, who told me that it was beginning to get harder for everyone she'd spoken with. She reminds me of what I've just told her: This is my first retreat, I don't speak any of the languages, including Buddhist, and I am alone in the Middle Hamlet.

Wednesday: I can hardly lift my body. I went into that semi-hallucinogenic state for two hours. Margot's arrival interrupted me. As I lay in my bed, not yet dressed, she taught me a bit more about Buddhism and its cultural adaptations. She encouraged me to come with her and the others to Bergerac. We walked through the farmers' market, looked in shops on the side streets, and stopped at the sound of every bell, the quickly established practice of Plum Village. There were many bells. I bought a washcloth.

Thursday: Writing practice with Natalie. Her instructions are "Keep your hand going; come from first thoughts; you are free to write the worst shit in the world..." Her first prompt was "I remember..." We wrote for fifteen minutes from that. Her second prompt was "I don't remember..."

I think of my mother, my neck, my possible paralysis. I tried to imagine the reality of the loss of my body- that I would not be able to brush the fly away from my eyes, that I would have no feeling in my skin, that John would have to carry me and that he would. I had never thought before of losing all sensation, of being so dependent, of my body limp... I stopped these thoughts then, as I am trying to do tonight. I don't want them. I need to keep away from the reality it may be. The chord is tightly pressed in the narrow column—no hands to hold a pen, just a mouth and failing teeth. I brought it on myself. I took a swan dive off the high hospital bed. I watched that moment, that decision in the making, my hands clasped behind my back, hand in hand so as not to break the fall.

I don't remember my father. I can't find him anywhere except for that curl in the nail of my left middle finger. Blake has it too. I hear people around me crying. If I can't find him, I want at least to find the grief of losing him. It was a grief I buried, not with him, but when I turned toward Charlie Boren, my psychiatrist at the Institute of Living.

Friday: It was six am and thirty of us watched Thầy walk toward us across the field. We had all received handwritten invitations for Tea with Thầy. At the door to the small hall, he slipped off his clogs, stepped through the doorway, and the door slammed after him. I startled. He came back out and went in again, closing the door gently.

We sat in a large circle. He asked us to enjoy our tea. I looked around, and for many of us, this was performance. He then asked each one to tell him why we had come. There were those who had left monasteries in the East after years of practice to take a different path. There were those who had suffered tragic loss. There was a vet from what we call the Vietnam War, what they call the American War. When he got to me, I bowed to him, as we all did, and he to me. "I have no practice, Thầy. I have no story to tell, really. A patient of mine—I am a psychotherapist—brought me a copy of Common Boundary, where you wrote about therapy and Buddhism. I read what you wrote, but it wasn't that. I saw the photo of you and knew immediately that you had something to teach me, something that I didn't know. At the end, there was a notice about this retreat. That's why I'm here, because I saw your picture." I felt a little embarrassed at the paucity of my motivation. Everyone else in this circle had much more important stories. After breakfast, we gathered with everyone else for Thầy's dharma talk. It had taken me almost half of the retreat, and then I got it, in a kind of "Aha" moment, that he'd been teaching Buddhist psychology. We sang a few songs, and then Thầy opened the morning's talk:

"No one came to the Buddha for his teachings. They came to him because of his presence."

The week before my patient gave me the magazine, I'd been traveling with John in Costa Rica. We were staying in a small hut a short path up from the Atlantic, and I dreamt in the lapping of the waves.

I was on a quest to find the iridescent orchid. I was alone in a cave that was pitch black and dripping water. I couldn't see my way. There was a soft voice of a man whom I had never seen, encouraging me to step carefully but to move forward. I found my way through by feel, touching the rocks, under, over, guided only by his voice. Finally, I came to a large opening. There was a flower, more like a tulip than an orchid, growing in the center of the clearing. As soon as I saw it, it burst into flames. The ashes held the form of the flower before they dropped away, and there, a small pink bud.

I am assaulted by my judgments. I must learn to lay out all the imaginable reasons for a person's behavior before me and not choose any of them.

The last night at the zendo, I'd walked like Quasimodo in the movies: stance wide for balance, heavy foot falls only an inch or so forward at a time, trying to pass through a neurological storm that threatened to throw me off my feet. I feared that if I tried to leave, I would crash through the glass wall; that if I tried to lie down, I would fall, floppy as a dog's ear. I walked that night, mindfully, right through it. I never liked to spin as a child. I did it, though, until I fell into a swirling heap, the sky rocking above me. At some point, this 'high,' shared by every kid in the neighborhood, smiled on by parents, turned into a nightmare. For me, leaving the steady plane of routine earth threatened that I would never return.

Thầy asked us to read a poem at the closing ceremony. I, who started this retreat alone, wrote and read two phrases, "We are apart; we are a part."

When I left, I was just beginning to learn how to walk and how to breathe.

Carl is in county jail. They called and asked me to see him because they were worried about his state. He has 'aged out' of the Center where I'd been treating him for six years. He taught me the reality of the attachment catastrophe, but his lessons were bleak and repetitive. He could not learn. I have no idea what he thinks about, but I know how his mind works.

The guard took me to his cell. He was a little, sad, terrified, homeless 18-year-old boy. He said he'd never felt so bad. He pleaded to go home, which, as had been the case throughout his life, was nowhere. I'd never seen him feel anything nearly as true to his circumstances as this moment. Every rejection, every failure, every loss, he'd collapsed under his history like an old roof under a downpour. He broke my heart, and I knew, all the same, that I was not real to him. I had never been. That was the treatment failure. I hugged him as I left, thinking now, in his despair, there is hope. I called the jail the next day, and the officer said, "Whatever you did was great. He's not depressed anymore."

I visited Charlie at the Institute in his second-floor executive office that floats in magnolia blossoms.

"I understand now that your response was," I looked around as if I'd find the word out there, "measured." He smiled slightly and said that it was good to finally hear me acknowledge this. It *was* poor judgment to swim across the Connecticut River with Marsha in April that year. But we were kids. But it was hot. We were unlocked. The muck we'd walked through to get to this little strip of beach was foul. I was a good swimmer. Marsha said she was, too.

ARLES GABRIEL

I called Arles in early November after a brief return to Westchester to talk with my uncle and with Kate, our caretaker. She talked about my mother's affair, an affair evidently going on before my father's death. She told me that my father gave my brother sleeping pills to keep him from wandering in the night. Hugh slid down the drainpipe outside his room and took my mother's car. She called Kevy a "walking rip," meaning, in Irish, that she was angry and "spoilt." She said we were all spoilt, running wild, and that our parents were too involved with themselves. Too much alcohol. Too many parties. Too little attention. My uncle spoke freely, as if to his biographer, about my father's long affair with his secretary. My mother once referred to a fling he'd had and had, at least to me, written it off to the nature of men. He also told me that my dad was involved in tax fraud. My mother once said that they were audited every year because my father turned into an agent for attempted bribery. I hadn't known any of this.

I told my friend, Eva, and she responded, "You went to Westchester to open some doors that you know you need to walk through."

I heard a door open, then softly close. It was ten minutes past the hour. I sat in the waiting room at the end of the long hall that had taken me, I assumed, past his office door. I folded my black pea coat over my lap and looked straight ahead at the wall. Then I tried to read the New Yorker with the torn cover. I heard a door open at the far end and footsteps approaching. I gathered my coat closer and shoved it, bunched under my arm, as I rose to shake his hand. His grip was secure. He was tall, lean, almost angular and dressed in black silk trousers, a black T and a black silk jacket. His greeting was warm.

It was his voice that brought me there, like a promise. I'd responded to a flier for a dream group for therapists. I would tell the dream of the iridescent orchid. He'd described his thoughts about the group, but I heard only the resonance and depth of his voice. I asked to be his patient.

I sank into his dark windowless office, two black leather chairs and a long black analytic couch, soft headrests at both ends; a smell of Twinings tea and vanilla; incense; books around the ring base of his chair—Adrienne Rich, Buddhism, Lacan. I sat on the middle cushion of the couch and laid my coat down beside me. The silence pooled around my ears.

"I am swimming slowly down into a translucent sea, circling around a Lucite pillar, no equipment but my body, taking air from within the water. No desperation; no fear; slow, steady, circling downward."

"Fetal fish." His voice was silk.

He startled me.

"I want to go beneath the story. I am trapped in my story."

"Yes, we shall go there, but I think first you need to tell me the story."

STORY

Age 5- Diagnosis: behavioral and learning problems. Treatment: Held back
Age 12-Thrown off the tall bay horse onto a rock. Diagnosis: None. Treatment: None
Age 13- Refuse father's bedtime kiss
Age 13- Father hospitalized. Diagnosis: Heart attack
Age 15- Brother kills elderly couple in a car accident. Diagnosis: Drunk
Age 16- Father dies. Diagnosis: Cardiac arrest; Cirrhosis.
Age 16- Disheveled. School counselor- Diagnosis: Depression
Age 17- Weight loss of 40 lbs. (three months). Diagnosis: Obesity. Treatment: Dexamyl
Age 18- Post wisdom teeth extraction tumbled down the concrete stairs. 10 days in the college infirmary. Diagnosis: Concussion. Treatment: Rest; Drop Spanish

Age 19- Date rape. Diagnosis: None. Treatment: Alcohol, Bridge
Age 20- Self-harm. Diagnosis: Schizophrenia. Treatment: Hospitalization, ECT; Thorazine; Stelazine; Mellaril; Amytal injections; Seclusion rooms
Age 20- Can't remember movies or childhood. Diagnosis: "Not ECT"
Age 20-21- Hospitalization, 1 year. Intake diagnosis: Schizophrenia. Discharge diagnosis: Emotionally dysregulated personality. Prognosis: Guarded. Treatment: Charles Boren, MD
Age 21- Raped. Diagnosis: "Any woman who goes to a man's apartment is asking for this." - my psychiatrist, Milici
Age 21- Overdose. 3-day coma. Diagnosis: Schizophrenia; Anorexia. Treatment: Hospitalization: Seclusion, Amytal injections; Residential treatment, 5 months. Thorazine, 1200 mg;
Therapy: Dr. Greenberg hands me a white plastic whistle on a lanyard - "Blow this when you get anxious." Thorazine, 1200 mg; 400-600 mg Tuinal hs
Age 21- Psychotic break. Hospitalized. I was in a bowling alley. Treatment: Thorazine; Forced feeding. Discharge: Financial. Return to Columbia
Age 21- Diagnosis (mother's): hypoglycemia
Age 21- Stomach and bowel pain: Diagnosis: Ulcerative Colitis
Age 22- Head-on collision, 80 mph; front seat, no seatbelt. Unconscious. Hospitalized. Diagnosis: Compression of the spine, broken ribs, concussion. Treatment: Discharge
Age 22- Self-harm. Young NYPD officer held my forehead together, his sweat, my blood flowing over his white knuckles. 44 stitches. Hospitalized for 3 months. Diagnosis: Schizophrenia
Age 23- Headlights on turnpike create visions in me: Neurology resident at Columbia neurology clinic. Diagnosis: Schizophrenia in remission; Treatment: Psychiatry
Age 23- (2 weeks later) Neurology clinic: Psychiatrist. Diagnosis: Not schizophrenia, Temporal lobe epilepsy. Treatment: Dilantin
Age 23- Dental clinic, Diagnosis: Abscess. Treatment: Tooth extraction
Age 24- Weight 83 lbs., Hospitalization. Diagnosis: Schizophrenia; Anorexia. Swan dive. Diagnosis: Concussion; 6-hour coma. 16 days gone. Diagnosis: Psychotic amnesia. Discharge diagnosis: Post-

psychotic depression. Ecstatic- I understand "Lucy in the Sky with Diamonds!"
Age 24- Hospitalization. Diagnosis: Anorexia
Age 24- Diagnosis (mine): Lock-jaw. Could not talk, eat, or swallow. Electromyography with German precision. Diagnosis: Hysteria; Anorexia
Age 24- Hypnosis. 2 sessions. 2nd session on the couch in my mini skirt and T-shirt. Instruction: 'Wiggle around.' Didn't. Discharge diagnosis: 'I can't help you.'
Age 24- Abdominal pain. Howling on the exam. GYN Diagnosis: Nothing wrong here; Hysteria
Age 24- (10 days later) ER. Diagnosis: R/O ectopic pregnancy. Appendicitis. Emergency appendectomy. Woman in the hall: "Now you are getting what you always wanted, you're the center of attention."
Age 24- (3 weeks later) Mount Sinai, Swallowing Disorders clinic. Diagnosis: Abnormal pattern seen only in grand mal epilepsy; Diagnosis: Tardive dyskinesia, severe
Age 24- Internist, Ray: "They tell me you will die if you are off these medications. You will definitely die on them." Diagnosis: Death weight 79 lbs.; medicinal poisoning. Treatment: Withdrawal from Thorazine, Stelazine, Mellaril; begin Talwin by injection, sodium amytal
Age 24- Married John
Age 24- Adopted his troubled son, Johnny, age 5. Yale. Diagnosis: Infantile schizophrenia (rare) (wrong)
Age 24- My dog, Trace of Treasure, dies. Diagnosis: Cancer. Treatment: Palliative care; Euthanasia
Age 24- Ray dies. Diagnosis: Heart attack. Cause of death: Suicide
Age 25- Columbia-Presbyterian Medical Center Diagnosis: Migraine
Age 26- Arrested during a sit-in at Columbia. Strip search; cavity search; jailed
Age 26- Dental clinic, Diagnosis: Abscess. Treatment: Tooth extraction
Age 27- Diagnosis: Pregnancy. Referral for genetic counseling.
Age 27- Diagnosis: Miscarriage.
Age 27- Diagnosis: Pregnancy, referral for genetic counseling. Counselor, Epilepsy Foundation: "So you're going to bring another freak into the world?!"

Age 27- A security guard threatens me with his cigarette. Diagnosis: Deja vu
Age 28- NICU: 5lb 8 oz girl, Diagnosis: Grand mal seizure
Age 28- 3-month-old baby girl, Blake, Diagnosis: Pneumonia. Treatment: Antibiotics
Age 28- 5-month-old Blake, Diagnosis: Pneumonia. Treatment: Antibiotics
Age 28- Held up at knifepoint in elevator. Diagnosis: Heroin addiction (his), Rage (mine).
Age 28- 7-month-old Blake, Diagnosis: Pneumonia. Treatment: Antibiotics.
Age 28- 8-month-old Blake, Tentative diagnosis: Cystic fibrosis. (wrong) Treatment: Leave New York
Age 29- Dentist, Diagnosis: Abscess, Treatment: Tooth extraction
Age 30- Dentist, Diagnosis: Abscess, Treatment: Tooth extraction - wrong tooth, a healthy one
Age 31- Johnny, age 12. Passed out, vodka. Diagnosis: Post-Traumatic Stress Syndrome
Age 35- Child neighbor, Molly, was sexually molested and hospitalized. Diagnosis: PTSD. Treatment: Foster placement
Age 35- Molly steals a car. Arrested in Florida. Diagnosis: Truant, PTSD
Age 35- Molly, a homeless, foster child, runner, joins our family. Treatment: Special school; Case management; Us.
Age 35- Sister, Kevy, hospitalized. Diagnosis: Aplastic anemia, Treatment: Palliative care
Age 35- Kevy dies. Diagnosis: Aplastic anemia, Childhood neglect
Age 37- Proud on the chinning bar. Diagnosis: Concussion; Treatment: Rest
Age 37- Johnny was arrested for assault. Not guilty. Diagnosis: PTSD, alcoholism
Age 38- Mother sick. Diagnosis: Breast cancer. Treatment: Radical mastectomy
Age 38- Dentist, Diagnosis: Periodontal disease, Treatment: Surgery
Age 38- Discover lump. Diagnosis: Benign tumor, Treatment: Surgery
Age 40- Neurologist, Diagnosis: Abnormal Babinski response;

Temporal lobe epilepsy. Treatment: Gabapentin. Referral: Dartmouth Medical Center
Age 40- Dartmouth. Diagnosis: Severe stenosis of the neck. High risk of paralysis. Treatment recommendation: Surgery. Treatment sought: Acupressure
Age 42- Brother, Hugh, hospitalized. Diagnosis: Chronic Alcoholism; Cirrhosis
Age 42- ICU, Hugh bleeds out. Massage his ice blue feet. Diagnosis: Cirrhosis. Childhood neglect
Age 42- Johnny is sick. Diagnosis: HIV
Age 44- Johnny is sicker. Diagnosis: AIDS, Treatment: Ryan White Foundation; Antiretrovirals
Age 44- 52- Johnny, Multiple psychiatric hospitalizations. Diagnosis: PTSD, Psychotic features, Bipolar disorder, Depression, Anxiety, Paranoia, Alcoholism, AIDS dementia. Treatment: Psychiatry, Polypharmacy
Age 49- Diagnosis: Post-Traumatic Stress Syndrome; Agitated depression; Dissociative Disorder. Treatment: Arles Gabriel

Arles asks me to slow down. I wanted to be done with it.

Retrospective diagnoses: Developmental trauma; dissociation; attachment failure; traumatic brain injury; epilepsy; hypoglycemia; hyperglycemia; hypergraphia; learning disability; mood instability; episodes of traumatic psychosis; no free-standing mental illness; 'emotionally dysregulated personality.'

❧

Being with Arles brings on the terror and the old forbidden hope. I may have felt this first with Mary when she was hired to care for Hugh and me. I was six months old, and my mother was in the hospital for two weeks after an emergency appendectomy. Mary was an orphaned eighteen-year-old on her own in DC and, to her, taken in by my mother and father. I still talk with her now and again. As we ended our conversation last Saturday, Mary said, "You is still 'my lil girl' even now. I loved Huey too, but there was somin' special 'bout you. I were wid you when you start walkin.' I say, 'You can do it, come to me' and then you does!" She described me at first as a happy baby, but then wondered about this. There was that night when I was left to cry, and she took me upstairs and put me in bed with her. The next day, I was diagnosed with mumps. Mary got very sick with them three weeks later. It was, as a child, the last time I saw her.

Charlie was the next to provoke this yearning.

Now it is Arles.

It is time to dress for the sparkling 12° day and take the dogs on the walk I promised them two hours ago. They wanted the comfort of my closeness last night. The wind frightened them and me too, until I had the image of John Muir lashing himself to a yellow birch and riding out the storm the way the tree does.

I am in an airport, I think in the Northwest. My family is on the departure floor. I am on the main concourse. There is a terrible storm with rain slashing against the pane-glass windows, thunder, lightning, and high winds. The loudspeaker announced the flight was canceled. I was surprised it had not just been delayed. Then they explained it was canceled due to small but severe and unavoidable storms in Idaho. I was walking with my mother outside. She said she knew these places in Idaho because it was there that she had lost her eye. I was shocked. I'd never known that she lost an eye, I'd never noticed, and she was saying it as if this were no news at all. I looked at her face. Everything looked fine, regular. She said she remembered that place because she had been unable to save her eye. It was false.

"Even if I am hit by a drunk driver, Arles, hold me responsible. Before Charlie, no one held me responsible."

He looked at me, nodded and, in a voice a little louder than I'd heard, but not loud, he said, "Have no doubt I will. Make sure that doesn't happen."

This was unfair, and the protest began. "But that wouldn't be my fault. I have to find a better example."

"No, you don't, Sebern. I will hold you responsible."

I sat in the chair across from him and turned the water bottle over in my hands, stood and paced, sat again on the chair, accidentally dropped the water, and kicked it across the floor. I went to get it. He swiped it off the floor.

"I want a drink of water!"

"Tough." He put the bottle beside his chair. "You will have to wait."

My voice echoed in a space outside the theater of provocation. "Is this okay with you?"

"Yes." He paused and continued. "But let me put it this way, 'no couch, no session.'"

I sat down at the edge of the couch.

"That's a start. You can lean back and feel the couch hold you." I slid back slowly, wincing.

"What is that?"

"I have chronic pain in my lower back. I just felt it. My sacrum."

"Your sacrum? When did that begin?"

"I don't know, Arles, it just hurts and has forever."

"Your sacrum, your sacred place," he said. I settled into the couch to ease the strain in my back. I liked the smell of the gray wool blanket that I pulled over me.

"This treatment (I adopted his word) will take a long time. Will you be able to stay in it with me? It's a big commitment."

"Yes, Sebern, I understand this. You have a long road." He corrected himself. "We have a long road."

"Are you sure? It won't be easy."

"Oh, yes, I know that too." He held me steady with his voice. "I am sure."

Last night I slept for two hours. I dreamt, although the state seemed in and out of dreaming- *I was with Arles in his office. It was brightly lit. He was wearing a white Oxford shirt with a rumpled collar and a red plaid tie. I refused to sit on the couch. He insisted. I asked to leave to go to the bathroom. In the hall, which was also a city street, I realized he couldn't tell me what to do, and I could lie down on this couch in the hall, which was also a bench on the street. I did and pulled the blanket over me, noticing it was like the one from my office, not from his. I was waiting for him to find me. I could see him in the office looking bewildered. He'd told me that he was redoing the alcove in his office. He will be putting in a master bed and curtains over the round window, and he told me that he was planning to hang a plant from the center of the window. The whole arrangement materialized. He said I had a choice: the couch or the bed. I fell asleep. When I awoke, I was being escorted to Clark Nine, the psychiatric intensive care unit, by a nurse's aide, a Black man. I was protesting, and he was being reassuring but firm that I had to go to this unit. I asked him to take me to Arles first, and he did. It seemed like a natural part of the process. He told Arles that I was having 'nookie' and that's why I needed the unit. I was stunned. I had no memory of this. I didn't know for sure what nookie meant, whether it was making out or having sex. He reported, 'Not only was she doing it, but she was doing it with someone not old enough to be a man.' I was stunned, ashamed and terrified. I had no memory of this event. I thought they were right—I was crazy. Not because of having sex in public, but of having sex with someone who was only a boy and not remembering it. I felt crazy. The aide motioned to take me up in the elevator. Arles said no, I was to stay there.*

After the dream, it felt as if I had broken a fever. But it's all slowly building up again as I imagine seeing Arles. I rehearse different scenes, trying for the best outcome. He is a piece I move on the board. He will fuck up his part. I try to predict his response. Provocation is the best predictor.

I was disassembling. I told him that I choked during meditation and had to leave the hall. Larry was speaking about the nature of insight. I apologized to him after the sit, and he said, "We all have bodies. We are mere tenants."

"Arles, I can't capture my mind. I can't glue it together with memory." I held my skull as a proxy. The session ran out.

"There are only two things I want you to do: feel your feet on the floor as you walk and pay attention to your breath." I was pulling on my boot. "Are you hearing what I'm saying?" he asked softly.

"Yes, Arles, I am. Thank you."

"And, Sebern... no insights."

Another shift had begun. I couldn't fight with him. Without terror, without fighting, he is not there. I whip something up. I am surprised when I can just sit and talk, and afterwards, I have no memory of being there.

I am going about making a safe place. He said something about my parents.

"I haven't had parents. I've had maids and therapists." He nodded. "But you don't know them, Arles! Don't act as if you do."

"That's right, Sebern. But I do know you. Their absence is a presence in this room, in what you just said, in you."

"Do you trust me?" I asked him. He took a moment to answer.

"At one level, I trust you absolutely. At another, I don't trust you for one second."

This was a perfect communication. I was surrounded. I looked for ways out, for breaches in the wall, in his tone or his words or his posture. I nodded then nodded again.

I told him about almost grabbing the pan I burned the other night. John had winced.

"It's a good thing you didn't do that," he said without empathy or alarm. "A very good thing."

"I am telling you the dangers of sleep deprivation!"

"You are threatening self-harm, and that's not going to happen." I didn't respond. "Did you hear me, or do I need to say it louder?"

"Yes, I heard you!"

"And what did you hear?"

I hesitated. "That you see me." I paused, still guessing. "That you hold me responsible."

"Yes, both right and what else do you hear?"

I turned further away.

"Look at me. What else did you hear?"

"That there will be consequences."

"Yes, there will be consequences."

I do not feel angry, but I turn on him.

"Fuck you, go fuck yourself!" and I don't even wonder about this.

I do not feel grief, but tears spill over. I feel no anxiety, but my shoulders are splintering. I have nothing to say and choke over my own stubborn silence. I slapped my flat hand hard against the tub wall during the third bath I took today. I sense the relief of my sliced wrist, but then leap across states to see that *if* I did this, it would change things with Arles. He would have to act; none of this would help.

"I asked everyone to write about something important to them that has happened between us, over the years." I was filling him in. "This is what she sent."

I handed him the narrow, pink, shiny card with a martini glass on the front. He opened it slowly with his large, careful hands. Inside, it read, "Happy 50th. Never too old for booze and sex! Make it a day." And she'd signed it, as she does, XXX, Mom.

He shook his head and watched me as he passed it back.

"What will you do with this?"

I shook my head. "I dunna know. Burn it?"

Little cuts, little burns, matches put out on my arm. It feels like the only thing to do. I am trying to keep Arles in my mind. I'm afraid to tell him and afraid not to.

"Are you fascinated by what my reaction will be?"

"I am like a hole dug in sand. You bring water, buckets of water, and it finds its way out in a matter of seconds."

I was startled when he got up, moved his other chair, and sat down in front of me—there was no way to avoid him. He ignored my demands and increasingly desperate requests:

"Please, back off. Please, go back. Please, you're scaring me!"

"I have no doubt it scares you. It should."

"Well then, push away. You're too close." I retracted my knees into my chest, my feet on the couch.

"No, Sebern, this is where I will be sitting. Closer, if need be."

I thought today of the power of a particular fantasy that I've had about nursing at Nell Carter's ample chocolate breast. I wasn't drawn into it. This is about the flat, hard chest.

I had been thinking of the damage I could do with the top of the dog food can before I accidentally cut my finger on the ivory tendon. The stitches are still in. I was frightened more than usual to see Arles that night.

He brought his chair close, leaning forward, and I summoned the courage to look at his face.

"You look serious."

"Oh, I am serious." But it was more, he looked worried. I have not seen him look worried.

He took my bandaged hand and held it almost too firmly. "I know you think this was an accident, but that's a lie." I tried to pull my hand away.

"It was an accident! I didn't do this on purpose!" He tightened his grip.

"There are no accidents in your life. This is dangerous behavior, and I am very worried for you. It is time, long past time, for you to be worried for yourself." I turned my head away. "Look at me, Sebern. This lie doesn't help you." I felt his hand around my wrist. I did not respond. After a long pause, he said, "The only good news here is that you don't believe it either."

I can, for a day or two, now hold onto his words and tones and that one facial expression. He talks to me of a forbidden appetite. I refuse to admit or submit to a yearning so old, so deep, so jagged. Yesterday, he would not be provoked, and he would not back away. He did not interpret or even challenge my wanting to leave. He simply said that I could not.

"I sucked my thumb until I was in college," I told him, filling in a detail of the hunger.

"You can suck your thumb, Sebern. It's okay." He sat back, and as he did, his foot touched the couch. It reassured me.

"What did you do when you felt Charlie's absence?"

I answered without thinking, "I ate glass." He closed his eyes and sighed.

"Of course, you did. That's exactly what you did," he said, shaking his head slowly. "You'll need to learn to miss me, not to enact it."

"I don't understand 'missing.' It's a concept."

"You will come to."

WILDING

"Last night I was leaving my office after my last patient, and there was a group of boys collecting near the firehouse. I suspected they were going to do a 'wilding.'" This tumbled out of me, anxiously. "I thought about going to the police, but there wasn't anything to report. Just my intuition, so I didn't. I saw in the paper this morning that a couple was 'wilded' coming out of Beardsley's. I feel terrible. I could have stopped it." He listened and then didn't pause.

"Tell me about the wilding in you."

I felt blinded in the beam of a floodlight, suddenly, irreparably, exposed.

She was eating from the dumpster, and when they went to catch her, she bit, kicked, ran, afraid she would never be caught. I knew her. It was not me. It was not me who lit fire to the tender flesh, a vindictive act, not one of containment, one of hatred. A hole in my arm. I knew I was not lying when I took no responsibility for the burn. Not me at all. Her.

Arles was angry. I paced. I threatened the stupid family sculpture. He grabbed my arm and yelled at me.

"Either you sit down on the couch now, or the session is over." The threat seemed suddenly overwhelming. He had my forearm. I arched and ordered him to let me go. Imperious. He repeated the terms. I felt the crumbling of resolve. He guided me, not gently, to the couch, and I sat, sullen, contemptuous, and relieved.

He pulled the chair right in front of me and sat down without his usual grace.

"Are you pissed?" I asked him, looking at my feet.

"You bet I am!"

I moved back on the couch. "I want to get this... but it's not *your* anger. That's your part in the script, the script that somehow I've written."

"I know this," he said, still angry, "and it is a profound problem. I am subsumed by the absence in you."

"At best, Arles, I hear a far echo."

"Cavernous, Sebern, cavernous."

I described the image of a two-family house. On the right side, there are people drinking and swearing, the TV is loud, a chair is thrown, and what furniture there is is rusted steel and vinyl. Beer, dirty windows. White light. The other side, the left, is painted warm colors, deep orange with waxed woodwork and Persian rugs. Soft music, Bach. One household knows the other through the shared wall where the stairs rise to the unseen second floor.

"I worked for QuikTrip Messenger Service the summer they were making *The Godfather* in New York. They built the Corleone family home on a soundstage in Harlem. I watched them put it up. There were stairs, but there was no second floor. It's like that. A set. An artifact. I watched too when they took it all apart."

"The gangster's home," he said, "both sides."

He held me steady with his voice through questions about my sleeplessness, about what I wear, about what happens when I wear underpants and when I don't. The light was too bright. As he went to turn it down, he made himself clear, "You will stay on the couch, and we will continue to talk about this."

Then came the footfalls in the hall. Squealing, my throat begins to close. He leaned forward, speaking softly but loud enough for me to hear, "You are okay, Sebern. It's okay. You are here. I am here." I fell back on the couch and grabbed for the blanket.

On Wednesday, I will leave for France to be with the monks and nuns and with Thich Nhat Hanh for ten weeks.

❧

As I walked through the Jardin du Plants, I knew that I could not be trusted. Every experience turns on itself, every moment falsifies the last. A thought arises, becomes a perception, then the opposite thought arises harshly, and my mind is canceled. I cannot predict myself. What does trust mean without prediction? I've been inviting Arles to witness what I think is a performance. I have been asking him to witness the truth of what I believed to be untrue. He has insisted that he is seeing the reality. I believe I have made him see the fabrication as reality, and on and on it spirals. Tonight, I hear his insistence as a gift of sanity. He sees what he sees, and I cannot distort it enough that he is unable to.

As I walked, I struggled with how not to lie if I'm asked about these scars, realizing that every evasion that was not a literal lie was one worse than that. So I will have to say, 'Can I tell you at a time I'm ready?' Just an evasion, not a lie. When it happened, Claude, the vet who crawled through the Plum Village night alert for the rustle of the VC, lifted my arm at my elbow and kissed the scars.

For seven hours today, I walked. Every minute, I contended with suicide. It was so dark in me that I couldn't see the reason for my death, just the need for it. I keep reminding myself that this too shall pass, think of calling Arles, wonder if I am mourning him. After seven hours of walking, I took refuge in Notre Dame. I had been so determined to get there, a hollow vault with tall windows. Plum Village, tomorrow.

I missed the dharma talk, the walking meditation and lunch in the Upper Hamlet. I watch as Arles slowly slips away, and I can't stop it. I thought last night that it was best to just let him go. The day I'd gotten here, I went to the clearing in the woods where we sit during walking meditation. Almost immediately, an owl swooped through, the largest bird I've ever seen, the wingspan of my outstretched arms. This is, a friend told me, an omen of death.

The sisters asked me to fetch Thầy for lunch. I knocked, timidly, on the door of his library. We walked back to the dining room together without talking. Throughout lunch, the phone rang, and no one went to answer. The machine clicked on. Thầy said, "They have to call; we have to eat."

At lunch after the bell rings, Thầy usually talks with the nuns in Vietnamese, and every once in a while, I hear my name. It feels like parents spelling so you don't understand until they come to 'cat' or 'dog.' When I was not at dinner last night—I had gone to get a bath and the only solitude of the day—Thầy, I heard later, asked where I was. When

I came out into the gift shop after evening meditation, he was sitting on the floor in front of a large tape deck, listening to one of his dharma talks. He grabbed the sleeve of my jacket with strength that surprised me and pulled me down to sit next to him. He used the phrase "killing time" on the recording, and I said, "That's really a terrible expression." He turned his face toward me and nodded ever so slightly.

Today is the 24th of June, and we are in the Lower Hamlet. It's likely that's how Thầy will begin his dharma talk on this day that we celebrate the 10th anniversary of Plum Village. I was ordained into the Order of Interbeing on Sunday, and after the ceremony, I felt the echo of loneliness. Thầy did not meet my eyes. He said this ordination meant that we would always have this community to protect us. He's been talking a lot about protection.

The moon filled half the horizon, and as it rose, somewhere, one of the nuns played her solo, melancholy oboe. I am as lost as a baby in a lifeboat. The waves are high, and the wind pulls the night in just behind it. The baby has stopped crying, as they do, from sheer exhaustion and hopelessness. I need the surround of body against body. I need to feel the sharp "No!" Where are your hands?

❧

When I returned, Arles was in London. When we met again for the first time in three months, I was glad to see him, mad in a murderous, truculent kind of way, and he was unrelenting. He took my pills, Nembutal, some Percodan and Fiorinal, and he will not return them. "You will get what you need from me. As much as you ask for control, you are constantly trying to undermine any control but your own." I think he said that, but he said a lot. I began many times to divert him with a hostile remark, but then I didn't dare. "You have gotten away with concealing yourself in every therapy, including with Charlie." I thought that nothing, realistically, kept me in the room. I didn't have to do therapy. "No one has stopped this bullshit." He is seeing what I think is a hologram.

"You make it seem like life and death..." I said derisively. He leaned forward.

"It is," he answered matter-of-factly. Then, softening his voice, "It is exactly that. Nothing less."

I felt the little urgent twinges of defiance. If I even flexed a muscle in movement away from the couch, even the slightest ripple of intent, he stopped me. I provoked him relentlessly.

"How big a penis does your boy part have?"

Bigger than yours, Arles. Bigger than yours. I didn't say that because I was stunned by what he was willing to say, because we had never discussed this 'other', because I was momentarily intrigued, and because it was funny. Then, for the first time, quite suddenly it seemed to me, he turned to listen, to try to understand and not deflect or ridicule the need I felt for a smack.

"I am not safe. I do not feel my skin. I don't really know that you exist at all. It wasn't even that you went away at Plum Village, or that you abandoned me when you went to London. I don't know how to make you understand this, but there are bodies in those interpretations. I don't have one, you don't have one, and there is nothing. I don't understand your words." I hear the tone of his words; I feel the timbre of his body. "I hear you when you're loud, and it scares me. I have too much control and then it..." I paused, "You and me, disappear. It's not what you said, some fucked up S and M scene in my head! I wish in a way it was, and then I could dismiss it too." He was so close to me I could feel his listening.

This morning, I felt the encroachment of a migraine and knew the Percodan was with him. In one corner of my psyche, I am in a full-blown tantrum, heels hammering the floor, fists flailing. In this scene, he sits in his chair, unmoved, waiting, and slowly I get that the answer is 'No.'

"There is," I said, recognizing this with slight despair, "no way out except out."

"No," he said, "There is no way out except in."

When I didn't respond, he asked if I had heard.

"Yes, I did, Arles." I wonder if he sees that something is giving way in me, a knot loosening because he will not let go. Tuesday, I insisted that the pills were my property and he needed to return them. This is all playing out on a stage. I am in the empty theater, in the back row. I am trying to tell the truth, but truth is itself a complex dissociative event. He ignored my protest about the painkillers and took up another thread.

"Is it the boy or the girl who drives 90?"

I looked into the driver's seat. "Neither. There is no gender. There is just a ball of affect—a little like how you might see in a Peanuts cartoon—and there's no object." He didn't interpret, and he didn't seem surprised. I can't get by. He gives me no choice. I must stay within the circle of Arles.

Hannah, my bipolar analyst friend with paranormal intuition, called to tell me the story of Jacob wrestling the Angel—an even match. Jacob pinned the angel and refused to let him up until the angel blessed him. I had her in mind when I said to Arles,

"You're like an 80-year-old woman analyst on the Upper West Side!"

"Sebern," he said with absolute confidence, "I *am* an eighty-year-old woman analyst on the Upper West Side."

Today, the wind blew clear. I walked for six miles and, in wave after wave, felt the beauty of being alive. Living today in that forest was a miracle. I embraced the slim yellow birch and kissed the bark.

"Why are you sitting there?"

"You have changed the frame of this relationship. It would not be safe for you were I to sit in my regular chair." I shifted to ease my back. "I want to make something clear to you. If you leave the couch, which you have some control over, the session is over. You'll be able to come back, but only if you stay on the couch. And if you leave, you will of course pay for the session."

I could not see how to escape this.

"Did you bring a knife?"

"No."

"A gun?"

"A gun?! No! Do you really believe I'd bring a gun?"

"You have been telling me." In my life of images, I was a sniper, being gunned down. People in the village expressed dismay to the press. 'Such a wonderful smile.' "You will not bring a weapon in here. If you do, you will not like the consequences. They are serious. Do you understand me?"

"No."

He raised his voice. "Do you understand me!?"

"I won't bring a gun here. I don't have a gun. I would never hurt you. Or anybody. But the honest answer is 'No.' I don't understand. It's not even that it's Greek; it's not even a language." I had to pull deeply to represent what I'd never known. "I get rhythm, tones, intonations and loud. I don't know really what we're talking about."

He sat back but not away. "You really don't, do you?"

"No, I really don't." My eyes welled up. I could not bear to sit. I could not leave. I pushed further into the couch.

Before I left, he told me about the poem, "The Panther," and last night, with a slight shock, I read it.

In the Jardin des Plantes

From seeing the bars, his seeing is so exhausted

that it no longer holds anything

to him. The world is bars, a hundred thousand
bars, and behind the bars, nothing.
The little swinging of that rhythmical, easy stride
that circles down to the tiniest hub
It's like a dance of energy around a point
in which a strong will stands stunned and numb.
Only at times, the curtains of the pupils rise
without a sound... Then a shape enters,
slips through the tightened silence of the shoulders
reaches the heart, and dies.
-Rilke

I shared the forbidden wish about playing with the pick-up sticks on the floor with him.

"You hate your baby parts so much."

"O god, no, Arles! 'Baby parts...' That's disgusting. It sounds sexual."

"Sexual?" he said, at first surprised. Then, "There is something very important here to talk about, but now it's a diversion from talking about your hatred. You are tempting Freud, not me."

In the dream last night, there was someone pointing to a picture. I couldn't understand what they were saying when they said it was a baby picture—it was from the back and was only the vulva and the rectum. It took me a while to see it. The rectum was just a slit. There was no bottom.

I leaned my head back.

"I don't think this can be treated, Arles. If this were all of me, you would not even consider treating me."

"It's a big enough part."

"I don't knock off banks!"

"No, you knock off therapists."

I acted as if I'd ignored him. "If this part were all of me, I'd probably be a gang leader," I thought out loud, a little pleased with my construction.

He paused for a moment.

"Yes, you are a gang leader. That's exactly right. The gang is inside you. I want only to deal with the leader now. That's not to say I don't want to know them all, but I'm only speaking to the leader now."

"I didn't mean that! What I meant is that you wouldn't treat this part of me because it can't be treated!"

"I can treat you," he answered, without hesitation.

The thought came to me as a voice between my ears. *There will be retribution for this.*

"You can sit on the floor for five minutes. Then you will do what?"

"I'll get back on the couch. I will. We need a piece of plywood for the couch. It's too soft."

I slipped hard onto the floor. And then it comes, impossible to hold back. I almost had to vomit. I could hardly breathe. He held his hand behind my neck, he held my forehead. I slapped my face.

"No! No! You will not hit your face." He gathered up my hands. He guided me up onto the couch. "You may cry and scream as loud as you need. You may not hit, and you may not bite." I started to pull away in a new seizure of crying.

"Don't turn away from this," he said. I folded my arms over my stomach, sobbing.

"I am *so* hungry, Arles."

"Yes, so unbearably hungry." He leaned toward me. "You want so much to be held, to be cradled, but you're afraid to take from me."

"No!" I yelled, looking at my feet, trying to slip them into sandals.

After admitting this hunger, rage begins to rise again. He sees it and, without warning, ends the session. I am shocked, and the state shifts, and I sit down.

"You were going to quit! How could you do that?"

He sat back too.

"No, Sebern, it was you who was going to quit. Do you see that?"

I met Bill, who owns the clothing store in the hall. At first, I didn't acknowledge it. He turned back and greeted me. Arles asked me how I handled this.

"He asked why I was here."

"What did you say?"

"I told him I was here for supervision."

"Well," he said, "that's true."

❧

I can barely adhere to the details of living: red lights, appointments, food. I am to the side of my experience, to the right of myself. Tonight is sleepless.

"It's not like underpants would protect me."

"A four-year-old wouldn't know this, though, would she?"

I can't sit. I know, desperately, even here alone, looking side to side, contemplating the cut, that there is no way out.

He wouldn't let me go to the DBT conference in Asheville, to meet Marsha and to socialize and impress around the pool.

"Halfway between the 19th hole and *My Dinner with Andre*. You aren't doing this."

He talked about Westchester, its perversity swallowed and embedded; a pervasive phoniness masking profound despair, leaving everyone there twisted by it. I want to argue, to defend, but there was no argument. I came from there. I told him about Zelda and Scott, Highland Hospital, and the Grove Park Inn.

“I’ve been thinking about Gatsby a lot recently.”

“Like going home, Arles,” I said, almost pleading, almost relieved, almost disappointed.

“You are home,” he answered flatly and twisted to pick his appointment book off the floor.

I started to protest, but I couldn’t. It’s true. This is where I live, in this office.

I took the pills when he looked away. He caught it. He said he was not angry with the part of me that took the pills; he was disgusted. Disgusted at the perversity, the cruising, the hustle. I heard it for a moment in the narrow zone that is his. This, too, I think, is not real; that I don’t really do the things I do. I have to hear the tones and register something in his face. I just began to dimly get that this might be real.

❧

“Are you scared, Mom?”

“I probably would be, but I don’t have enough energy.”

I look at her while she sleeps. After five units of blood, there is a hint of pinkness in her cheeks. I see her true innocence, a confusing innocence. When her cardiac surgeon arrived to inform me first of his success, then of the tumor, I tried to stay attentive to his assurances and to my own reaction. I cried, but did not know why. It was not recognizable to me. I was suspended in the threat of her death. At the moment she dies, I will, I think, finally have an experience of intimacy with my mother. I do love her, but it is vaporous and distant, until she closes it suddenly with an attack. She forgets to ask how I am. She does not ask what I do or what I feel. She cannot imagine the effect of our shared history. I await her death, hoping then for a moment of absolute connection. I encounter my voracious hunger. Little is different whether she is alive or dead.

Blake called about her grandmother. "I need to see you, Mom. I need you." I noted my very slight nervousness and opened my arms to her, wanting her to feel it all. But I have no fierce attachment to life, which, I guess, can only be as strong as attachment to another. This is thin in me. When I talked about my wish for drugs, Arles said, "The hole feels too big, doesn't it?"

I wondered today how people really bear a conscious life. I feel at the edge of another siege. As I walked across Washington Street to the garage at the Floating to drive home, I had a glimpse that this history, these symptoms, this behavior with Arles, the fury, the terror, all of it has meaning that I either dismiss or try to defer.

I put myself through a terrible ordeal, through a death perhaps singular in nature that I could not abide. Over the day yesterday, when I had not heard from him, I came to believe that Arles had been killed. The tragedy of his death dwarfed my terrible need for him, a graceless, voiceless need, suddenly insignificant. I watched the belief gain on me as natural moments for calling came and slipped away, swallowed by the darkening day. When he finally called, after 10, I cried like a small child and told him how scared I'd been, how relieved I was to hear his voice. I went through it all: bargaining, being good, no stealing, no drugs... Had I told him how important, how special he is? I have no wish that he die. Immediately, I suspect this. The part of me that is attached, young and present, that mind would be lost. There is another part, the face he must hold, the one who flies off the couch, throws things, dematerializes, and flings herself into the walls. And the knife. Who's the woman who loses her way crossing the street in a death-defying feat? The woman who twists to bite his hand? Is this a woman at all? Does this feral child wish his death?

There is a long gasp on the phone: "I was so scared, Arles." He grew quiet, then closed the distance of hours.

"I do understand, Sebern."

"Do you?"

“There is much to understand. There is much that has gone unspoken that must find words; there is much that has been understated that must be stated.”

I feel at the edge of the shadow world, a whole body of knowing not yet known. I could not have done this any sooner. I hung up. I noticed the calling back of all the bargains. What is this reality that exists truly only in its own negation?

I have a cold. A rare event for me. I am not entirely immune to the ravages of my own life. Thank God he is not dead.

My mother is recovering from a heart attack that damaged one-third of her heart.

He usually waits for me to begin, but not today.

“Why didn’t you leave the number in Boston, where you could be reached?”

“I thought that would be being dramatic.”

“It was ‘dramatic,’ Sebern, not to leave the number. Your mother had a heart attack. This is real. This has meaning. This is important.”

“Oh, yes, I see that.” I didn’t.

John laughs when I ask him if I have an exaggerated startle response. I’ve asked Arles whether I've had a kind of routine, hard life. He smiled, shook his head slowly and said, ‘Oh, no.’ These are genuine questions. I turn my mind back and the scan reveals wealth, privilege, plenty, the smell of my father’s handkerchief as he tells me to ’blow’ to free myself from another clot of tears, piles of gifts at Christmas, Ginger Ale and sherbet for sore throats, playing with Kevy, my own room where the bedspread matched the curtains, my dog Tracy, the trips out west. Is it true that the third floor of 40 Stewart Avenue darkens after Mary leaves? Is it true that Hugh and the new boys tied me to a tree that day when I was six and left me there? Did the older boys really ambush me with a hail of stones, laughing as they hit their chubby little target? What grade was this, first or second? I have no emotional memory. I believed that I had to make up a story to justify the symptoms. I was startled yesterday to read something John Mack wrote in an article on abduction experiences: "It is difficult to conceive of a post-traumatic clinical picture which arises entirely from within the psyche." In a sense, this is what I wanted to believe and wanted Arles to believe. That is, no meaning.

Friday, someone knocked on his door.

"Oh, no, no, no," I whispered, wildly looking for a place to go.

"It's okay. You're okay. I'm here. I'm not leaving. I'll be right back." He went to the door, opened it narrowly and slipped through. He came back in and closed the door softly.

"They are here for the first time, and they're early," he said as he approached the couch. "You are safe here." He pulled his chair a little closer. "Breathe, Sebern. It's okay. No one will hurt you here." I looked away and gathered up my coat.

"This is your time and your place. Don't leave yet."

Tears rolled over my cheeks, and I pulled my coat on, one arm all the way, then the next. When I am not there, he is not there either.

I dreamt of him most of last night. I was considering buying his house. As I walked up the stairs leading to it, there was a tattered black kitten: dirty, mewling, with big black eyes. I avoided it, thinking he would want me to take her. I looked around, and the linoleum in the kitchen needed replacing. I thought the cost of the house was too great. I wouldn't buy it.

I told him the dream.

"I think you bought the house. You are experiencing buyer's remorse."

"I stood looking at this tree ablaze with its death, flooded by the divine and knew that had I had a gun, I would've shot myself through the mouth."

Arles is worried. I feel no imperative to live, no attachment to life. I could die of my own carelessness. It had been gaining on me, like a fever, pale, and hot.

"Please, don't put me in a hospital, Arles." I plead mostly out of embarrassment, not really from an assessment of my own safety. I didn't care.

"I don't want to have to consider a hospital," he said. He insisted that John be with me. He asked in detail about my weekend. When I had no plans, he said I must call him and tell him the plans I've made. He must hear from me each day. He authorizes sleeping pills, but the bottle must be brought immediately to his office. When I bring them, he spills them into his hand and counts them out. He reminds me how serious this is and why we are engaged in it. "I will, without hesitation, call John and if I can't reach him, the police, if you don't follow every one of these steps."

I followed every one of these steps. He was in every one of them. He was, briefly, in every breath. Then it was memory and reminder and humiliation at the idea of the hospital and, finally, its futility.

Eva looked at the baby pictures. I am four months old. "I can hardly stand it that this is you." She noticed not only my face but how stiffly I held my body. I'd shown Charlie these pictures on my recent visit with him. After a brief search through clinical descriptors, he said, "It's bewilderment, that's what you're feeling." He handed the album back to me. "These are too disturbing. Put them away." Arles calls them horrifying, but he will not put them away.

"This is where we are, Sebern, exactly here. These baby pictures are irrefutable. This is your mother's look too, the look of anaclitic depression."

"They have to go back. I promised her I would return them."

"Your mother will never get these back." I imagined having to deal with this on the Cape and began... He cut me off. "No, Sebern, never. They stay here with me." I felt a bracing deep in me let go. I felt my back on the back of the couch.

My mother never missed them.

The experience of no harbor; the experience of clutching for Arles in blind terror when FedEx knocks on the door; and the photographs, I cannot undo these. I try, the photo session is just one moment in time; the man at the door, well-rehearsed drama, so well rehearsed it becomes real, but this script is beginning to fail me. I feel a new kind of hopelessness. I am hopeless that he will win the battle for control. I asked him if he had seen hate in my face.

"It isn't hate. Hate is too relational. You can look like a wild animal."

When I told him how much I want to cut, he took my hands by the wrists.

"You are very angry at me. You will not cut yourself. You will learn that I exist."

This is not the cruelty of abuse; it is the fact of absence.

I brought my tea to the office, but he took it. If I want to drink, it must be milk.

"You will learn to take from me. You do not need to provide for yourself. In this regard, you cannot provide for yourself." I feel like a million slippery fishes. I want to dive back into the sea. I am unable to surrender and unable to fight.

Yesterday I sat in a retreat at Cambridge Insight Meditation Center and, after a while, settled into it, into myself and into the soft play of a dreamy sadness. I heard Arles' voice, its tones and inflections, and at moments my own sharp response, and at others the sense of being filled in by his attention, his hands.

"This is not *your* world, Sebern. I am in it now. You have been quite successful at arranging your life so that you are in control. You made a conscious decision in your life that there would be no other."

"When I was five? When did Mary leave? Is that what you mean?" He didn't say anything. "Is that the right answer? Is that what you're saying?" He didn't answer my question.

"I am attached to you, Arles."

"Then why do you pull away?"

"I know, but I am." He doesn't nod, and immediately I know the twist in this, that part of this is a con, and I challenge him as if there were no con at all.

"I *am* attached to you!" He holds my wrists tightly, ignoring my complaint.

"There is a snake deep in you, a profound part of you," I asked him to let go because I needed to adjust. He laughed almost warmly, "Oh, you don't have a clue how much you need to adjust!" He didn't relax his grip.

CHAPTER 2

It is a year to the day that I began this therapy. He was so soft-spoken that I often couldn't distinguish what he said. He sat in his chair at the end of the couch, surrounded by books – ever-changing titles, consumed, it would seem, like so many cups of tea with honey. I have the idea to capture the high points. But the high points in therapy are never the high points, and the drama, the true amazing drama of it all, is embedded in the slow, subtle shifts beneath the surface, the deepening; the cleansing of aquifers, not the tidal roar of disturbance. So, what is to be said? He speaks to me in a loud, clear voice, so I can feel his voice on my skin. He sits with his knees inches from mine or on the couch, demanding that I tolerate not only his closeness but his surround. He does not let me leave... and so.

It is Thanksgiving, and we are going to see my mother. When I asked her how she was doing, she started to cry. The third time in our lives. She is scared, exhausted and vulnerable. When I asked her to try to arrange the procedure on a day I could come to get her, she did not protest. She softens within me, and I feel a touch of my own fear and real tenderness for her.

She is facing more surgical ordeals. She enters the hospital a week from Monday, and this time, I fight not to acknowledge my yearnings for her life and for her painless, quick death. She seems sad, scared and stoic, all but the latter as undercurrents. She will take the bus to admit herself to the hospital, and I will pick her up to take her home; when and under what circumstances cannot be known. My poor little mother. I took a bath in the clawfoot tub upstairs in her house, to immerse myself, to feel its protection, to find a dimension, to control the pressure on my skin. Subtly, as subtle as the undercurrent of my mother's moods, I lose my skin.

When you become aware that this moment contains every other moment, living in the present moment is not so simple or stripped down as it appears.

On Tuesday, I brought in the native carving Marsha had bought for me when we went to Port Townsend. He asked me what she saw, this sad lady with the weathered face. The artist had dropped tears in her eyes. "The death of children, grinding, unrelenting poverty and the slaughter of whales." The latter I dismissed at first as a poetic flourish until I remembered the totem of whales—the historian, the archivist, the one who remembers.

"Your mother's death is the most important event of your life," Marsha said. She is sitting, gazing at the Olympic Mountains, and I am lying in my bed on the other side of the country, watching the gentle fall of snow. I am filled with the grief that is at the center of my relationship with my mother, this predator of empathy, the one who renders my experience meaningless and then erases it from memory. What can ever change this? I am disabled, but not only by the mother, the unraveller, but by the destruction of cells committed to continuity and construction. Neither Marsha nor I can trust memory. I have imagined Arles holding my head to contain this process of annihilation. She is not like the schizophrenic mother who takes her children to the carnival to help them forget that she just accidentally ran over the family dog. She is the mother who intimates that we never had a dog after momentarily noting its loss.

Any relationship other than that of the engaged mother and the receptive infant betrays the need. There is no adult equivalent. No adult capacity. This relationship with the therapist is the most proximate. Last night I called my mother. The news is not good. The tumor is malignant. I have moments of grief that echo in the deepest hollows of loneliness. I will visit her before her next surgery.

I am here to care for my mother. It's the middle of January, after her ordeal that began in September. She is weak in the aftermath of the surgery to remove the malignant lobe. She minimizes the near-disastrous drop in blood pressure that delayed the surgery. Her surgeon cautioned me not to tell her that she nearly died when her heart stopped. He wants her to be confident and proud of her strength. Today, even though she is weak, she is happy for me to go out to Nauset.

"You couldn't call my father's death an accident, and it wasn't called tragic," I thought as I walked back along the beach. "But what else does someone call the death of a forty-four-year-old father? You are killed by a train that jumps the track, or the bullet meant for someone else, or by your ambition, or your father's approval, where's the difference?" It's all an accident; the heart bleeds, the heart bursts, the heart breaks, the heart stops. Do we reserve 'tragic' to describe only those events in which the victim participated, not at all? They argue over suicide or an accident. Is there, particularly when there is a question, any doubt at all?

Last Thursday night, I saw a grave digger, steam rising around him, snow falling, preparing the grave for the morning, the scene backlit by the headlights of his truck.

I sat alone in the meditation room as the moon rose over the patient wing of New England Medical Center. The city sky darkens, but never grows dark. It is reflective. The surgery was to be over at 4. It was twenty to 7 when Dr. Daley arrived in his street clothes. Perhaps he was too bloody to come in his OR fatigues. The operation started at the same time my wait did. I sat, and during my meditation, I knew that I wanted her to live. I got a brief glimpse of the absence of her, of her back disappearing through her bedroom door. When Dr. Daley arrived, I was relieved at my relief.

❧

"Nothing happens here or will happen here that you do not want to happen. But that does not mean that you are in control of this therapy. You are not." He sat next to me on the long analytic couch, and I moved to the far, rarely occupied end. He laughs easily,

"You really are impossible." He told me to sit back where I had been. In response to my silent refusal, he took hold of my arm, and I slid over the leather close to him. We sat there in silence.

"Is that your hand, Arles? That is *your hand,* isn't it?"

"Yes, this is my hand."

"I knew that..."

I drew the outline of each finger with mine, then looked at mine.

"What is the color of your mother's eyes?"

"She has brown hair." I thought a bit. "They must be brown. Or maybe hazel."

"Don't you think it's odd that you don't know the color of your mother's eyes?"

"Yeah, I guess."

"Perhaps you have never looked at them." Even now, sitting with her, she 76, me 50, I cannot bring my eyes to hers.

"What color are mine?" I didn't look up. It was a humiliation.

"I know the color of Blake's and Jakob's."

Sam tells me of the study of infant monkeys separated from their mothers. The cortisol levels that sustain the infant through birth are brought down when the mother cradles her baby. In these monkeys, they never come down, keeping them in a state of hypervigilance, often unable to sleep, or maintain a consistent temperature or play with other monkeys. This is the state Arles addresses in this radical therapy. I can, with effort, gaze at his hand, but not his face.

I am fearing the permanent loss of the fighter, but by that afternoon, she has returned, more ambivalent, but there she is, decked out in blue jeans, leading with her chin and snarled lip. He is undaunted at her return, maybe since he never seemed to recognize that she'd left. I warned him.

"You better be careful, Arles."

"I better be careful? You have that wrong, Sebern."

I told him today that I wish I could just see all this, not have to experience it. Last night again, I was overtaken by an almost neurological terror and rage I could not control. I kicked my legs; I cried out, strangled cries. Pieces of my body flew off.

Arles has the flu. Beneath the flu is his exhaustion. I am part of it. I try to reassure myself that he has not gone far. I finally knew to pull the heavy quilt over me. It was all I needed. I calmed down. Just before the quilt, I had the image of trashing his office. In the image, he stands by, unable to control it.

"What kind of holding are you missing here?" he asked. Hot tears rolled down my face.

"The horrible news is this need is beyond anything you can soothe. It is not a normal need, not a need. It is beyond remediation." I could only begin to cry. Part of me is struggling to understand, to find the words. How did it happen? He sat next to me, gently insisting that I look at him. He held my face and kept holding it, soothing the eruptions, "Go away from me, get away from me, don't touch me!" I didn't jerk my head away.

"Shhh, shhh. It's alright. I am staying right here."

Last night, I spoke about my new patient, and he asked, "Does she, too, have multiple others that need taking care of?"

"Multiple others," I agreed, warily, "not multiple 'alters.'"

"I was very careful about my choice of words."

"She was brutalized by a man at the direction of a woman." I lost ground and stuttered out, "This breaks my mind."

The air changed and the light. When he said he saw this, it all stopped. It was not repression or suppression; it was another innate intelligence, a biochemical switch. Held to the spot by his voice, wrapped as much as possible in myself, I said, softly, "I want to go."

"I know that was a frightening thought, but it's ok to be here. You can talk with me about it or not talk at all, but you are safe here."

I stayed there, muscles alert, but without thought. The time came, and I walked out into the freezing night.

I came to Arles, who was sitting turned away from me. He turned toward me, and after a moment of taking each other in, he smiled and said, "There is good news; the baby is born. It's a girl!" I was very happy for him (in a way that does not come easily to me), genuinely delighted. I hugged him. That's wonderful, Arles! And I kissed him on the lips.

Marsha called this morning in a state of anxious exhaustion. She had her first suicide attempt. We spent two hours talking about this. She said one thing that was very important for me and for my patients to hear. "The fantasy of the suicide is that now others will understand, in a way they had not before, just how awful it's been. No one has that response. Instead, everyone says, 'I knew it was bad. I wish she'd made it.' Then they feel angry." Before we got off the phone that morning, she said, "If you kill yourself, Sebern," she hesitated searching for the words, "I will kill you!"

I borrowed the Infant Mental Health Journal from Arles, and when I opened it that night, I found my Christmas card.

Otto Kernberg's house burned down in Scarsdale. He lost all his writing on the aggression on the borderlines and aggression as the problem, in the fire.

I don't know what happened, but sometime this week I blew out—fists, teeth, spit. I lost track. I felt sorry.

"I will never do that again." I was humiliated and made a somber promise.

"I think you might. I think you honestly do not want to do that again, but it is not a matter of morality or of will. It is not that domesticated."

"Please don't let me hurt you, Arles. I couldn't forgive that."

"I won't let you hurt me, Sebern."

"If you weren't stronger than me, this therapy couldn't be."

"But I am."

We sat together without speaking for some time, and then I said, "Even when I look at you, I don't see you." It came as an accusation and as an affirmation.

He responded as if it were neither. "Yes, that's right. It will take years before you'll be able to see me."

The photo album lay out on the black leather ottoman. "I want to make a ritual of it and burn those pictures."

"Oh no," he said with a gentle alarm. "No. Lest we forget." He picked it up. "We are exploring the outer reaches of the birth of a psyche. This is uncharted." He closed the photos gently within the faded pink silk binder and laid the album on the table beside him.

I stopped writing this to prepare for the worst winter storm of the century. I filled the tub, moved wood to the stove, distributed candles, cooked lunch, took my bath, set out pots of water, cleared the first snow around the door and brewed tea with honey. I took Elsa for a short walk before I came crashing down on my knee on the ice. Well-trained now, I noticed the thought before the fall, "If an account of this therapy were to be well written, it would be written by both of us." The wind is blowing powerfully, and the snow is thick and light. I don't expect to maintain power. The wind penetrates the walls and into me. There is nearly five feet of snow. This life-threatening snow became my safety, though. I am safe when I am unreachable.

I spent last week in Durham at Marsha's brilliant course on DBT, easily separated this time from home and from Arles. I remember very little of the Tuesday night session except that I entered angry and recalcitrant. He said I was already gone and angry about being allowed to go. I was unreachable. Out of nowhere, he took my wrist, turned it up and smacked my hand so hard it stung. Multiple contradictory responses jammed each other. I thought to be outraged, but wasn't. I thought to protest, but felt no protest. I was angry that he had the gall to act outside the contract of my provocation. I didn't expect it at all. I looked and then held my right hand to my chest with my left.

"My hand is redder than yours."

"As it should be."

"I guess I've been pulling for that for a year."

"Now will you remember me?! Touch your palm when you begin to forget, Sebern." He had no regrets, no second thoughts. He had not lost control. At one point that night, he said, "This is your last conference for a good long time," and that old feeling, the crease in my belly, came. "You will call me from the Ramada when you arrive in Durham and on Friday night, and as soon as you get back here. And you will leave the phone number of your hotel."

❧

After four nights without much sleep, it becomes sadly clear. I sat up in bed. I cannot continue. This level of therapy is a mistake, his and mine, a kind of arrogance or irrational hope. This broken attachment cannot be fixed. Understanding it does nothing. There is nothing for me to attach to. At this core place, I have no capacity to change myself. All change and all limits to change relate to attachment. Like a severed limb or a congenital deformity, this reality is to be known and accepted; in the language of the trade, sealed over. This would be regrowing the amputated hand.

I was taking two kittens up to my place. One got there safely, and I am coming up the outdoor stairs, perhaps carrying another. I see a door carelessly swung open. I catch one of the kittens, and it falls a great distance, repeating what had happened to the mother cat. It is a tiger kitten. I looked through the railing to see if it was moving or dead. I hope that she is still alive because she landed on the body of her dead mother. I hesitate somehow, strangely, but then run down the stairs. I pick the kitten up carefully so as not to break anything or hurt her and try to see if she is alive. She makes a little sound, perhaps a weak cry and part of her moves, but the rest is rigid. I don't know, but then, given the stiffness, I decide she is dead. I'd lay her down on the other cat, now both clearly dead and walk up the stairs with the weakened railing.

My mother was in bed when I arrived last night. On the way, I'd stopped to visit Solo, my former patient in foster care, at the Department of Youth Services detention center. I brought him an Easter basket, with jellybeans, chocolates, a stuffed bunny, and the *Autobiography of Malcolm X*. He looked four years old, lonely, on the edge of disaster, with no way to comprehend. As I left, he was standing in the grim hallway, holding the basket in his sixteen-year-old hand, his big dark eyes sad and scared. When he'd first arrived in my office, he told me he had nothing to say. Words seemed impossible for him. I asked him to make a video of his life and tell me what he saw. He looked at these frames in his head and began to talk about a desperate life in a forsaken ghetto of Boston. He wrote to me at Plum Village and, in the 'longest letter I've ever written,' told me of his love for his brother and for me. He wrote, 'I would die for my brother.' I wrote him back and asked him if he dared to live for his brother. I told Thầy about this. I think it's how I got my dharma name: True Right Speech.

I gathered my mother into my arms, warming as I do to the sweet scent of her face cream. Tomorrow is Easter.

❧

He sits back in his chair, both of us resting our arms on our heads, attentive. He talks about my fear of looking at his face and seeing the wrong look. "This is my fear of fragmentation," I said, catching then that it's not only a memory, it's also now. He nods slowly. I exist only in my knowing that I am in his mind.

He was insisting on emotional connection, on reciprocity, on the reality of him. I told him I was getting uncomfortable.

"Good." I got up and, attempting to avoid his hand, knocked over a vase of pink tulips. He ended the session. Later, he left a message.

"I will see you on Friday. As for your parting gesture and remark: in the field that is being constellated here, there are no accidents, only consequences." That night, *I dreamt of a wild cat in my backyard, a cheetah.*

Like amber in the glacier, grief is held in deadness. I have just begun to cry. If this part of me is not dead, but frozen, then there is hope. It could melt in the heat of his hands. The picture changed again. This dead/frozen/amber was not the end, not the bottom. I was holding against nuclear fragmentation. I look into his face, and it begins. Tears slip down my averted face.

"Arles, there was nothing you could do. I could barely make it from session to session; my only safety was here. I organize my existence around you. We did everything we knew how to do to contain the perpetual state of being blown into bits, and it was not enough." In October, with the added threat of my mother's death, I gave in. "I don't only re-experience it as it was then in the infant's blank mourning, but I experience it now."

"Yes, I see that. I have been here with you."

"These babies don't experience grief, do they?"

"What baby are we talking about, Sebern?"

I turned away. "It's just an honest question, Arles."

He only paused briefly. "No, they don't, at least not what we can recognize as grief. The grief is in the deadness."

He asked me a question, and I couldn't figure it out. I couldn't put it together.

"It's okay," he said, "You have put a lot together today." I started to cry. I felt his kindness. He wanted me to just rest, but in some state of agitation, I started to put on my shoes. He took my hands tightly and talked me through the seizing, nameless fear.

I took his hand in both of mine. I felt his hand, his fingers with my fingers. I made a joke about hands as partial objects.

"There is nothing partial here," he said, folding his hands over mine.

"It is true what you have seen. I can have all this insight, talk deeply, make connections, and never change how I relate to you."

"Right."

"But I don't know what else to do. What can I do?"

"Who said anything about doing?" And there I was, caught in being.

I talked about shock treatments and my long tenure in seclusion.

"Do you recognize what a nightmare that was?" he asked me.

I shook my head. "No, Arles, you don't understand, it wasn't. Seclusion was the best it got. Even still."

"You weren't alone there, were you?"

"I think whenever I was or was for too long... Oh, god, I was so alone there."

"Were you about to say that you'd find a way to get their attention?"

"I'd never say that! It wasn't about that at all! That's a dismissal!" I hardly paused. "Unless you mean like a wounded animal."

"Yes, Sebern, that's exactly it. That's the nightmare."

"There were four seclusion rooms around a central one that also had a bed. In a room they kept locked, with a lot of equipment, towels and other stuff, there was a huge bathtub with straps and a cover they could snap on. They let me take a bath in that, once. It was like I was a little kid." Arles listened as my voice rose with the delight of reminiscence. "They let my mother visit me there one evening when I was the only one back there. She'd come from dinner at the 21 Club." I looked up at him quickly to see if he knew this reference. He seemed to. "She brought me steak tartare."

I heard what I was saying. "Do you think I am sick, Arles?" He did not answer quickly.

"No."

I rested. I am beginning to get that his face is not a creation myth.

❧

Last night and the one before, I lay in a four-poster bed in Seattle, and I dreamt. *Three tiny abandoned black kittens. Their mother was absent, nowhere in the dream, and I had forgotten to tell them to come on this trip. I was horrified at what I had done when I saw them huddled together without food, never having grown. In the second dream, I went to where they lay on the wood floor, thinking now there were only two, but finding only one. She was weak and almost weightless. I fed her with an eyedropper – mother's milk from me, somehow. It took some patience to arouse her appetite, dropping the taste of milk around her mouth, then, suddenly eager, she sucked the eyedropper. The second kitten walked over to me. Most of her left side was rubbed raw. There was no skin. I thought this one would die too, and I shouldn't even try. A waste of time. But I couldn't let her die, and I fed her too.*

MARSHA

Until she begins to talk about the soul or allows a gentle moment of tearful grief, Marsha renders her humanity and all others like a puzzle reduced to learning contingencies and neurons. She discounts mystery, but then there is a mystic depth. Her external mood never wavers. She wakes up talking and drifts off listening to NPR. She wears the white coat of her science, a science discredited by scientists, with humble pride. She has no snobbery. We accuse each other of certainty, but embedded in our certainty is the certainty that nothing is certain; that we are most likely, not certainly, wrong.

She does know a lot. She has the capacity for desire and believes her ambition has been satisfied by the treatment she has developed and the book she published. She does not practice, but she does take long retreats with her beloved teacher, Wiligus, and takes pride in her koan status. I open my mind to it but find it hard to see her, as taken as she is by distraction and motion, as a senior student. Like me, she takes comfort in the material, it is the only trusted embrace. She aches, deep below the ample shapely flesh, beneath the broad scarred bones. She has no patience with attachment theory—"there is no data"—not even her favorite photo of herself with her mother when she is three or so and reaching for her as her mother looks away. "Your favorite picture, Marsha?" This discussion dies.

She is funny, opinionated, and non-dogmatic. She loves her students as fiercely as any mother loves their children: protectively, expansively, harshly. She demands they scrub behind the ears and takes over if they've missed a spot. She takes no credit for them, but they are like children, forever "my students," regardless, I assume, of their age, independence, or status on the globe. She is generous, big-hearted in her way, but she is wary of her impulse toward spontaneous generosity. She praises God for coffee, flowers, and email. She reports sudden "joy attacks." She was born to teach, and she, like others, breathes in and out thousands of unnoticed times a day. She forgets, and despite a deep empathy—we talked about this—she is insensitive and can leave a wake of small miseries behind her. I looked back at the saleswoman in the soap store after Marsha concluded the sale, and she was looking confused and angered. I tried momentarily to imagine how Marsha had insulted her. I looked at my friend, oblivious to any pain she'd created and then back at the saleswoman who caught my glance, smiled, and shrugged.

I love Marsha, and I loved her the most in the deepening night on Camano Island when she dropped from her constant, almost chipper register into tears. We'd been talking about the situation in my neck and the worst of the dire prognoses.

"If what happened to you happened to me," she said, "no one would care for me. No one." I wanted to protest, to reassure. I wanted even more to taste the tears, to have this moment, the silent moment of silent tears, no comment, no understanding, nothing but the candlelight and the love that held us there. I am grateful for that moment. It eclipses all others on the island.

I felt an inarticulate loneliness being with her. It is I measuring distance and time and miles from Arles, and it is Marsha, happy, content and deeply lonely, too. I made strawberry shortcake for her that was hopelessly flat and hard and earnest. I hesitated at one point, remembering slicing strawberries and sweetening them as a treat for my mother. She'd said, "Did you ever think that someone else might prefer them whole?"

I gathered shells for Molly among the rocks on Puget Sound. I thought of her broad smile, her black leather, and her sweet-smelling baby. Jakob is just two.

The loneliness and sadness that arise and plummet may require radical acceptance. Radical acceptance may indeed be the only possibility. Marsha asked me what I desired, and I had no answer. She asked if I desired at all, well, I did, and I again had no answer. I am pulled limb from limb by desire. Desire as ambition, no; desire as inspiration, no; desire as greed, no. But even in this absence of desire—which is like everything else these days, the sequela of broken connection—even in its pitiful or glorious absence, I feel envy disguised at first as irritation at Marsha's perseverance on money and siblings. She has much of both.

The kids sit on the sidewalk on every block between here and the University and pretend to be bitterly content with their costumed emptiness, with their enraged hopelessness, their street-chic despair. And I hear myself repeating, "How does one live without the love of one's mother?" I sat on dumpsters once. I belonged there. I am grateful that I don't miss Arles.

Both of us are in the practice, and I, in part, because she introduced me to Zen. We have been taken by many to be pinnacles of mental health. "The graduating class of May, 1963," Charlie said. Were this our college, this would be our 30th reunion year. Her struggle is, for her, mostly done. Mine just renewed. And we jostle each other in the ways we think about our histories. We have no shared language. Instead, I gratefully consult with her on DBT and feel exhausted that I am initiating the Center's conversion to this model. I smile at her and appreciate her energy, her intelligence, her deep moral concern, and her compassion. What else is there to know?

We talk of the Institute, which is our childhood together. She uses our conversations as memory.

"You told me you were a strong swimmer."

"Well, I think I was, or maybe I thought I was." She paused and looked curious. "Why did we do that?"

I laughed, but her question made me lonely. "There are different theories about that, right? At the time, it was simple for me and maybe for you too. It was hot, and it was a long walk back through the mud that stank. It was a more appealing plan."

"I remember that I was caught by the current and that I called out to you. You yelled to me to float, not to fight."

"You remember that? I'm so glad." I waited, but she didn't ask. "I made it into the eddy around the first abutment of the bridge and was able to rest. It must have been freezing, but I don't remember that. I remember losing sight of you. You were swept down the river."

"I floated and did the backstroke. I was a mile down."

"How did you get out? What happened next?"

"I think it was men working on telephone wires who pulled me out. They'd called the ambulance. I don't know why, but the ambulance took me to the Institute, not to Hartford Hospital. That's all I remember."

She didn't ask.

"I made it across to the next abutment, rested and then to the shore. The two others, the one who picked the lock on Thompson Two—remember that?—and another, shorter girl who'd walked back across the bridge was there waiting. We were terrified that you'd drowned. But almost immediately, there were police there. They took us to the Institute."

"Do you know what happened when we got back?"

"We weren't on the same unit. Do you remember any reaction from them, from your doctor?"

"No. Do you?"

"Oh, yes!" and I began... Her phone rang. It was a call she had to take.

❧

His absence is stark. Time that drags its feet on this continent is racing sprints for Arles in France. I do hope the sun is warming his marrow and that his sleep each night is deep, untroubled, and long.

I'm glad he's back. No doubt I missed him.

I tried to pull away after I wiped my face with my sleeve.

"Haven't I suffered enough!" I screamed it, I pleaded.

He held my hands tight at the wrist, his fingers over mine. I sat when he said to. He waited for me.

"This is not suffering, Sebern." I looked up, suddenly confused. "This is torment. Suffering is different. Suffering is grief. Your mother turned grief into absence, sucking meaning from experience, sucking experience from experience, leaving it lifeless as though it had not happened."

Nieves called here at 9.

"I took half a bottle of Aspirin and I'm going to the store to get more. Goodbye. I am outta here!" The phone clicked off. I called the beeper. Tess, Art, and the police went to search for her. A store clerk confirmed that she'd bought Aspirin. At 11, she called me from a payphone and after a few minutes- I feared they'd disconnect us- she told me where she was. She was scared of being arrested, of being thrown out of the program, of dying from the pain in her stomach. She was only minutes from the residence. Tess went to get her, and by midnight, I was at the hospital. The dose was lethal. She was alive because she vomited. She was on a heart monitor, and her stomach was lavaged. I looked down at her in her hospital crib. I felt such sorrow for what this girl has been forced to endure. Her wanting to live is extraordinary, not her wanting to die.

His smell is gone, overtaken by his long absence. He comments on the undertone of contempt.

"Because you don't recognize this in yourself does not mean it isn't there!"

I stirred.

"You left! You left me here in the dark." He acknowledged how hard this was for me, and I sat retracted and unforgiving.

"How will you get from the position you are in to the bread in my hand?"

I'll suck your dick, I answered in my head, as if that were his request.

I described the one that was here last night, cold, demanding, and ruthless. Tight black pants and shirt with a gold chain, running numbers and trafficking in girls and child porn. This one sickens me. I see him for who he is. No one in his/her right mind would invite this creep into their home. I'm glad he threw him out.

The twisted braids of characters have faces and ways of walking, a tone and tilt of the head. Arles experienced my flight into hatefulness; I experienced a sudden takeover, not of the pitiful call girl, but of the solitary, brutal pimp. The self that is organized and living off the hatred of women. Sex is degradation and humiliation. It is pornography.

I was crossing a bridge over a wide, deep gorge. I assumed at first it was open and used by common traffic. With closer attention, it was clear that it was only a footbridge. Planks were missing at some places and, at others, enough space to fall through to my death. To get across, I need to step from steel girder to girder. Arles was at the other end, encouraging me. He had made the crossing.

This is not about "healing," a paltry "as if" metaphor. It is as if this is an illness or a wound. It is as if there is a cure to this disease. It's the wrong vocabulary. This is about being known and knowing. It is about being held, being said to, being re-scripted, being brought up short, and being brought up. It might even be about being brought to life. Wounds and healing are incidental. I trust Arles. I trust him to require of me.

Last fall, I stood before a tree, inflamed and discovered an early death. This October, I discovered a black disc. I felt it for at most five seconds. No one could stay there; it would shatter the mind. Arles asked how I was able to keep breathing. On the phone, he said, "You have glimpsed the tear in the universe." His soft voice surrounded me. My sobs became hiccups and then evaporated into stillness.

I had a flashback. I don't know what else to call it. I saw him from behind my mother's back, looking around her legs. She had a sweater on. She was talking to a Black man who was at the front door, insisting that he wanted to see Moses, the man who lived in the attic of our house. She was scared, I could feel that, and she was attempting to dissuade him, but gave in and let him come in. I felt my pelvis pull apart. This image scares me. The black disc evaporates me.

I saw Arles emerging from the background of the sky. His body was outlined by stars at the knees and elbows, backlit enough that I could recognize its long, angular shape. A sitting figure. His face came, then faded, but it was mostly, as he put it, "Arles in the sky with diamonds."

I feel an almost magnetic pulling apart. My voice and tone sound odd to me, cloying. I called again, this time a 10-year-old dumpster child heading home for a shower and a cruise in the men's lounge at the yacht club. I haven't felt that persona for a long time. I simply want a clear note from him, a clear 'I'll be back, take care' message, but there is a zero on the machine. When it does register a call, and my heart begins to race, it is a call for help from me.

I begin the ramping up, the slow, steady symptomatic push.

I had another image a few days ago, arising from some river of unbeckoned images, of a breast shooting bullets. When spent of its ammunition of lead and milk, it collapsed into a scar.

I withdraw the contact beneath the surface of my eyes when forced to engage eye to eye. Arles is determined to re-pattern the molecules of aversion. There is nothing else to be done. I have lived in the secret pathos of nothing there, of no other, long enough. And, of course, I don't believe any of this.

Our dilemma is profound. I either stand outside the divided house, just believing its reality with a hand on a sophisticated hip and rip off the therapy, or I move into it, own it, filled with hate and indifference, wrap myself in dark isolation and become absolutely unreachable. Arles doesn't know how to approach this. I asked him if he was discouraged.

"It is beyond discouragement; this is monstrous." He paused. I could feel him looking at me. "Bring the part here that wants to change." I turned my head away. "You crushed whatever maternal opening there was in your mother! You can not look elsewhere entirely for the source of this problem." He was angry. I looked at his face to see if it was true. He caught the edge of my eye. "I want to hit you in the chest, to break your sternum, to destroy the cage."

He said things on Friday like "You have to want to be here." This gives all the power to the criminal. He saw it. "Forget that. You will be here whether you want to be or not."

Friday night, I felt a throat-closing panic when I glimpsed the utter desolation that lies at the root of this. Something of this order is beyond healing. It *is* monstrous. But there is a body.

When he turns away, it moves through my neurons like a grass fire, and he stands by like a toothless farm boy with an empty bucket.

I knew today, as I climbed the fire escape stairway to the waiting room, what the feeling is that captures people with anorexia. In one moment, such sublime control. What a strange notion, "sublime" and "control" butting up against each other.

There is a battle between presence and absence beneath my ribs. And where am I? Am I just the battleground, the neutral, worn-out field? Do I weigh in on the side of one or the other? Where in this war is the existence of any Other?

Arles felt my mounting alarm as I fumbled to put on my new shoes. He took them and stuck them behind his chair. And then it begins. I double over on the long black couch, retching, choking in the sauna-like heat of this body, the silky long moans, the fathomless keening, without images without memory, and I say almost inaudibly, "but she's just a little child."

"Ok, it's ok, now, shhh, it's ok. Look at me." His voice was warm like pudding. "Open your eyes now. Look at me. Look at the ceiling. See these walls. It will help you know where you are... Look at me," he repeated, and gently and slowly his voice settled into me. It was his office. It was Arles.

I covered bear prints with my own today as I stumbled through the fading gold light to the cathedral walls of Windsor Jambs.

I left him a phone message that I would not be coming for the extra session, and that I could bear the cancellation.

Sam told me today that the weakness and compensation of my pelvis, and the pain at the sacrum, were like those of a child raped at an early age. The image came again; no more tonight.

"When I didn't come on Monday, I was... it's... inexpressible. You no longer exist; I don't exist; it is as if all there is is echo." Even then, I could not look up for fear of what I'd see. "It's the white-hot center of nothingness."

"This is an ontological crisis," he said, taking it in again more deeply. This acknowledgment, with all its power, understates it. It implies "being" a form, a past.

"It's your hands that establish you, until the sting disappears. Then..." I stopped.

"Then? Try to put that into words; what happens then?"

"I know, I have to do this differently..." He interrupts me.

"What happens when the sting goes away?"

"I am embarrassed, Arles. I don't want to say this. It's humiliating."

"Forget the humiliation," then his voice softens, "Tell me what happens."

He did not interrupt my long hesitation.

"A free fall begins that doesn't end. It stops... if I hear you, or catch a look at your face, but it's when I feel your hands. I was desolate on Monday, and you were sucked into it. You exist... as a photograph exists."

"What about my hands?"

"They remain."

"How?"

"Through the heat on my skin. The heat and the smell that comes with it. I desperately try to recall you... I can only find you in my resistance to you."

He nodded and leaned forward.

"I am going to give you something to resist." He was matter-of-fact. I knew he was going to forbid the trip, so I was planning to go to the desert. I felt flawed and humiliated, and I pounded my face with my hands, entering, as if drumming, into a trance. I heard him say *No!* sharp and loud, but I was beyond that. He took my hands hard in his and held them as he sat down next to me. I broke into terrified, choking sobs. I felt his hands, not my own. He cradled my head until I could hold it up again on my own.

Chapter 3

Marsha arrived in the dark and pouring rain to a welcoming glass of pinot grigio and our perfect Christmas tree. We ate and talked mostly about her and her important projects. As we were parting today, she told me of her love and fearless loneliness. She holds me as deeply as she knows how to and I find her easy to love, if not always to be with. We had brunch at Swift River with the crew from the Center. She was, as usual, bright, and generous with her time and experience. I hope they liked her, and I imagine they did.

I told Arles about wandering through the Nature Store and seeing a toy made of bamboo sticks. I had the urge to buy it. It is a construction toy with joints to hold the pieces in relation. In the seemingly irrelevant ramble, I suddenly realized what he'd known all along: the meaning of the pick-up sticks. I brought them to him at the beginning of our work, the scattered bones of a psyche. No coherent self except vaguely in the activity of picking up, of being collected, of being held in his hands. Gently treated, calmly, thoughtfully considered. One black stick is worth the most points and always seems deeply buried, piled over, and difficult to claim. I remember how excited I was to buy them. But they weren't perfect enough, so I lacquered them each several times. I gave them to him, and he received them warmly, saying only, "Thank you. I will take good care of these." The black stick. I have held this aspect like an analytic bauble, a trinket, or an artifact, not to be taken seriously, but to be taken in by, to be fascinated by. It is a real part of me, and perhaps too, the colored sticks, thrown around, desperate. Why does this remain so challenging to believe? Yesterday, in the midst of a transaction at a store, I realized I had shortchanged them. I didn't say anything. Later, as I looked in a store window, a woman asked me if I'd dropped a five-dollar bill. Without thinking, I said I could have, which was true. She handed it to me and said, "Well, then it's yours." I knew when I saw it that it was not, and I grabbed it, like a starving orphan would a piece of bread.

As I was leaving his office, I picked up the container of Pick-up-Sticks. He took them from me, put his hand on my shoulder, and bent slightly to look me in the face.

"We will play with these together."

He didn't like my tone.

"I don't need you to teach me manners!"

"Oh, yes you do!"

"I've had enough, thank you!" I pushed the milk container away. I fell into a stubborn silence and lay there in the cold pool of my own vacancy. "I am not here, Arles. There is no impact."

He sat silently a little longer. "This is like the massacre on Long Island. That is not an exaggeration."

He ended the session.

We talked about him cutting the session short.

"So, you feel you are being punished for something you cannot control."

"I know I have to, but..."

"How does the killer feel about being thrown out?"

"The killer?"

He nodded. "Yes, the killer."

I didn't turn away this time. I could answer this.

"Enraged at first, then he doesn't give a shit. That part of me gets harder and colder. The connected part is enraged at being thrown out, too, but rapidly it becomes desperate, fearful. It's catastrophic. She decides to shape up, to do what you want. What do you want?"

"Do you 'shape up' when you feel my hands?"

I shook my head. "I try, but I can't." I broke down.

It's 10 below zero. On Christmas Eve, in a cacophony of misery, I knew I couldn't continue this life this way. There needed to be a drastic change. I awoke with some sense of possibility. Neither John nor I need to be condemned by our shared inertia. I prepared breakfast, fed the animals, and made tea. I was hopeful and felt the warmth of the day. Then John gave me his gift, an emerald and diamond ring. I felt crushed. Unwilling to destroy Christmas, I slipped it on, hugged him, and said, smiling, "I gave you a T-shirt."

Last night, the black cat was back in my dreams. *I am in a bedroom, sitting on Eva's bed, which is just a feather mattress with a flowered sheet. At the head of the bed, there is a cage built into the wall. At the bottom of the cage, a black cat paces. She is half-domestic, half-wild, a small panther. I am playing with it. At some point, Eva reminds me that this cat is mostly wild. The cat bares its teeth and growls at me or hisses, and it scares me. I turn my attention away, and when I look back, it is pushing its way through the mesh, as if its bones are infinitely flexible like those of a mouse. It was out, all but its haunches, and I warned Eva that it was escaping. I went to the nurse's station to let someone know.*

I was trying to ski around Elsa, who'd stopped urgently to scratch, and I fell hard, forward, no arms to break the fall. On the first day of this new year, I gave myself a concussion, a compression of the neck, and a torque in my lower back. I went to see Sam late Sunday night. I'd been shy about coming, afraid I was being dramatic. "This is a serious injury," he said, "I am very glad you called. It needs immediate attention." He worked on me for an hour in our shared silence. "It will be at least two weeks before the bruise and the haze, nausea, and exhaustion begin to fade." I pulled on my boots. "You are like a Beckett character, Sebern, who says, 'I can't go on. I must go on. I can't go on. I must go on.' But at a profound level." Driving home, I took a series of wrong turns, but finally recognized the small back road through the woods to Plainfield. A car had passed through the snow, and I followed the track, only at moments aghast at my decision-making. I was hypoglycemic and hadn't asked for food, lost and now on a road steep and winding, difficult in the summer, treacherous in the winter. There were no houses for miles.

Arles did not hold back. I started to cry: cold, wrapped in my coat, muffler circling my neck twice. His reaction built like a prairie storm, slowly, steadily gaining power, trying to drive home how serious this was. He did not have to say again that 'there are no accidents in your life.'

"This is the last time. This is the last time you fuck with your life!"

"I wish that were true, Arles," I said this as a fact, not as provocation.

"It is."

I felt no defiance. I will accept whatever he does. He has to stop me.

"How likely is it," he asked, "that you will fall again skiing?"

"Probably close to 100%."

"And what did the neurologist say about your neck and falling?"

"He didn't talk about falling. He said that I had to wear a seatbelt even when backing out of my driveway."

He waited, and when I didn't go further, he said, "You don't get it, do you? No more skiing, Sebern. I forbid it. You have no judgment. You follow excitatory pathways. I am your judgment, and you will listen to me."

"I want to end this. Today." I said, looking toward the door.

"What do you want to end?"

"My first thought? You."

"Right," he said.

I commented on his impatience, and he showed me the paper clip he worked between his fingers.

"I come toward you tidally, a tidal wave of desperation and when it recedes, I am left scattered and mute on the sand; the wave leaves behind bone, bed spring and broken shell."

He leaned into the gap between us.

"What will happen if you are successful in destroying this relationship?"

"It would be the end of me."

"The sun would fall out of the sky." I know this is true; it cannot be believed. I want this never to have begun. No one looks for these places in themselves. There is a part of me who wants to tear these years out of the fabric of time and rejoin my life as it was.

❧

The new girl, Terry, told me that I am the first one "to get it." She feels my respect for her and my seriousness of purpose. She has spent most of her life in residential placement and now ours. She said that when I went away, she didn't feel angry, but "Like a machine with a part missing. I felt lost." Nieves let the fight slip, lay on my lap, and began to cry stinging tears, a meager beginning, the slightest opening to a universe of grief. Billie, also a therapist, blows our relationship apart in her rage at my going away. She has no protection from the part of her who would hurt herself to hurt me. Back with me, she begins to settle into the reality of us. All through our session, I was aware of our compelling parallel processes and wondered if it was just that she has more courage. She radiates in her renewed connection, and together we appreciate that she can feel her fear and see her distrust and still begin to open to the possibility of loving and living her life within this deepening awareness. She looks at me, wide-eyed, really, "You are the first person ever, ever in my life, not to go along and let me do whatever I wanted. I am amazed you were right. Until last week, I was so angry you wouldn't just let me go." This woman, who has fought to be free of me every session, is amazed that I did not give up. Nieves says almost the same and thanks me from that wide-open, beaming heart of hers.

This is about Arles, about what he has given me that I now give to them, about what he teaches, about his confidence and his willingness to take this on. Last night I told him of my difficulty sleeping and my disappointment with the Halcion.

"Halcion?"

"Yeah. Not that great."

"When did you get that?"

"Ahhh, last week."

"Who prescribed them for you?" His tone was light, and I entirely missed what I was saying and what was coming.

"My regular doctor."

He leaned forward and took my chin. "What the hell did you think you were doing? What was this about?"

At first, I tried to twist away. I had to catch up with what was happening.

"You forgot to leave any of my pills for me! You promised, and you forgot!" I could feel myself ascending to the high ground in this accusation of abandonment, in the reality of his forgetting. He loosened his hold on my chin, but he held my face between his hands.

"I understand how this must have felt to you. It would have been terrible. But it's no excuse. There is a phone. I am reachable."

He took his hands away. "You are faithful, no, fiercely loyal to the absence in you; the absence of your mother, and you will not abandon it or her." He paused briefly and continued. "If I need to, I will call your doctor. You will get what you need here, from me, for now, for quite a while yet, only from me."

My heart breaks when I read of a woman, 69 years old, who steps out of her home somewhere near here. Her door lock freezes. She goes to a neighbor who hears her but, afraid, calls 911. Police come an hour later, and the woman is dead from the killing cold. The neighbor said if only she had called my name. It is heartbreaking, the stand I take just outside the door in the embittered cold, not knowing his name.

He went to the bathroom. I was splitting off. As I went down the stairs, heart pounding, I felt like I was running away from home, my thinking pushed to the outer edge of my brain, drawn away in dissociation and momentum and fear; drawn back by hearing, feeling his anger, knowing the certainty of it. The duel was fought out in my escalating heart rate. I hid around the corner, afraid of a scene where he would come looking for me on the street. I hid because I couldn't go forward or back. I hid to collect myself. His anger penetrated the dissociative swirl, my fear of the certainty of his reaction, the inevitability. I turned around, fighting to hold onto my mind, fighting to remember that he could, would, help me with this. I stood outside his closed door, wanting to run again. I knocked so softly that he might not hear. He opened the door quietly, took my coat, and then my hand firmly in his.

"It wasn't me. It wasn't me!"

"Yes, it was you! And it is you who is going to sit here with this." He sat me down on the seemingly endless black couch.

"Do you know I am here yet?" No answer. "Do you know I am here?"

"Yes."

"More than that, Sebern. Do you know I am here!?" His voice was getting louder. I shook my head almost imperceptibly.

"What are you trying to do?" No thoughts come. "Think! What are you trying to do?" I tried to think. "You are trying to kill me off. Just because you use a silencer doesn't mean it is any less lethal."

I felt an indentation in the thick air between us and tried to stretch away. When I looked at him, I was startled that he was so close.

The session was over. I wasn't free of the dissociative pull. It felt like the lining on my nerves was peeling off. I wanted to burn myself.

"I have been so damaged," I whispered.

"You won't stay that way," he said with a hint of irritation or maybe resolve.

"It is a world of grief."

He had my hand. His voice softened.

"It is not grief," he said. "This cold emptiness lies above a crying so deep it frightens you." He holds, and he holds against what I cannot bear. "It is going to be very painful to let go of this nothing, this mother."

I have an image of myself, age indistinct, with my arms wrapped around an egg of air, arms and legs, and he is pulling me away. The harder he pulls, the tighter I clutch. I saw for a moment that Arles was saving my life. It seemed epic, like Satan and the angels. I am in that fight over me, unable to take sides.

Winter dark, the fall, the concussion, headache, migraine, flu, and the constant backdrop of subzero temperatures have weakened me... But today is my birthday, and today it is predicted to be 55°. I want to turn away from what haunts me. I will rest today and again tomorrow; I will regain my strength.

"It is a very real grief, this loss of self-construct, nothing abstract, nothing less than losing someone you love," she said.

"Pray for me, Eva."

"I'm not worried about you," she said. "You have never been more alive, more available."

I want to quit this therapy. Arles is convinced that an entire autistic system is breaking up. I laughed when he said "breaking up is hard to do." I am startled when he makes a reference like this to a reality outside here. How does he know this song?

"I want to sleep through this."

"You can't sleep through waking up." He paused. "When one finds the right teacher, either in meditation or in analysis, one learns truths that are unbearable."

"Memory is relationship, isn't it?" He agrees, and we both know that this is the problem. I imagine opening the door and on the other side... nothing. I looked directly at his beautiful face and told him the truth. "As long as you understand that even when I am holding onto you for dear life, I don't feel you."

"That's okay." When he says, "It's okay, it's okay," it's a lullaby.

"Are you my friend, Arles?"

He answers without hesitation, "Yes."

I walked into the empty sunlight. I passed people engaged in existential distraction: piercing their noses, buying a dog, working out, throwing up breakfast, doing yoga, calling their mother—it's all an effort to distract.

"I caught something about my sleeplessness. Part of my mind separates from the rest of it and watches over me, and it keeps me vigilant and awake. This is not good news."

"No, Sebern, it is not, but it is what you must know."

"I lied to you about the sleeping pills." I went on, "I need them. I need to have them."

"What happened to you after this 'successful' lie?"

"I don't know what you mean."

"How have you been feeling since then? What have you been telling me?"

"I don't know exactly. Alone, though."

"Yes, because you have been. When you 'got away with it' you felt I'd abandoned you and you fell into the white noise of absence, the no man's land that so terrifies you. It is a barren refuge."

A new child has entered my life through the clinical door, Merrit, whose life until age 13 was unparalleled for neglect, terror, brutality, and sadism. Talking about her at her psychiatric review, I felt the press of overwhelming sadness and the horror of this child's life. I said the only goal I have is to give her me. She is terrified by the dissociative diagnosis, almost as if the diagnosis, not her child's life, is what dooms her.

❧

Johnny has descended into panic: surviving, recovering, plummeting. He has been asking John about his grandmother and his birth mother. He sent me a feather bed for my birthday. Molly is approaching her acupressure practice in fits and starts, and it is easy to see her capacity for distraction and sabotage. Blake was here to celebrate St. Patrick's Day at the bar where she used to work, see her friends and sleep long and deep in the bed of her childhood.

Today I walked with a twenty-pound pack for three miles, one mile straight up. I finalized arrangements with San for our retreat into the Sedona desert with Anne Dellenbaugh. She will bring binoculars and a knife. I have no reason to hope that Arles will give me mine. I have only one credit card left to pay off. Elsa can no longer walk with me for long. She does for a while and then guides me home to care for her hip. She lets me massage it. I have lost my walking companion of 11 years.

After the backpack training walk, I took her in and then went snowshoeing for an hour in the mealy snow.

Merrit asked me how someone feels full. As if I knew, I said, "By prediction." You feel full even when you are hungry if you can know with some measure of certainty that you will eat again, be held again, that needing comfort will be comforted.

He challenges me to remember, or at least to know that I don't want to, at the same time, he cautions me when we talk about Merrit that memory is not always a gift.

I leave Friday for the desert.

The first day, now three days ago, was hard. We hiked 61/2 miles first in mud, then up and down arroyos. My pack bent me to the weight of my own sustenance. I struggled with balance, with caring for my neck and my back, with acceptance. We did not make it to our campsite the first night. The rain kept up with us. We set up the one tent we had and the long sheltering tarp in a small meadow atop a bluff. We awoke surrounded by red cliffs and a single bluff that they call a witness. The sky was cloudless. Our campsite was at the top of a steep, rocky uphill climb that I felt I could not do, but I did. One foot after the other, eyes only one step ahead, thoughts only one step ahead. In the wilderness, care for myself is so clearly care for everyone. We arrived at Airport Mesa and dropped our packs. I have never seen any place more beautiful than this. I thought, "Here I could be a hermit, here I could live alone in a high dry cave."

I found the horseshoe crab constellation last night, the crossbow and two shooting stars. The big dipper drips over my head. Anne came to give me the prophylactic pills for Giardia, and, for the first night since putting myself at some remove, I found it difficult to sleep. It is people, not wildcats or wildfires, that keep me vigilant at night. I have kept an imperfect silence and have walked into the wilderness alone.

We are camped in a red canyon, on a beach of Cedar Creek in Sycamore Canyon. It is filled with the song of a single canyon wren. I watch a hawk in an apparently aimless glide and, after five days here, begin to feel the clots of emotional exhaustion—long hours on a long couch, holding and being held as my mind opens. I sit in the grotto in the side canyon, a place to pray. The whole land calls to prayer, and my heart is opening.

In one more minute, I will lose the sun on this rock. The canyon is deep, and the walls are high. A small, sweet moth flutters around my nose. The toads on the cliff sound like tiny jackhammers.

Anne has said "No" to my solo hike to the Taylor Cabin and, were I her, I would have done the same. My disappointment rose in my throat, acidic like tears held back, and I was not gracious. I felt ten and spoiled in my disappointment. As I lay here, breathing it out, welling with tears, regretting treating Anne poorly, wishing still she'd let me take the risk, I hear Arles deep in this desert. He is saying "No" too. He knows of my close calls. But risk is not the impulse tonight. Tonight, it is to open to the universe, to the desert, to me and the desert alone. I will apologize for my petulance tomorrow.

I swam in the cold, clear pool naked and opened to the vast silence. I want to be alone here. I can tell the time by the sun on the rock. I made the acquaintance today of a short-horned lizard. It will be hard to leave this place. I cannot comprehend how I was ever afraid. Every day I have walked alone for hours, surrounded on all sides by red cliffs, deep green trees, white petrified sand dune cliffs, and the arching cloudless sky. The grass of the Mesa is blue-green-silver, and the flowers are yellow, purple, white, and Indian paintbrush red.

I have thought that the references in feminist ecology/spiritual literature to earth as mother were grasping, somehow, their problem with metaphor. I realize here that the problem is mine, it is the problem of profound motherlessness, it is the problem the earth faces.

I hang wash out, dripping the red earth from Arizona into the brown soil of New Mexico, and the laundry will dry before I'm done with this entry. Doing laundry and hanging it out pleases me.

I realize that I have learned to set aside worries. I don't think of home or of the JCAHO audit or John's illness. I stay pretty much where I am. Part of this peacefulness, a good part, is feeling Arles's presence lodged somewhere in me.

When I told him that I slept well out on the ledge away from the camp, he said, "You were among your own kind."

Sam thinks I came through the trip strong and with more damage done by the sleeping drugs than by the fifty-pound pack.

I dreamt of Blake as a three-year-old, sleeping with her, all knees and elbows and champagne hair. The dream felt as close and as warm as memory until I saw it, and then she was startlingly white and, until the end, unknown to me. I mourn the small death of ECT and the tragic theft of brain cells that allow memory. What an arrogant desperation, doing that to a twenty-year-old girl.

I dreamt that I was driving into town and all the trees were gold, with many bare spots. It was a beautiful color, but then I realized with a shock that meant it was fall. The spring buds were leafing into a dying foliage, and it made me want to cry.

I dreamt of a whale caught in the harbor where the boats put in. The water and sky were gray and cold. I am swimming into the forbidding water, knowing there is a whale that could attack me. I can't see it. I lie across the Styrofoam surfboard, and my feet kick into the body of the whale, the body of the beast I cannot see.

Charlie Boren's cancer has been cut out. The surgery was successful.

I am up against this stony, cold center in me. I might have held onto my connection for the entirety of the vacation, but Arles going away and being sick and needing to change his schedule and threats to Charlie's life broke the thread. Yesterday, he pulled away to tell me I could defeat him, that this part bored him. I know this must be true, but I can only imagine it vaguely. I was astonished when I confronted Norman, my young patient at the Center, about his impact. He did not have a clue. He asked vacantly, almost innocently, if he did have impact, and of course, my affirmation had no impact. When I insisted that he get sheets for his bed, he bought black ones, and of course, the staff let him. I wrote in his case note that if we were ever going to treat this boy, we would first have to make him up. It's the same for me. Arles asked me to write from this place.

"There is no one there, no one to write for."

"I am there, write to me."

I told him about the conjoined quintuplets.

"Which organs do they share?"

"Heart and stomach." Integration is impossible. Parts need to be killed off to rescue other parts. All parts are facing inward, seeing only themselves. "The risk of treatment is death to all; the risk of no treatment is death to all."

"And yet a choice has to be made," he said, pragmatic, like a surgeon.

"I know this is only a construct."

"Constructs have the deepest reality; they construct the psyche-soma."

I am trapped by language. The metaphor locks us into a sense of inevitability, even law. I asked him to take me into his universe where the laws are different. Attachment laws. Integration laws. There is no operating under the present ones. This monster cannot live, no matter how big the heart and stomach.

He has rejected my notion of compliance. I think, however, that compliance is the only route. When I arch my back, it is my universe. When I don't, I get an intimation of his.

So much now is about the face; the look; my wanting to scream out to the baby who smiles at his mother who is about to let him drown. I can't bear to remember this, but I cannot look away. Oh, Johnny.

I acknowledged that what he said was true. "I am not absent. Your mother's depression covered her absence. You 'received that,' now you recreate it. You can't feel anything about your neck unless someone else is feeling it for you."

"Black holes, Arles, are constantly created, but not by the wishes of stars."

He sat back in his chair. "You don't trust me."

"That's not true!" I cried out, "I trust you more than I have ever trusted anyone!"

"That's small consolation, isn't it?"

Yesterday I lay on the warm sand at Nauset and slowly drew my hand across the surface of the earth, here where it dips into its deepest unconscious. I felt it. I patted it. I wondered what it would be like to really feel the body of another. I felt the wind and smelled the sea and was happy there, loving Nauset Beach as deeply as the hopeless Sylvia did. I, though, will survive myself. On Friday, when my crying let up, he asked me if I knew the story of Tear Drop Tea. I shook my head. He told me the story of a bear who wants to cry, so he thinks of all the sad stories and songs he can and cries into a teacup. He makes tea from his tears and drinks it.

"I said to myself, 'What will you feel like when you leave not knowing you were held?' This is the voice of a supplicant hoping for an answer. I hear nothing. It's answered with a deadpan." He was struck by the expression of expressionlessness, the face of the depressed mother.

"What do you see in Nothing?"

I shook my head. "What's known," I answered finally.

"And what do you see in me?" I wanted to flee. He answered when I didn't, "In me, you see 'want.'"

There was a man in the dark, backlit hall. He said, "You are the devil." I didn't know; I was disoriented; I couldn't see him; I looked for someone on the stairs. He repeated himself, and a voice within me said, "I am not the devil." He said, "No, you are a good person, just like me." I moved past him once my eyes adjusted. He called my name, and I turned around. He asked if my name was Sarah. I didn't know him. I don't remember saying anything except "No, my name is not Sarah," feeling an almost subliminal panic that he'd asked my real name. He didn't. He thanked me for talking to him, and when we got down the stairs, sat down in front of the Coffee Connection to a waiting cup of coffee.

❧

He squirted me with a spritzer he'd been using on the plants.

"You'd better keep that handy," I said, barely breaking a smile. I sat on the couch and tugged my shoes off. "There are tidal surges between anxious yearning and a withdrawal into emptiness."

He pulled the chair up in front of me. "We are now wrestling with your 'autism,' and we are right where we need to be." I liked that he said "we." I hate it when he, in his own autistic habit, says, "It's good that" or some variation. I hate it.

"You have a theory, and you have fit me into it."

"Maybe you showed it to me."

I said, at some point, "The sociopath wants to take over and blast you out of that seat!" I can feel the crawl of this in my brain. He grabbed my hand and smacked it.

I pulled away so hard I broke the seal. "That was hate!"

"No, Sebern, that was love."

He took my hand, and he covered my stinging palm with his hand, like a compress, like a bandage. I dropped deeper, and I moved between sobs and whimpers and the high-pitched squeal, begging to leave, insisting on my right. He held me there. "I know you think you're going to die," and a ripping cry acknowledged him. He tightened his hold.

He kept me waiting, and when I said I hadn't eaten, he bought us both chili and a soda. I liked eating with him. It was trust. I couldn't eat much. I put it aside on the couch.

As he ate, I described my voice.

"It has four positions, in my body, in me; in the container of my body, but disembodied; coming from behind me and through my mouth; and coming from in front of me. This voice is the voice of my mother. And the choked off cry of the pig, the high-pitch squeal that I hate."

"Where does that come from?"

I knew immediately and answered, "In me, disembodied."

"And the deep cry?"

"In me, from my body. It is warm."

"Is the other cold?"

"I don't know."

"Is there a shiver in it?"

"Yes."

Five days ago, two of the girls I treat ran away to find their mothers. Merrit, brash, street-smart, and bright might find her way back unmutilated. My fear mounts every day for Terry. I woke with the thought of her raped, left for dead, enslaved, and trafficked, disappeared into the salt mist of early overwhelming trauma. She is four and wandering alone. I pray for the kindness of strangers, but that's not what these kids attract. And at the same moment, I felt nothing, held back from these feelings like a mother at a fire scene. These girls, all of them, are motherless. Terry's mother is fragmented across fifty-two personalities, loving her daughter when she knows who she is. Nieves' mother was arrested again for heroin; Merrit's mother is sunken in by depression; Rennie's mother gifts her daughter the heritage of incest, and on her birthday, panties with the crotch cut out. Their mothers, too, were motherless.

He is not a person. He is a surround. His office is the rest—the arms, the atmosphere, the predictable weather, the environment that could be mother.

A black kitten, very thin and somewhat weak, was nonetheless sauntering through the basement hall of a school. I recognize that she has been weaned too early, and she is starving.

"What do you focus on in the dream?"

"The thin haunches."

"What attracts you to a hollow at your belly?"

"I like the feel of the curve of bone. I like no belly, no evidence of need. The image came from the TV. A Holocaust corpse being lifted onto the back of a truck."

"Yes, you have many images of the Holocaust. Like Sylvia Plath."

"That's true, I do," and I immediately say, "It's appropriated, exaggerated."

He paused and then said, "There is currency in this notion today that reports of the Holocaust are exaggerated, that it is all made up, that it didn't really happen."

Today I cut a bough from the apple tree. It was infested with tent worms. I set a crumpled bag beneath it and lit a fire. The wood released a sweet perfume, but I had to watch as the worms scrambled futilely to save their lives. An imagined terror? What else could they feel? I felt true pity and sorrow for their plight and for mine, for the choice of one life over another. I am confused by the real compassion in me and the me that watches beatings or rape as both the aggressor and the dissociated victim, without compassion. Merrit and Terry are both back, more than that, they had nowhere to go, but they were rescued.

I saw why I have not forsaken the image of swimming in the aqua sea. It is an image of immersion, nearly effortless, in the truth. The truth has threatened to tear my head from my neck and my mind from my body, but this does not dissuade me from knowing it.

❧

It was Johnny on the phone, identifying himself with a now characteristic wariness, awaiting my annoyance that it was him. Then the hum of lubricated small talk.

He'd called to say, "I need to save my life." Something snapped inside of me. "I am going to an AA meeting at 7 AM tomorrow." He was drinking vodka as he said this, as much, he said, as a fifth a day. "It will be hard," he said, "because I like it. It stops the pain."

"You have been in terrible pain, John."

"I have been in pain all my life."

"Yes, I know you have." When I asked how he manages this, he didn't know. He slips further into his alcohol haze, and when I talk about therapy and our willingness to help with it, he rambles away. I bring him back, and he tells me of his own premature death. His liver has been enlarged for five years, and he has changed doctors to avoid the implications.

After he had said three times that he wouldn't live long, I asked, "Do you have AIDS?"

"No!" I could hear him swallow. I kept my silence. "I have never been tested. I am so suggestible that if I test HIV positive, I will develop symptoms immediately." Both he and Sean had had partners with AIDS.

"All I ever wanted was to be normal. This all started when I found out I was gay."

"Oh, Honey, no. This started when you were a baby when you were abused by your mother."

This came as news.

"Do you want to know, John?"

"Yes, I want to know everything." He was drunk by then. I had a moment after hanging up where I felt the slow sulfurous rot of his brain and body.

Johnny called. He went to AA. He continues to drink and talks of his American flag and his need to be normal. We knew his sexuality. We accepted him. We didn't realize that he felt our acceptance as a betrayal of his hope to be normal.

Arles has relied on the hypnosis workshop, but there are conditions. I may not be a subject, and we will not miss session time. I hadn't thought about being a subject.

"It is important that you not learn some things before you're ready." Hot tears spilled over, and I said, almost in a whisper, "This could be true."

Yesterday Merrit called me from the hospital to tell me about her multiplicity. "Why did this happen? Why is one mute? They don't just threaten. They do things." She wouldn't tell me what. "What will happen to me? Who will I be? There are some I don't mind if they die. There are others I want to keep."

The next call was to Dr. Newman at the emergency room. After speaking with me, they decided to section Nieves. She had threatened to kill me. She was escorted into my office, trembling. She asked if she had frightened me. "Oh yes, you did." She broke into sobs and threw herself into my arms. I held her. At the end, I took her to Emergency Services. Yesterday morning, she called to tell me she wanted out of the hospital. I reminded her of what just happened and told her I wanted her in.

"What is ego strength if not the arms of the mother?"

"That's right, Sebern. Perfectly said."

I was in the wilderness. We came across a stack of lumber or something covered with a tarp, and there was a baby on it and another in a stroller beside it. The baby was slipping off, and I grabbed it by the foot and took it into my arms. I went to the door of the house behind a stack of stuff and knocked on the window in the door. I could see in, and there were many, many babies and young children. My knocking was being ignored. After several tries to get access and get care for this baby, I just opened the door and saw even more children being taken care of by two teenage girls. There were six or more small children (like a litter) at a wooden table waiting for food. They looked physically good, surprisingly well-cared for given the number of them and the age of their caretakers, but they were hungry and angry. There were more in the back room being dressed. No one paid attention to me or the biracial baby I was carrying.

At her evaluation for admission, Nieves told the worker, "I will go into a hospital if Sebern wants me to." I said to her through the interlocutor, "You must do whatever will keep you safe," not sure how to make these decisions when she is both my patient and my murderer.

That night, Arles moves as I move, blocking the way to the door. He makes himself known in empathic opposition. He leaves me room to move only in my most adult self. About the rest, he has constructed a crib of his ribs.

We lost our appeal on the Northampton house that we bought on Marsha's financial advice on Camano Island, and the medical imperative from my neurologist. Even a whiplash could paralyze me. I have to minimize driving. My mother is here. She is old, and she is no different. She insists on a solution to the house that is untenable. The second time she says it, I say, "I don't want to talk about it." She snaps back at me, and I apologize. She snaps again, and I let her have it, reminding her that I have just received the news. Three times I say, "What a hard week," and she doesn't ask. I am hurt and enraged. It will pass, and one day I will grow up.

Last week, Sam said my body hadn't felt like this since I was nearly hit by the truck in Shelburne Falls. My hand was on the bumper as they slammed on the brakes. This week, he brought the MRI images up on his computer to illustrate his belief that I had shattered the C2 vertebra that now presses on the spinal cord. Hundreds of fragments he thinks of at the point of impact. I was shocked, and even looking at the evidence, this event is not real.

I walked around Bass Hole in the misty gray evening light, and I recognized the familiar death wish, habitual, not casual. It is not an instinct. It is a reaction. This baby turns toward her mother, and her mother turns away.

I relapsed at 8:06 this morning in the empty three-quarter Cape, my schizoid mom burning a Corntastic in the toaster oven a floor below. Arles had given away my hour. I negotiated it all, the false talk, the false values, my mother commenting as if surprised by her own perception and proud of her insight,

"Mothers are important to their progeny, aren't they?"

"Yes, very."

As aware as I am and as unwilling, I slip out. Arles had sent me off without him. I was back at the edge of a place in me I cannot go.

"This is not me," I cried in a deep, soft, unfamiliar way. He recognized this. "I wish that you could feel what I feel only for ten seconds, no longer. No one, no human being, no creature, should ever have to feel what this feels like. But I want you to know, but only for ten seconds." He asked me to tell him, but there are no adjectives. I try. "I am in a landscape with no horizon." He leaned toward me, closing the small distance between us.

"I am learning this, Sebern. I have an intimation. Your mother's emptiness is too much for you. No more visits to the Cape for now."

I pushed back. Organizing around the sociopath, I'd bought a knife. He took my hand and, before I could curl into a fist, smacked it.

Then he held my hands as if in prayer. "I know why you needed to buy the knife. Do you have it with you?"

"No."

"You will bring it next time." I looked away. I could feel the feral child muscling up in me. "No, look at me." I turned my face toward him, but not my eyes. "You will come on time and bring the knife." I nodded slowly. "You need to come to know I am here."

"But you weren't!" I screamed. "You left me! How would I know? Someone else ate the breadcrumb trail..."

He nodded. "That's so, Sebern. It is too soon for you to remember. Do you know now, right now, here?"

I shook my head. "Nothing is substantial. Just to make it from second to second, I act 'as if.' I move into the 'as if persona,' as if I was all right, as if I was normal, as if I was not tortured. It was she who went to the men's locker room." I recognized the odd pitch of my voice, a distant monotone, a drifting cadence, only when he reacted with impatience. This boy(s) has been my protector. They are fleet, agile and good with knives. They will humiliate or kill. They mock. They assault tenderness and decimate empathy with vicious attacks that would silence anyone.

September 1st was my tenth anniversary at The Center. Most people were away, but I got a bouquet and a moving card. My program director asked to hug me and said, "You have truly enriched my life."

We are getting frightened calls from Sean saying that Johnny has threatened to burn down the condo. I can't respond except to speak with John and the girls with kindness. If he is seized enough, Johnny could do this.

I howled, torn in the teeth of frenzied predators, and suddenly, without warning, it stopped. The silence that follows is confusing, empty, and brutally sad. I obey the state. There is no feeling; I am not bereft. I am wide-eyed, open-mouthed, startled, and subdued. He comes quietly and sits down next to me on the couch, careful, I think, to disturb nothing. I was five years old, and I knew the hopelessness of old age, a loneliness that moves forward in time and expands to make the universe.

I left a message confirming my appointment for tomorrow and asked him to bring a straitjacket. This morning, I woke to a raw, cloudy day, and I flew into a rage, smashing my fists against the glass door and then, after slapping my head hard with both open hands, accidentally laid my hand on a hot toaster. When I was finally able to calm myself, I became aware that this is all hormone-charged, but the intensity is insane. What sense is there? I had wanted two beautiful days. The forecast said I would, the man in Saint Paul said I would, and when I awoke to gray skies, I felt ready to kill. Arles reminded me that I've been talking about my rage at Kevy's birth. When he helped me see all this, I cried out, desperate that he might not know.

"But I didn't kill my sister!" He reassured me, almost as if I were still three.

"No, Sebern, she died of internal causes."

Is there a suicidal rage that is not homicidal? Yesterday morning, after the dangerous fit, *I had the dream of giving birth to a baby who was arched across my womb, of telling the Haitian aide that I was afraid of all the blood and shit that would come and her reassurance that the room could take it, it was designed to.*

I could not leave my bed that morning. I wanted to suck every molecule of comfort from the smell of my pillow. Is this really about Kevy?

"Unconsciously, persistently, you are attempting to destroy the treatment," I asked if there was a recognition in that statement of how much

I've changed. He said, "Yes." I asked if there was an understanding of the validity of my worries about him, of his contribution. He said, "Yes."

"Well, then I think you're right, and I hate this. I am imprisoned, kept away from you." Too much has been said, the assault of voices screaming at me, insulting me. Cold, degrading, alarmed, and I can't bear it. I go mute. He asked me what I was feeling.

"That I want to want you to sit next to me, but I don't." The voices of derision got louder.

"Tell me what is happening," he paused. "Be honest."

"The voice is the demon voice telling me to get away, and I twist in it."

"Yes," he said, acknowledging these voices, "They will want to take you back, to repossess." I caught the progression. The terror is first in the muscle. It builds in my stomach, and only then is there a thought—'I must get away.' I twist and stare like a blind girl. Seeing but not seeing, both eyes white.

"Most people get off this stream of consciousness, Arles," I said, covered to my chin in the gray blanket.

"Yes, Sebern, they do."

"But I can't."

Sinead O'Connor sings a song I will play at Thanksgiving for Arles. It begins, *Thank you for hearing me*; It ends, *Thank you for breaking my heart.* This therapy, this practice, is about breaking the heart. There is no other way. A patient of mine gave it to me.

❧

My first call was from Nieves, at the hospital for blood tests, scared. On Monday, we will learn if she has AIDS. If she does, she would've gotten it from her uncle when he raped her repeatedly between the ages of six and ten while her mother looked on. Yesterday I watched the sunset in her hospital room, hating to leave her, feeling a desperate urgency to get out of there. Johnny's was the next call. He was calm, thoughtful, and mature. The night before, eating out, he'd experienced chest pain and sweats and feared a heart attack. At the ER, he was diagnosed with a panic attack, and he decided to admit himself to the detox unit. Last night he spoke with John for two hours, about his terror, about seizure and stroke and about his resolve. After the third call, this from Billie, torn apart by early abandonment and feeling every minute of it, I left for the fourth day of the trial of Merrit's father on multiple accounts of sexual assault. On her. She is shattered, so early and so unrelentingly. I don't know what can be done, what I can do, what she can do. I try to sort out how I feel, but what I feel sinks into a barely audible static.

I told him about Merrit's father sitting on her chest and forcing her to take his penis in her mouth.

He was quiet, then he asked, "Who did that to you?" I feel like throwing up.

"No one did that to me!"

"Who told you to say that?" he asked, softly, the chair already pulled up close to the couch.

My eyes are white, pale blue and opaque. It is as if a magnet has cleaned the disc. There is a *hole in the memory* more than there is *no memory*. The getaway builds up first in the muscle, only then an impulse, but how does the muscle begin? In response to what? I doubt everything except perhaps what I should, the doubt itself.

I left shaken, oddly spacey and sat for ten minutes in the dreary stairwell before doing the descent. I didn't want him to find me there, to have to deal with me. I don't know what to call these states. I can force myself out of them. I can more or less allow myself to slip into them. They draw me like a slow, powerful intravenous drug; a sedation. An invitation out. Or in.

"Arles, I have found my way out. I know another place to live, an everyday place where I seem to join real time, a place that is without interior; I lived there last week. It wasn't without feeling, but there was no depth, and I felt in synchrony with regular life. I felt no terror, no rips, or tears; my sense of being was seamless with the time it was being in. Perhaps it's atavistic—it took no will to live; no consciousness outside my own dailiness." I could hear his breathing.

"I know you want this, Sebern, or some version of this..." He trailed off, or I interrupted.

"I came in here two years ago with pigtails and freckles, naïvely asking to go beneath the story. Now I feel humiliated by such stupidity."

"The decision," he said, "feels like yours, but it's not. You are not on this journey."

"Who is?" I asked, confused momentarily and then derisive.

"The psyche needs to do this."

I am afraid for Merrit. This time, though, I think he will be convicted. I am afraid for Nieves, sick in the hospital and lonely. Marsha is visiting, knowing what she knows well, knowing nothing of what she does not know, exhausted and in that, less exhausting. She asked me to make her coffee and bring it to her in bed. I did so gladly. I don't know about this really, but I love her more all the time, almost for her self-centeredness, her tenderness.

Merrit's father was convicted. I would have been outraged had he not been, but it all tears me up. I feel like vomiting. The program manager said, "Well, now Merrit's healing can begin." Will Merrit's healing begin? What does healing even mean? What happens in this complex system? What happens to the part of her that identifies with him?

Arles greeted me in the warm November night with energy, humor, and love. I could talk about the horror of the week, the desperate human tragedy of that trial. I said to him that all I wanted to do was weep.

"For whom?" he asked.

"Them, me, all of us." I was crying. "I was not strong enough to be at that trial. I was not 'other enough' to be at that trial."

"Yes," he said, "that is more right than 'strength.'"

There are, Sam says, knots on the knots, and I am exhausted.

I am looking out at the sheets gliding in the breeze, into the gentle morning that embraces my exhaustion, that eases me out of the hard, hard week. Nieves does not have AIDS. Merrit's father is in prison for twenty years. Is Merrit in prison for life? No, I refuse this. We are in different stages of house arrest.

❧

I returned from four days at the Silver Spring Holiday Inn learning hypnosis, surviving there, perhaps in a constant low-level dissociation, a sinus infection, a vacated city center, no hot water, lousy food, elevators that did not arrive, a room crowded by anxious psychotherapists and assorted others, and one beautiful woman from Eritrea. Some system of defense, bombarded by trance, disintegrated. I have vivid, disgusting imagery of myself: a fetus, skin you can see through, large brown eyes, hardly a nose or ears, the mouth, the opening of the inside to the out, no lips, no backside, legs hardly visible. I came back from the training broken open and spilled out like an egg.

"You will not lose your mind. You tried for years to do that, and you couldn't. I won't let that happen now."

In a sense, I rehearsed not only saying what was true, but being in it, a true person. He understands my dilemma of self-construction.

"Symptoms are a compromise. They are about continuity. They are the only trace back to the truth, the only memory." Then I asked, in the voice of a very young child, "What makes me up?"

Our sense of self is at least in part a sense of continuity over time, a narrative built on interpersonal memory. How could I "make myself up." There is no one to confirm or provide facts or stories other than my mother. Everything she has told me she has either idealized into a lie, told as a lie outright, or she subsequently contradicted.

One day, I will make a sculpture with pick-up sticks. I will make a whole body.

I yelled at him, turning what started as a shameful apology into an angry affirmation.

"Yes, you have to fight for me! I do need you to fight for me!" After the hypnosis training, every door slammed open. I was back in the barren landscape. I arrived with a quart of chocolate milk. He did not embarrass me with interpretation.

"Symptoms are my only memory," I said.

"They also will keep you from remembering."

I persisted.

"What if I could sleep at night? What would that mean? We know what it means that I can't, or we lean into my absent memory in a certain way. Right? Without symptoms, I would have to rely on your memory, I would exist only in the universe of your memory."

He stepped out of the argument that was pending. "This is," he said thoughtfully, "a perfect description of the mother-infant reality."

This idea entrapped me; it meant dependence on his holding me in his mind. If he forgot, I would no longer exist. My mother's mind does not hold me. The awful images came at me relentlessly, they were fetal, deformed.

I entered the office and sat quietly.

"Do you remember our session, Sebern?" He asked me in a way not to jar me, but he did.

"No, not really."

"It was pretty rough, Sebern. The trance induction and these states of opening are connected. This week is the beginning of coming out of trance, and that can only happen here." I can feel the protest rise and collapse. "You can finish the training only when you don't have to go away to do it."

"I'm due back there. What am I going to tell him?" I was beginning to object.

"The truth. Right now, this is too much to know."

Monday night, Merrit set a box on fire outside the door of the residence. I could barely keep attention to the necessary activities of living. I called my hypnosis teacher to tell him that I would not be coming. He said I sounded sad, which was approximate. I did not sleep. Merrit was taken to the hospital for assessment.

Wednesday, I worked with the staff to ease their fears of this shattered child. She had no intention to burn down the house. It was an episode inside her head. They receive me well, and tensions are eased before I leave. I go to wash my hands with the black soap that smells of his hands and count the hours.

I talked with Arles as though the early week had not happened. Neither of us seems to notice. I can't stand up straight; it bows my neck. I cannot get off this rotation on my own axis, in a glass box called therapy.

I spoke of communities, of his, as I imagine it, the company of intellectuals and artists, genuine artists. I added, "a small community."

"And yours?" he asked.

"Mine is of people who think about how to keep a kid from burning down the residence." I got home to a message on my machine from Tess: "The girl's residence has burned to the ground. The boys' is not habitable. Arson. Two suspects." Both are my patients.

I went to the police station to say goodbye to the new girl. She was sure that I hated her, and she tried desperately to put the best spin on all that had happened, in the language she had learned growing up in these places—psycho-babble. For four days during the investigation by the arson squad, none of us knew for sure who had done this, but most bets were placed on Merrit. We found housing for all the kids in a down-at-heel motel out by the traffic circle. Clothes were donated. It was, of course, all played out in the papers that I did not read. I made no press statements. The sergeant, an expert in arson and arsonists, looked at the remnants of the basement rec room and said the fire started there. He questioned the two girls each several times. In my office, Merrit was crying and pleading, "Sebern, it wasn't me. Please, you have to believe me. It wasn't me."

"You set the little fire three days ago, Merrit. What do I make of that?"

She looked up at me, eyes filled with tears, "I know. It looks really bad, but honest, I didn't ever want to burn down the place. Ever."

"I think most of the house staff think you're guilty, Merrit."

"I know, they hate me, but *you* have to believe me!" She sobbed, both angry and almost pathetic and by the end, I believed her. Then I saw my new patient. She had no history of fire-setting. She denied having anything to do with it. Looking at me without flinching, she lied. Both of these girls were supposed to be on one-to-one coverage: the new girl because she was new, Merrit because she'd set the box on fire, but then someone on staff is out sick, or looks away, or gets scared and doesn't say.

As the police investigated, I talked with the staff about what we knew and how important it is to know exactly what we know, to refuse to engage in rumor and if the kids elaborated on this, to firmly but gently correct them, to remind them what we know and what we don't. Mostly, we just don't.

The investigator told me there was no question, the new girl had set the fire. I went to Thornes just before it closed in time to buy her a teddy bear for company in her next homelessness. No one wants an arsonist.

"Is this really for me?" she asked, her face crumpling into tears.

"Yes, it's really for you."

"I never had a teddy bear," I think that's what she said. It was all muddled in sobs.

There is a rainbow halo around the waning moon. It is the winter solstice, and we are mourning. Elsa went into kidney failure. Blake came from the city, John cut his workshop short, and we went to her. They carried her in to us on a blanket, and when Blake lay down next to her, she wagged her tail weakly and gave us her clear Elsa smile. The vet talked of the short life of dogs as a reminder to live every day, to take nothing for granted. She, too, was close to tears. I took Elsa's head in my hands and kissed her between her eyes. I thanked her for coming into our lives and asked her to go gently. She did. I held my hand on her heart, and I felt it stop. She was gone to become, the vet said, a greatly needed guardian angel.

"Elsa's death," I told him, "can open a door for me, a door to a world of grief."

"Yes, and what will allow you to walk through that door?"

I shook my head, "You."

Chapter 4

The nor'easter took out three trees in one spot and the door off the hinges. It was Christmas this year; 78 mph winds, slashing rain. The internal erupts here and on the Cape. No one is reported dead or injured, but I feel both. I'd hoped to be past this. My mother is a surly ghost. She served roast beef, and again I ate it, not wanting to stir up the smooth surface of things, wanting only to get by, quietly enraged at her, at her pretense, this exercise of Christmas. I am at the end of this string. I want nothing of this charade. I became absent too. Two ghosts, one surly and oblivious to the wreckage all around her, the other surly but subdued, all too aware. On our return today, I entered the house without Elsa, and that grief hit me again, like a tree crashing onto my head.

Words go away. Since Christmas on the Cape, I am garbled and tongue-tied. I feel neurologically disorganized. I am clumsy too. Sitting tonight, I felt as if there were landmines placed around the pericardium, and if I move wrong or too quickly, I will explode my heart. I want to lie on my rug and hold my dog and feel the slight disappointment in her response to me.

I want to feel differently about my mother. I want to love her again, cherish her for both of us. It is only when I am with her that she is not alone, and I am not with her. She said nothing about Elsa.

I thought tonight of John Cotton, the psychiatrist-in-chief at St. Luke's hospital. His spacious office was on the ward, Clark Eight, where I was first admitted in the early spring of 1962. I'd left my college abruptly, but after many broad hints and finally, in a kind of terrified aimlessness, I took the train to Miami. Early in the morning somewhere, I imagine, in South Carolina, in a fit of agony for my mother, I spoke with the porter who'd brought me a pillow and a blanket from the sleeping car. He said, "It's okay now, honey. At the next stop, I'll wire your mother. You can sleep."

My grandparents told me to stay right there at the station, and they came to pick me up.

I had no intention of returning to college, and the psychiatrist told my mother that they would only consider re-admitting me after a year of psychiatric treatment. I was allowed on the campus only to pack my stuff into the Ghia and leave. My mother dismissed this recommendation, focusing on hypoglycemia, until she asked her social friend John to see me. A month later, I was a patient on his unit. One night, I found his door unlocked. I went in, closed it softly, dialed my forbidden friend Bobby, and we talked for an hour. She told me that Milici, my doctor and hers, was talking to me when I was sedated for shock treatments. I'd told him of our pact. "Shhhh," I whispered, "They are in the hall." I swung my feet off the oak desk and slid down under it, telephone on my lap, pausing our conversation only when they opened the door in a frantic search for me. I suppressed my gaiety until the light flipped on, then off, and the door pulled shut. She told me that he was threatening her with Bellevue, and she'd told him she would die first. They returned ten minutes later; my struggle was feigned. I'd kept talking with Bobby mostly because we weren't allowed to speak. I think they finally noticed that Cotton's extension was lit up. He'd read me the riot act more than once, perhaps even after this, but when I didn't improve after ECT, he twisted collegial arms to get me a bed at the Institute of Living. I wonder if he believed what was so often the summary evaluation, Prognosis:

Poor. My mother drove: me, heavily sedated in the back seat of her station wagon, my brother up front with her, Chu, my favorite nurse, in the back with me, to Asylum Avenue in Hartford. I was there to see one particular resident, Charles Boren. Word had come the day before through the porous walls of the unit that Bobby had hung herself.

I know my parents as caricatures, flattened into a cartoon by memory short-circuited by absence, by years of fictional construct: theirs, my siblings,' my own. I know no more really of the reality of my father's character than my friend knows of her father's tenure in the CIA. There are no fewer lies stringing my family together, just no patriotic rationale. He, too, may have been a charming crook, a fraud who, in his way, loved his children. The thought occurred at the slippery edge of the cliff overlooking the Jambs. There is no such thing as a happy alcoholic, another family myth, unquestioned until two hours ago, my arms around a tree, my cheek pressed against the rough bark. I know nothing, and I have no way to learn.

I became aware suddenly that when I hear voices in the wind, I prepare for my own death. In the deepest infrastructure, I inhabit a savage world of murderers, terrorists, thieves, rapists, and con men. When the sun goes beneath the cloud, I feel fear.

I have no memory. I am rooted to a tissue of lies.

There are moments now with Arles—they almost feel captured on film —where I am. Just moments, but moments as precious as they are exceptional. Ephemeral. He likes me. This feels new in the way I feel it. I know nothing of being loved that is different from fascination, or awe, or idealization. All of this is brand new, unexpected, and unchoreographed.

I feel dumb in these unconstructed moments, as if I'm there, openmouthed, innocent of expectation, without guile. And even as I write this, I am aware that the lie comes to me without angst; the truth requires exertion. The lie is as smooth as quicksilver, as effortless as reflex.

I held the journal in my lap. "This is my only memory."

He stopped me abruptly. "Have you copied it?"

"No."

"You are playing Russian roulette with our relationship, with your sense of self. Copy it by Monday and give me the copies."

"Oh, oh, ok, ah, yes," I said, "Thank you, I will."

'It's been three years,' I hear myself saying. 'It's alright that I'm changing.' Some molecular structure is reorganizing. It is how astronomers know there's a black hole there, through the intimation of factors. I look forward to time in my attic room, quiet and alone, able to lock the door and pull the blinds.

I am here. My first night at the new house on Elizabeth Street. I turned a Rune: Algiz, "Protection," and it told of newness and fear and fortitude. As I sat to write in this journal, the phone rang. It was Arles. "To let you know you are remembered and that I know how to reach you." The night will bring what it brings, all easier now.

"The terror is very real, and it also serves the terrorist. It is used to savage connection."

"I don't cherish the terrorist anymore. I don't want you to think of me that way."

"You don't 'idealize' it anymore." I heard this when he said it, as a misunderstanding or an addition to my word "cherish," but it wasn't; it was his contradiction. I do cherish it, still. I don't like it, but hold to it like a soft, frayed blanket smelling of childhood. I sat bundled in my coat, my long scarf wound around me, like a refugee.

"I am as cold as a Russian winter."

"Yes," he stood over me. "Take off your coat."

"I just said I'm freezing, Arles. Turn up the heat!"

"It's plenty warm in here, Sebern. Give me your scarf." I looked up at him, wary, preparing to defy and slowly, as if the wool were heavy, I uncurled its many loops around my neck. I bunched it up and put it in his outstretched hand. He put it under his arm. "Right, now your coat." I unbuttoned it carefully and slowly pulled out one arm, then, even more slowly, the other. I lifted it toward him, and he swiped it off my finger. He laid them down at the far end of the couch, then sat down next to me. I felt the weight on the cushion, and then, without any warning, came the sharp, sudden integrity of his hands. That night, I felt the reality of a body. That night, before I said goodbye, tears in my eyes, I was just beginning to feel where I end and where he begins.

Wednesday night, I was there with him, close to sleep. Thursday night, the terror rose in me. I felt weak, helpless, not up to the simplest conflicts or concerns, afraid, bewildered, and guileless. I couldn't sleep even when John hung the shades, the protection against being seen when I could not see. I heard the footsteps of my tenants and, repeatedly, I reviewed the situation with the locks. The walls seemed thin. It was the third floor. I recognize body memory, and then my mind wipes it away when it finds no image, no character, no name, no face, no words. I feel in a kind of draw. "Blank memory," he called it, like blank mourning. A whiteout.

Eva told me of her dream that morning. *She saw that I was sitting in the refrigerator*—did she call it an ice box?—*in the house in Plainfield. She thought this was odd, and I would not answer when she asked me why I was doing this. I closed the door, and she went to the living room to tell John. He shrugged his shoulders, more helpless than indifferent. Eva suggested that at least they would want to time it.* We spoke of it as the wind caught us outside the restaurant door. 'Attractive nuisance' was her thought. Is this me? How do I enter the cold core and stay warm enough to begin life and incubate a self?

I thought the door was locked. I thought someone was coming. It was pitch black. My bed was at the end of a long hall. There were no footsteps, just John's voice. "Prepare yourself, they are coming closer. There was one in Ossining." He was telling me about earthquakes. I looked around me, wondering what he thought I could do in response to that warning: move off the third floor? Live in the basement? How would that help in an earthquake? I became resigned, but resigned with some fear. I saw this house, well, this story, collapsing on me, crushing me. The dream is caught in a restless sleep. I remember another dream image from Thursday night. *I am trying to get through many layers of cloth to get to the breast and, once finding it, seeing that it was mutilated.* Does Arles know of my breast tumor, nine months after her cancerous breast was removed, the incision that would not heal, the incision on the line between breast and nipple?

Merrit has reached new depths of grief, yearning, and sorrow. They ransack her. She is ashamed of feeling this and terrified of the power she gives her foster mother by loving her. She called me tonight, feeling like she wanted to explode. She wants a connection with me to help her bear the anguished separation from Tess. (I almost wrote "Arles," but of course, it is all the same.) I will see her tomorrow.

I cried with Arles, soft, deep, broken-hearted, but not broken. He met me there with his own softness and spoke of these three years, this exceptional exploration. I lose most of what he says because he says it quietly, and I send up a kind of white noise. I fled into last Wednesday's persona of confidence and falseness. Every word began to feel hollow, and he seemed little more to me than a canyon wall throwing back the echo. He said after a while that he had two alternating responses: exhausted despair and wanting to beat the living daylights out of me.

It is being left alone. This is the unbearable pain.

❧

My mother tripped over a duffel bag carelessly placed on the airport floor and hurt herself, possibly ribs broken, a swollen hip. My cold heart was flooded with protective love, fear for her fragility, and empathy for her that I was glad to feel again. I don't want my heart further lacerated or further neglected, myself the perpetrator. It is April 1, and she is 79. There are flurries. Today I listened to Tosca by the fire.

I came into the bedroom of a friend, and she was showing me her baby. She herself stood off to the left, almost out of the frame. The baby was on a bed with a white bedspread. She was beautiful, a biracial girl with dark curly hair and large dark eyes. Her expression was pleasant, but unchang-

ing. I picked her up and saw that she had a penis. I said to my friend, "This is not your daughter, this is your son." She said, "No, look more closely." The penis was, in fact, a long fold of skin, and I put my finger at the lip, and there was her vagina.

"Finally," he said, "an opening."

❧

Suddenly, there appear four horses grazing through the succulent snow, and now I see in Amelia's sculpture the disfigured but beautiful Japanese face, the face of Hiroshima. I have stepped outside on the deck to see the horses and to loosen the nest of snow from the eaves. I did this barefoot without any discomfort, my soles warmed by the red boards of the deck. It is mid-April in the New Mexico desert. The sun remembers this. Large patches of earth are already cleared, thirsty, no doubt grateful to be drenched in this white storm.

I cannot will anything: not my sleep, not my progress, not my attention. I can only practice.

Arles had asked me what I hoped for in New Mexico. I stumbled around, embarrassed, thinking I should have an answer. 'I don't know' would have been fine. He would've just nodded or said 'Um Hmm.' I said instead, 'opening,' and this is not a bad answer, but it failed because it is not particular to New Mexico. What I realized once here is that, beyond the essential quiet and solitude, the vast silence, there is here, inherently, spaciousness. Spaciousness is my New Mexico quest.

I wrote to Blake:

My dearest child, I love the silence. I take it into my pores. But I have that too in Plainfield. This landscape provides spaciousness. Spaciousness is one of the goals and the gifts of this practice. One teacher said he looked so deeply into his own heart that he saw outer space. I am sitting several times a day to look deeply into my own heart. During one sitting, I started to cry. This, of course, is not unusual – the tears come with my awareness of turning in, ever more, and how this may affect the ones I most love. It could so easily be felt, as my turning away, as not caring, as refusing to mother. I don't think, in one reality, that this is at all true; and in another, it is. This journey consumes most of my energy, most of my thoughts, most of my time. It may be revealed at some point as a self-centered delusion, unreal, unimportant. I don't think so, but... it was when I thought of you that I cried. I can imagine you wanting sincerely to reassure me that you feel my presence and you would do so lovingly. But I know that I will never leave this path, so that for us to truly walk together, you must join me. You must be unafraid of your fear. You must be willing to deeply engage with the truth, at least the truth of me. You have said you can't bear to know. There is, of course, a part of me that can't bear to know either, and I, perhaps more than anyone, have taught you this fear. I talked to Eva and Arles about this, and each said, "like the child of a Holocaust survivor." I have wanted to protect you, my most precious daughter, and I will never tell you what you cannot bear to hear. But until we can share it all and are engaged in the deepest knowing together, we walk on different paths, close but not touching.

I love you as much as life.

Mom

Last night I sat under the desert sky until the cold entered too deeply to ignore. I wanted to climb the roof to have no obstruction. I wanted to accept the obstruction. I wanted to rail at the obstruction. And then, suddenly, instead, my heart tore open to the suffering of all hearts and to my own. I thought that, in any one unit of time, there were billions of moments of suffering. As I lie here awaiting sleep, I know I am nothing but particles, particles of everything else.

It is not the loneliness itself. It is when it is insinuated with anger and fear, like ribbons of fat. This is when I try to swallow without tasting.

I thought about Arles today, about how gently he soothed me last week, how he held me in the crook of his voice, swaddled me in soft tones. He coaxed me, "What is your fear, Sebern?" He anticipated me. He knew the fear was as old as my ancestors. I will be forgotten; he will forget, and I will break apart; he is my skin. Something in me is letting go, something held deep and tightly coiled.

Last night, after the long ride back from Santa Fe, a difficult, agitated sitting and a brief time under the clear star-crowded sky, I lay down on my little bed and cried. I cried tears that moved through like cleansing rain. I cried for the relationship of me to me, for the degradation, the contempt, disregard, and willingness to injure. I relate to no one else with so little compassion. I remembered a moment when Arles, at the end of his patience, remarked on my pervasive, unrelenting self-hatred. I laughed and said, "I don't hate myself." I have so deeply learned hatred that it is my nature. I am held in it like two wrestlers, exhausted, their grip as much a mutual embrace. They stagger, unwilling to let go even though the crowds have long since gone home and the referee is there only for the overtime.

I met Charlie for lunch at the hotel on the plaza in Las Vegas, New Mexico. We both ordered chicken salad. He asked about my neck, about Johnny and about the fire. I noticed the soft shock of being remembered. When I reminded him of the way I injured my neck, he cringed slightly, his bright blue eyes darkened, and he looked down and back again. "Sebern, you are immortal. You should have been dead twenty times." When I told him of my intuition that his cancer would not return, I took hold of his hand, and he did not withdraw. I told him that he and Arles were my 'Midwest bookends' and of Arles's appreciation of him. "Arles and I are brothers," he said unselfconsciously, and I remarked on their great differences. Charlie would never have been able to take me to these depths. He appreciates this journey and gives me perhaps more credit and Arles less than is due. Arles is the exceptional one in our relationship. When I talked about Marsha and her attachment dilemma, he said that my understanding of people impressed him. He talked about us both. "The two of you worried us very much." Neither Marsha nor I know that we worried people, that we even made a dent in their awareness.

He took the check and said he had to go. I walked him to his Jeep. "I love you, Sebern, and now it's much easier for me to say it." He kissed me on the cheek and accepted one from me.

I saw a coyote who ran from me sideways, a rippling mixture of fear and curiosity. I saw antelope in the low desert, heron and wild turkeys. My skin turned brown, and one of the beautiful bays nuzzled my cheek with the flaring black velvet of her nose. I read about mindfulness, and slowly, I slowed down.

The week before I left, I had a dream. I remember only one image. *My face was wrapped in plastic except for my tongue, which stuck out through it.*

On my way up from the airport on 91, I saw Arles in blue jeans and cowboy boots, and I broke open to the deepest moment of love, perhaps the purest I have ever felt. I ached with it, like the opening of a deep vein in a rock, a fault line. I watched myself move to close it up, but thought instead, "I'll see him tomorrow. I will tell him of this awesome experience of loving him." It left me in a muted state like the end of a sunset. I drove home in the cold rain, open-hearted. He'd left me a message. He would not be here tomorrow. "Something unexpected came up; someone important is in from Europe."

When I couldn't contain it any longer, I exploded at him on his machine and only many hours later could I find it in me to apologize, as much for my need as for my rage. That night I dreamt *I was walking on a back road and saw a white cat running behind a tree, trying, I think, to hide from me. I was delighted to find her. It was Meep, the cat I thought had been taken by a coyote. She tried to run, but I caught her, and I swept her up in one hand, bringing her to my chest. Everything about her was fine except for her eyes. They were circled as if burned, looking through me, an unbearable look of a terrible secret history.*

Sadness creeps along my arms just under the skin, to my neck and down my body, into my knees, building intense pressure between muscle and skin. It seeps down into the cells, it diffuses through the blood, it covers the organs, it closes my throat. Arles understands me, but he can fail at critical moments to estimate the raw pain, the critical disappointment, the slipping of fingertips off the high ledge. He chastises me for "false maturity," but demands of me that I not really experience his abandonment as abandonment, to "grow up" about it, to posture a resiliency that I don't yet have, that comes only with time after time of predictability.

He stood with me on the porch the following Wednesday. In the throes of agony impossible to contain, I flung my head against the brick wall. "No, no, no," he said, both urgent and soft. He cradled my head, and I let my forehead drop to his chest.

Yesterday I held a day-old lamb, the tiniest of three, orphaned, and after a minute or so, she just relaxed all her muscles and fell into me.

He opened the album. He said, simply, "Awful." He held the photo tenderly, watchfully. "This is a suicidal baby. These photos could be used as a Thematic Apperception Test of attachment failure."

It was the tenth anniversary of Hugh's death. I traced his face with my finger. I described his hemorrhaging on every breath, his final flaunting of the life force. "He told me that if he survived this, he would do as I'd asked and stop drinking. I wanted to believe him, but I didn't. I nodded my head and said, 'Survive this, Hugh.'" I did not describe how I wiped away blood that erupted on every breath from his nose and his mouth so that it would not pool in his ears. I watched his eyes lose color; they were hardly blue anymore. The color left in his face came from broken blood vessels. I rubbed his feet and hands, pulpy and cold. The doctors came to me. I was the one to make the decision to stop the blood transfusions. Our mother was twenty-five miles away, not on her way.

We three black kittens were doomed from birth. All of us were bloated with hunger; all of us took blood revenge. All of us preferred our own deaths to hers.

I had intended our conversation to be some kind of acknowledgment of the anniversary of Hugh's death. It ended with me screaming at her, "God dammit! When will you get it that I am just trying to protect you, to care for you?!" She accuses me of betraying her. I love her with a passion reserved for children grown in the culture of absence. All of us fiercely love our mothers. We hemorrhage with that love. We blow ourselves apart. My madness is testimony to the truth of her. And the meaning, the reality of it, that she attempts to destroy.

I was in the City the Friday they released *Ordinary People*. I knew she'd want to see it with me, but we had made no plan. I took the last seat at the matinee performance while she was still at work. She went to see it the next day on her own. As we sat down to our supper in her high-rise apartment, she asked me, "Didn't you feel just terrible for Mary Tyler Moore?"

❧

It is a downpour. A week ago, James, a former patient of mine from the Center, called to tell me that he is working now and attending night school. "I look people in the eye now." We had worked on this for months, eye contact that hurt him to make, and on his handshake. He said he missed me. I learned of Carl's arrest for kidnapping on Tuesday. After a high-speed chase on Rt 2, he crashed his stolen car outside the front gate of Concord State Prison. The cop was smiling when he told me. I feel this boy's terror more than my disappointment or my failure.

Arles is on vacation this week. Somewhere, I feel that life is not worth living. This is a very early decision. I've managed it—when I have—by leaping over time, by finding the next event to fix on. Now and Then becomes a suspension bridge over the chasm, over her withdrawal, over her unbearable absence. It's only next Monday. There is no life until then, just movement. It is only a week.

"I will be fine," I said.

"You'd better be," he said.

On return from a four-day conference on trauma and dissociation, I dreamt *I was standing in the bathroom, and a bullet shot from outside shattered the glass of the window, just missing my head and lodging in the wall. I knew this had happened before, and I was afraid it would happen again, but I didn't tell anyone because I was not legally living in the house. I was not supposed to be there. Someone, I think it may have been Kevy, persuaded me to call the police. I called 911, but didn't think it was really an emergency until I said, 'Someone tried to shoot me,' and then I knew it was. The dispatcher was a woman, and there was some confusion about my address. The police came. Kevy dealt with them. They made some kind of investigation that I tried to ignore as if it were going on behind me, and they said they would do their best. Kevy came to tell me, "You'll be relieved; they found nothing." When they excavated the site of the bullet hole, there was nothing. I was relieved because now it would not be in the papers. I was also confused. But what about the shattered glass? What about the bullet hole?*

The atmosphere of the conference was dense with its subject and corrupted by a fascination just as dense. The humor felt condescending and degrading even to those making the jokes, not to mention to their tormented patients. Many of them were organized, understandably, around attacks they'd received or feared they would. It felt to me that their thinking was interrupted by it; that, perhaps, they needed to address their own victimization before they could get to that of their patients. They seemed to share a kind of voyeurism, an aggressive, but disguised, response to their patient's dependency and little understanding of neglect and attachment rupture. Their attendance made them important to themselves. Many made themselves experts. A few were, and they were, frighteningly, already demigods. I often found myself staring at this crowd, trying to decipher what brought them to this work in their flowered cottons and pumps, their sharp summer jackets, their rumpled shirts. Merrit is in crisis, 200 hundred miles and worlds away and afraid that I would be mad, that, even worse, Tess would.

Their strange gaiety, like a cocktail party, closed in on me. I tried to understand, but everything began to lose meaning. The sky was gray, the air saturated, and only Tess's liveliness kept me from sinking into the swamp it was.

The dark bruise, like a fingerprint on my arm. I don't know where it came from.

Eva and I talked. I revisited her remark of months ago, that she has 'learned to be nurtured by her mother's intent.' I said I thought I needed to learn to be nurtured by my mother's belief that it was her intent to nurture.

"I don't believe it's possible. You can't be nurtured by that. You cannot be nurtured by your mother."

I sent Arles a Father's Day card. Just a man's hand beneath a baby's bottom. He thought the card was beautiful.

❧

"I didn't know how to get out." I was almost breathless. He sat down next to me...

"Was it real, Arles?"

"It was real, Sebern."

I knew I was crying. I knew I was hard to contain, and I knew that at the end, I shared something that frightened me as soon as I said it.

"I think this is the fear of ending therapy."

He shook his head slowly, "No, I don't think so."

I was howling. He asked me how big I was, and I wanted to show him the little space between my thumb and index finger, but instead said, "little, little, little."

"It is all there is. There is horror in my head. Oh, God, Arles, they went after my body, and they got my mind."

"Describe what's happening," and again, there are no words. I pressed his hand down on my skull as if he could reach that featureless horror through the hard bone of my head. I knew these facts even while I didn't know them at all.: Time, place, size, age, event; the present became background, eclipsed, imageless, even, for the most part, bodiless. "Oh, God, oh, God, it's happened again!" A hair in my mouth. I swab it off my tongue, close to retching: a black pubic hair. I looked frantically toward the door. I couldn't get away. No one—I must have known this—could hurt me at that time; what time? And I felt an assault without end, no description, no substance, everything, everywhere. Refuge does not exist. When I can sense him, feel the wall of his side, this moment drops back, away from now, into another time.

Many weeks have gone by like this. But after this session, I had no more pain in my back.

On Wednesday, I was a totality, undisturbed, impenetrable. I was a man in a white suit, ultimate confidence, posing as serenity. I was untouchable.

"It took four days for you to be re-inscribed in your mother, in her absence."

I decided that I had to put an end date to therapy; one year, and it would be a good idea to cut back. I was now much better and suffered nothing more distressing than your average neurotic.

"Now I understand my reaction," he said. "What you are saying is not true, but it's the swagger. I just want to smack you."

"I tried not to swagger."

"Yes, I saw that too, but nothing could hide that walk."

"I want to leave."

"I'm sure you do, but not now." He gathered me up, and perhaps then the saying became true: all hell broke loose.

❧

I was in the water by 6:45, swimming quietly so as not to scare the heron perched on the crest of the stone at the center of the lake. She was almost three-feet tall and serene even as I got closer. Then she flew inches above the water, turned in the mist and back toward me to another rock out of reach. Noble, alert, but unafraid, the survivor of prehistory; the trajectory of the unconscious, the flight of a dream. I slip my suit off and launch myself deep into the lake, playful in my quiet approach. She allowed me even closer before abandoning her perch and me. As I turned back, I saw a form in the water, swimming an impeccably straight course. At first, I imagined it must be a beaver, but they never swim straight, and then I saw the shape of the head. It was a tawny doe taking the cool shortcut, shore to shore.

On my way down the mountain, I experienced it, sudden and unexpected. The world turned menacing. I felt a near psychotic dread. The fragmenting began, but was not so complete that I could not try to think why this was happening. Was it because I was going to see Arles? No, clearly no. I have been looking forward to our time. I became aware of an old fear recurring, or an old construction: as the time to see him got closer, it meant the end of the session was also close. Was it the weather? They had just forecast severe thunderstorms, and there had been some cracks of thunder. I realized recently that trauma survivors experience these events as recapitulations of terrible forces unleashed, natural and beyond their control, ordinary so that no one sees what's happening, coming out of the blue like an alcoholic rage. The weather made its contribution, but it was not the weather. The interview? Claudia Brenner talked about being stalked and shot at while she and her partner were camping on the Appalachian Trail. I shut it off, saying clearly to myself that this is not good for me to hear, then, chiding myself, turned it on again. I was disorganizing; the world outside me was distorting in some way that is hard to watch—through all senses, though, not just visual—twisting and mesmerizing. My only strategy was to get myself around normal people, doing normal things. I was very aware of their states, the people at the beauty parlor where I was having a pedicure. It was not just to see that the strangers were benign, but that they reacted to the weather as weather. I paid attention to my feet, to the sensations of warm water and massage, to the ease in the muscles of the young woman's face. I did the same study at the gas station and in the parking lot. No one else was frightened, and this helped me collect. I had the thought that just stops me: after Hiroshima, life went on. How can it be possible that life just goes on? What other possibility is there? What about memory? Finally, I knew. It was about their being shot while naked in their tent. That detail of their utter vulnerability; their trust in the goodness of place and time, their innocence; the shame of their innocence. I wish I had never heard it.

I told him of the state in me, something more than fantasy, a capacity, and it made me sick.

"I don't want to be in that camp," I sobbed. "I don't want to be there, I don't want to be either the shooter or the shot, the murderer or his victim." He had asked me about the murderer's state. I asked not to talk about it. I think he understood that this time was different; my relationship to that part of me was no longer one of appreciation, aggrandizement, guiltless pleasure, but of near incomprehension, repulsion, and fear. At some point, he took my glasses, and I anxiously surrendered my keys, my only weapon. He was quick to take them; he knew the danger I was in. All I knew from then was a descent into imageless in-body terror, covering my head, a contortionist, as if I could find a posture that would enclose me, protect me. I took my keys back. "No." He lifted them from my hand and offered me his arms and his voice instead as my protection. I described the cold that spread up under my rib cage. He said many times, "I'm here." "It's me." He soothed me this way, as he does, trying and usually succeeding in finding the edge that keeps me from dissolving into the state, while also not stopping the discovery of the state. This is actually a hallmark of his being with me, pushing my experience of each state to the edge of tolerance, and when I go over into it, he helps me return. He has allowed me to experience myself as a sociopath until that becomes no longer a state, but a reality and then, he reminds me somehow that this is not me.

The crying I do is not like regular crying; it is saturated, desperate.

"Am I destroyed?"

"No, Sebern, you are not destroyed, and you will not be destroyed."

"I want to tear my face off."

"I know you do." He held my hands. My shoulders dropped. There was a long, empty silence.

"I've had a hard time."

"Oh, yes, you have."

"Do I scare you?" I'd seen the darkness in his face at the beginning of the session.

"Do I seem scared to you?" I shook my head, uncertain. "Don't you think you'd know if I were scared?"

"Yes, I would. These are forbidden trails I am walking." I looked around blinkered. "It's your hands, Arles. Not your words. I know where I am in your hands. I know where you are..."

"Hands are the first language. They are the language before eyes, before faces."

Like an aperture or a pupil, I close around a single point of focus. I pull in to conserve energy. I have no creativity except whatever I use to create myself over and over, in that pinpoint of energetic focus. It feels as if I barely make it from breath to breath.

❧

We talked about the new admission, a 15-year-old White girl with a history of repeated hospitalizations, with stitches in her forearm. Sabelle. She has been diagnosed with multiple personality disorder, and I'd taken her on to my caseload. I'd only met her briefly on intake the afternoon she arrived. She held a small pumpkin, hollowed out but not carved, at the center of her chest. Where had she arrived from? She was a pretty girl, with large blue eyes, downcast, chestnut hair only slightly snarled, jean shorts and a sweatshirt. The psychiatrist had read her records. He said, looking at me in a way that was meant to shut down disagreement, "I will order the sleep-deprived EEG, but she will of course need to be on medications." I could feel the muscle tension of the group, anticipating me. Our nurse told me later that I rolled my eyes. I thought that I'd found a professional chord. "Can you at least wait until you meet her?" The group was nervous, and they took cover behind him. Sabelle would be, by history, on meds.

"I realize that they made you very sick, but..." I interrupted him.

"They make everyone very sick, Arles! They are toxic. They make no one well. They are at best chemical restraints."

"Yes. And all too often that is the only restraint possible."

Merrit was, I think, hit by a car. She does not remember anything before coming to, in the middle of Route 9. She told me that she may have run into a tree. What would that mean? She can't tell me. She wasn't there. She has three stitches in her forehead and, likely, a concussion.

It was that cold May evening, chilled through, when I realized that my mother had no empathy. I had made a discovery of great importance. But I didn't recognize it, like finding an odd fragment in your yard and being slow to realize it is a tooth of a Paleolithic man. A missing clue in the evolution of one's own emptiness; the explanation of the atmosphere of an echo.

I scoff at the line "There is no infant without a mother."

As I walked there to see him, I tried to understand the state of no desire, no urgency, the state that could/would sit with him conversationally, that was solid and clear, spacious, and sane.

"You are not organized within yourself, you are 'about' not 'from.'"

He is going again next week to Belgium. I do not feel numb. I feel nothing.

❧

It is an agony to be here. I cannot love her enough. I cannot free her from her stone courtyard. I search wildly for safe subjects to protect her from the injury of knowing. Her innocence tears at me; her dead eye pierces the skin of my heart. Our secrets hang in the air between us, taunting me; hers are invisible to me and leaden; mine are mostly about her. I try to breathe into the silence between banal spurts, and occasionally we find something to say that holds our interest for a few minutes and does not threaten to tear the heart out of the love between us. I looked at her tonight. I refused to be afraid. I crowd around the naked baby who is repeatedly losing her mind. 'She means no harm. She does the best she can. This is forgivable.' It is her innocence that devastates me. I am exhausted by my attempts to protect her, unrelenting and unsuccessful. I would do anything, I can do nothing. Nothing but keep the silence wrapped in layers and layers of lies and gossamer omissions. The only end to this particular agony will be her senility or her death. I cannot bear to hurt her, and of course, I will.

My uncle is dead. His lungs filled with water, he sank beneath the gentle waves, and he is gone. My mother went deep inside herself, and she was unreachable. She cried several times, but it was mysterious. What of it is about him, about herself, about my father? She did not respond to my touch. Not one muscle acknowledged my presence. She did not touch me. I feel compassion for my mother and the dawning of the deepest grief, not for me but for the baby I was. She was as stiff as vacated.

I was very glad to be there for her. I want only to tell her how much I love her, but it is for me as if a sock were pushed down my throat.

Eva and I spoke about our mothers.

"You know," she said, "how people speak of being with a dying child, helpless to make a difference, the incomprehensibility of that. That, I think, is what it is to be with our mothers."

❧

"I am beginning to change my attitude toward this baby. I am beginning to use a different pronoun from 'her' to 'me.' I am beginning to experience a forbidden empathy." He was vigilant about the movement of my fingers over her face and her hands, ready to restrain even the merest impulse toward disfigurement. He would've taken my hand away. He would've protected me. "If you really got close to the reality of this picture, it would break your heart."

"It does, Sebern, it breaks my heart."

"You have to come back," I said, "I have places to go, and I can't go without you."

"I agree. You do have places to go. I will be back." We have a glimpse. We share a vision of a realized life in the life and mind of the other.

There is no growing up fast. On Thursday, after many successful efforts to maintain all of his messages on my machine, I accidentally erased them. The shock of what I had done registered in my belly. On Friday, I began three days of migraine that even Sam could not stop.

Walking softly today, I become aware that I am unable to truly taste the air without him with me. I am steady, but orphaned, my sense of being held in abeyance, wanting to point at him, my finger like a gun: stay away from me; wanting to throw my arms around him; wanting to take his hand and say, "I am so glad you are back."

It is something about being understood and being reduced or compressed. It is as if when Arles gives experience meaning, it loses its significance, its meaning. There are times when what he says adds to the body of identity, but mostly it reduces it—I am just like everyone else. His words, like warm water on a sugar cube, make me disappear. He will destroy me by understanding me. I hang like an orchid with roots in the air, a delicate thing that cannot survive being planted in the soil. I told him this.

"You are not like everyone else, Sebern."

When I left the session, I didn't feel that way anymore. It wasn't that I was braver; it was that I was safer.

I dreamt last night that I was at a play and that the seats were zafus.

I awoke that morning in a bad mood and discovered a new bully, eight or ten, but this one was a fat boy pushing his way into my head. He was not going to kill anyone, but he was jostling for space, for recognition. He wanted to be dealt with. Arles did acknowledge his presence.

I held my fingers like a piano player at the sharp edges of the flat, wide wrist bone, feeling it.

"Have you ever broken a bone, Arles?"

"My ankle."

"How?"

"Playing basketball."

"Did it hurt?"

"Oh yes, that kind of pain registers forever." He looked back at the court. "Why do you ask that just now?"

I realize only now that I began the session by telling him of the possibility that Merrit, as an alter, had broken her own bones. I am trying to say something about violent dissociation, the unspeakable memory lapses from childhood. It seems impossible; I try to stay with it—the colors in my mind fade to pastel, and I mingle into the muted sunset. And still there is this fat boy with a crew cut wanting to get what I get. This persona in me is the bully, not the scaredy-cat on the playground. And where is the agile, ratty ten-year-old? I left my session, stopped at Essentials for the black soap, slipped off the cellophane skin, and rubbed it on my hands.

In Belize, I discovered a new relationship to time. I have described this sense in the past when away from Arles, of keeping my head down out of the assault of time, waiting it out. I have also known the position of pulling time along behind me like a stubborn child, dead weight. Ahead of time; beneath time. In Belize, I rested in the current of time. Neutral about it, having no thoughts about its speed, I drifted in its flow like a sunfish. Mayans drew time as a crocodile with heads at both ends. One head is skeletal and smooth, and it swallows the sun; the other opens its fleshed-out jaws each morning to let it escape.

When I return, there is no reaching me. I am weightless and compressed, held in a kind of dissociative enthrallment, untouchable, muted, glazed, motionless. I have images of trying to curl into Arles, but I can not do this. I am rebuffed by the fact of his bone, his separateness. He and I are accidentally inhabiting the same space, still, voiceless beings, huddled into our own disappearance. And then he is big and dark, indistinguishable from the room and the primitive art. I am dark too. In my dream, the light, like Jerusalem, like Belize, is so unrelenting that it drives you into the caves, or so slight that the only purpose seems to make clear the reality of the dark.

There is something to this sense of Arles' diminished capacity. It is true that we have been on a journey together, a journey that requires him to find, re-find, name, and hold, to turn toward these places not only in me, but in himself. I have no longing, just the determination not to move, not to be. He asked me if he was present to me.

"You are in me, in my cells. Your cells are interwoven with mine." He entered not through my mind but through my skin. It is this metaphor, this sense, this fact that organizes me. His tones of reassurance, "It's okay, I'm here," have become the lining on my nerves. But, no, not present to me.

Who knows what this night will bring? Merrit is asleep downstairs after an episode of stark terror, in and out of dissociation since 5 AM today. Her voice was little, her courage remarkable, her experience, both internal and historical, so terrible, I can only come to the edge of recognizing it without beginning to black out. When she came in, she was clutching Tess. She pleaded, "Sebern put me to sleep." She was frightened of her state, frightened of her need, apologetic, appreciative, exhausted.

"It's okay, you're safe here," I said to assure her of the reality.

"I'm not here." I knew this was true.

She recognized what triggered this—her bed on the floor, the man coughing in the next apartment. She finally fell asleep, but woke up terrified. There was nothing else we could do. I remembered Arles and imagined that he would do this for me. He would tuck me into the guest room; he would do everything he could to harbor me. He said when I told him, "You did the right thing."

God, I can't stand what happened to this child. She does not suffer from a sickness. She is not sick. She suffers unbearably.

Chapter 5

This evening was the service of reconciliation and forgiveness at Weston Priory. I am here on retreat. Thirteen Benedictines monks and their guests. The prayers are simple, and many are beautifully sung. They wear blue jeans under their robes. One prayer is, "No matter how gray or how old, let me be little," and I think for a moment that my endeavor is holy. I left Arles to drive here, feeling Merrit's agony and Tess' pain, and Marsha's stark loneliness, echoing beneath the exoskeleton of behaviorism. Maybe, among them, Tess has permission to feel what she feels, but little of that. I am beginning to experience permission from the laying on of hands.

After days of indecision following my uncle's death, his ashes were buried in New Paltz with no one attending but the yard's owner, the same man who had dug his grave, as we would for a hamster or cherished dog.

It is Christmas Eve, and I have just walked up the hill in the frozen, starless night. All ambient light is tossed back by the deep snow. The bell began to ring. The Brothers are welcoming, and they seem to love their venue of song. My alarm is set for 3:30 to arrive at the main kitchen by 4:30. Morning vigil on Christmas, I am told, will be a full house and then again, for the Eucharist. I will receive communion tomorrow because they will be delighted to give it to me.

Perhaps the true encounter is never with the causes of fear, however justified or overly determined, but with fear itself. But I have needed someone to know and say, "this happened" to skirt psychic death. Who could that be?

I want no other life than the one I have, the one I have had, and the one I will have.

"How can anyone feel God, truly love God and truly receive God's love," I asked, "without being loved by their mother?"

"Yes," he said, having thought about this himself. "We need our mothers to bear the face of God, to make its brilliance, its vastness, bearable. Our parents are the domestication of God." But then he stopped this conversation. "How are you doing?"

My tears fell freely. "I am fine, and it feels as if this mystical place is barren. I am led out into the desert, and I can't bear how alone it is."

"*It* is?"

"Right." I corrected myself. "How alone I feel. It's ontological. I am weak when I open to this, as weak as the baby who has surrendered. When I asked to look at the photos, I hoped to see the spark. Her eyes are almost dead, her body is rigid."

"The terror *is* the spark," he said.

Today I protested. At one point, I stood up, my coat on, and he stood up and gently but clearly told me to sit. I stomped my foot and said, "I don't want to!" I could feel his smile, and I looked, and I laughed and then cried and refused. He took my face in his hands. He told me of his friend and that man's daughter. "He was trying to get her into bed. She said, 'I don't want to be a tired little girl. I want to be an animal that bites,' and she bit her father." I sat down.

I was moving back in time, and then, even though he had made time travel possible, we could not go there and stop it from happening.

"If you'd been there, you wouldn't have let this happen; you won't let them hurt me." Before he could answer, I saw the clock, and I flipped back into rage.

Johnny is crashing into terror, the terror of dying at his mother's hands. I am torn up by his unrelenting pain and his imminent death. He is driving to visit his foster mother today, trying, I'm sure, to snuggle in, to be little and safe. When I turned toward him this morning, he cried in relief, and I think in gratitude. I was grateful for the inflow of kindness I felt for him. Some cold veil of protection has dropped between Johnny and me. When I think of him—that in itself is different, I am no longer putting him out of my mind—it is with empathy and tenderness. His words are in my head: "I don't think dad knows how bad it is; when I feel like that, it's like I'm going to die." Then taking a drink means holding onto life. I hope his therapist is halfway competent. So few are.

I took the Peter Pan bus home from Eva's after spending the weekend at her new home with Barry. A lot of it I just watched. I was taking in the dailiness of life, the spreading of the comforter, the soup on the stove. It is a fascination, the wonder of an alien as I begin to drop into the reality of living a life. I am not studying how to make a bed. I am absorbing that there is living one's life. This is it. It is not an activity to be finished with so that we can really live; it is the profound and holy act of living. It was ordinary, comforting. I took a seat at the window to read an interview with Pema Chödrön on her relationship with Trungpa, her most important teacher. She was certain about what she'd gotten from him without needing to rationalize or even understand or line up this certainty with his terrible, unenlightened behavior. Or perhaps it was that it all did line up for her, that she needed all of who Trungpa was to learn what she learned. More precisely, she needed all of who he was to her. Reading this, I felt a new level of security with Arles. He is who I think he is. He has taught me what he has taught me, and he is a person struggling in the rare struggle, the fight to be fully conscious and deeply engaged. All of his failures, perceived and real, are just what they are, and they are, in a mysterious way, part of the gift. My certainty in him allows me to bear my uncertainty in him. His failings then become gifts; his absences, now—I can't believe I'm feeling this—part of his presence and part then of the deepest holding of this therapy.

I am exhausted in the battle between knowing and not knowing, the possible futility of the effort, the humiliating and degrading voices that call me a liar, a skeptic who knows my susceptibility to suggestion, that that very susceptibility may be evidentiary, coming up against the white wall of no memory over and over again, the somatic sense of catastrophe repudiated by my mother, by the mind that refutes everything it says, and the part that wants it to be true, the final justification of this long life of seclusion rooms and dreams of them. What is the unremembered, private injury? Arles says there is agony in my voice, but I don't remember. Marsha thinks invalidation is the central factor; it surely was for her. But for me, it never remains as domesticated as "invalidation." It is annihilation. I am now the perpetrator of this, and I don't know how to stop. Short of Arles saying, "this happened," there is no way. And he can't know any more than I.

Tears were streaming down my cheeks. "I don't want to tell you; I want you to tell me in little bits, so I know you're there." He understood. "If it was as bad as it seems it was, even by four months, how come I was not a disturbed child?"

"You were too scared to be."

I could not follow him.

"Flashback is not the same as memory, just as a nightmare is not the same as a dream."

I asked from deep in the hollow,

"What am I doing wrong?"

"Did you hear me criticizing you?"

I fear the trust I've given him, nothing less than the power to annihilate me. All he would have to do is say what my whole constitution is arranged to hear, "I don't know what all the fuss is about. Nothing terrible happened to you. This is psychodrama."

"Why would I make this up, Arles?"

"I don't think you have, Sebern." He was trying to help me understand that my experience, while not of memory, is of flashback, that, like a nightmare, it has meaning. He was not preparing to destroy me. I moved from thought to thought like a hunted frog, not daring to go underwater. He spoke of my dream this morning.

I remembered as I came awake, *"The closer animals come to living on the land, the better their memories. It is as if when the evolution process is being lived 'at sea,' they cannot remember. Everything each day is deep gray water, and there is no demand on memory. But when you crawl out of the vastness of the sea and must negotiate the hard surface beneath you, then you must remember."*

He thought it was right that memory was needed on land in a way it is not at sea, that it was particularly needed when you moved out of the forest onto the savannah. The memory of who is part of me, who is one of mine, whose territory it is, what is safe, who is safe, this requires memory. I don't have it.

Part Two

Chapter 6

NEUROFEEDBACK

Kathy, Peggy, and I were in a supervision group some years back that came together to discuss object relations theory. Everyone in that room, six therapists, was scared, mostly of each other. I was a late arrival, and I departed after a few months. When we met for dinner a month ago, Kathy told me that she'd been sorry that I'd left, that I had been a breath of fresh air. But it wasn't about that tonight. She wanted to tell me about a discovery she'd made, something that was called "neurofeedback." She asked me to imagine that I could treat the kids at The Center by having them play video games with their brains. "Really?" I said to myself, "This is high-tech snake oil." She leaned across the table into my skepticism.

"I know it sounds bizarre, but it seems to work. I'm getting a system." She picked up the little creamer and settled back in her seat to lighten her coffee. "Would you be willing to be my first," and she smiled, "for want of a better word, 'subject'?"

"Of course. Sure. I don't get this at all; it doesn't make any sense to me, but if you think this is a thing, sure. Why not?" Our target would be insomnia.

Kathy's system, a Focus 1000, arrived last week, and yesterday, I spent the day with her reprogramming my brain. She put an electrode on the top of my head and one on each ear. It was work that was not about effort but about persistence. Four sessions, almost 2 hours in total, getting just perceptibly better at raising and sustaining the green egg and a tone close to "OM," the reward for changing my brainwaves. I didn't feel much of anything. It was a plaything, a novel way to spend time with her.

Afterwards, we talked at some length about her very troubling patient. I tried to help Kathy give her what I think she needs: Kathy.

What are his positions? I no longer see him out at every point of the circle around me. I no longer visualize this surround. I feel it. Maybe this is an infant sense of being embedded in her mother. There is no mother yet, out there. There are moments of emergence that startle me, and then, as quickly as he came, he is absorbed again into the background, mine the only mind, undifferentiated. This is his developmental position.

Arles takes meticulous care in positioning himself during the press of my somatic experience. He stays balanced on the thread-thin line of neutrality. He could easily weigh the ambiguity in favor of "knowing" that that is still unknown. He could say, "Look, all the evidence suggests." If he did, any relief would be temporary, and then I wouldn't trust him. He would have been duped. Now, I experience him kind of in the shadows, deciding this is false, made up, dismissible.

"What if, after all this, we found out there's nothing, no traumatic event, nothing done to me, then what would you make of this history?"

"You need nothing more to explain your history, Sebern, than what we already know."

"But I hear the undoing, the unrelenting psychic annihilation of my mother's mind."

"Exactly. That is what I am saying."

"I think I said some time ago that the greatest injury and greatest fear was that I had been and will be forgotten. I am confused by that now because there is no mother to forget me, just empty space where I think she should be."

"Yes," he said, "By the mother who never asks about your neck."

I am a little worried about what happened on Friday. I don't know what... it appears as a gap... whether this is a neurological or a dissociative event. After the session, I ran an errand at Ted's Boot Shop. As I left the store, I got very dizzy and felt pulled to the right, almost staggering. For several minutes, I had to lean up against the cement wall to establish my feet.

On Monday, when I told him, he asked if I was frightened. I started to cry.

"I don't know, I don't even really ask that," I told him about the bone spur in my ankle and my belief for over a year that this was psychosomatic. "I have never known what is real." He wanted to hear about these episodes of physical pain, of unattended pain. Then he came back on Friday. I asked him if I had had a bad episode.

"Yes, very bad."

"When you say this," he asked me to speak a little louder, "it is taking my head in your hands to keep my shredding psyche within the skull. You are making something real out of nothing ever real. I feel terrible things in my body, some like pin points, some diffuse, a pressure, like a memory, but I see nothing. It wasn't that I couldn't see, it was that I would see nothing. It isn't the endless landscape with no horizon. It is almost as if nothingness was back but now contained, like the inside of a cup, this is the 'nothing'. There's something behind it that shapes and contains it. I think that's your body." I looked over at him. "But then you can fade away. You feel that as my annihilation of you. But this fade is not me destroying you. I am entirely passive, powerless. It is a kind of crib death."

He held me in his gaze, his chin in his hand and nodded slowly.

We looked at the death mask I'd made at the workshop on the echoing vacated third floor of Thorne's Market.

"Does that look like a white girl from Westchester?" He laughed. "It's male. He looks sad and tired, but with a kind of composure."

"Is that what I look like?"

"Exactly!" I hadn't recognized this. It was him, him, pulled through and out of my cells and fashioned in papier-mache.

He told me he had held me on Friday. It has something to do with the door.

"Was it holding or a restraint?" He thought about this for a moment.

"Friday, there wasn't much distinction."

"I don't remember." My eyes filled with tears.

"I remember," he said gently, fatigued.

My mother delivered quickly. My father was relieved that they made it to the hospital in the blizzard, afraid he'd have to attend to my birth in a snow bank on York Avenue. He was glad it was a girl, and my mother was open either way. She knew she was about to be left alone. She has told me about watching submarines going out of the East River. World War Two. She did not tell me about feeling torpedoed; I know this only from deeply knowing myself.

"If I knew a way to give up, I would."

"Do you wish you hadn't been born?" I hesitated before I looked up at him.

"No, I don't wish that. I don't even wish that I hadn't suffered so much. But Monday is my birthday, another marker of the depth and length of my fight to surface and to breathe air. It's not over yet."

"I know, Sebern. It is not over."

I brushed his face accidentally as I got up to leave, but I hardly felt it, as if my fingers had gone numb. I told him about Merrit's last session. Tess held her as she always does now and spent 20 minutes teaching her how to whistle. She gave her lessons in a French accent, which met with our peals of laughter. Each touched the face of the other. One small child and her adoring mother.

"Do you think it is true that your birth was not celebrated? Where did the orchid come from?" The dream image of the iridescent orchid, the long, dark, sightless search, the flame, and the ash that drops away, revealing the perfect pink bud.

"My mother was the close and slippery channel into this plane. Perhaps, miraculously, she did give me that. But she didn't celebrate my birth." Arles waited. "I have been looking so hard for her, wanting her so much, I could not find you."

"Yes," he said, "That's right."

At one end or the other of a sentence, Arles said, "When your father died," and I felt a strange shock. He saw it.

"There is a part of you that doesn't know that, isn't there?"

"My father did not die; he may have disappeared..." I stopped, "Of course he died... I know... I knew it at the time. The coffin was closed... How do I know for sure? All of it feels unreal, a life lived on stage sets, the coffin, a prop of death... That I usually see as empty. Everything is flattened out, cardboard trees and gas lights. I cannot make anything real of this childhood."

"Don't turn away from this. Stay here. You are real. I am real."

"Do you think this is because everyone was just hollow, that only real encounters were the moments of betrayal and rage?" I paused, quickly exhausted by hypotheses. I looked over at him. "It is hard to live a life believing that you will destroy those you love."

"It is unspeakable," he said and went on. "It's not where you are right now, but it is very important that you know that you did not kill your father or Kevy." He waited for a response. "Did you hear what I said?"

I nodded slowly, then just as slowly, shook my head.

"How is it that I am like this again when just a short time ago I felt such pure love?"

"Yes," he said, "what about that?" He sounded patient.

"It is such a powerful feeling. The most powerful feeling there is."

"Yes," he said, "that is true, and it was an open channel to your heart. For me to feel that way, your heart must be open to me."

"Yes," I said, softly, surely. And I started to cry. "Do you know what 'carrari' is?"

"No, I don't. What is that?"

"It's a poison that acts only on the heart. It stops the heart."

He said, "Curare" and spelled it.

"Right, like 'cure.'"

"Yes, like in 'cure'."

"The open channel is like the blowpipe that the poison dart travels through. From my mouth to your heart." I crawled into myself; I needed to cocoon inside my own skin. "I would rather live without you than risk killing you. You said living with that fear was unspeakable. It is a constant. It is always with me. I can't keep an open channel. It is too dangerous. I would rather live forever alone."

The equinox is passing. I have not opened to their stories of dark rituals that Sabelle, at least, is so close to telling me that she trembles. Merrit goes even darker. There is the threat of murder. These girls were tortured. So far, in this turn of the earth, they are alive and managing their terror.

It was rainy and cold, a typical March weekend. We began on Friday afternoon and continued through to Sunday morning. I wanted to stay in by the fire in the country, but I drove the hour to Kathy's place in Great Barrington through downpours. I had four sessions, three were recorded. They each lasted thirty minutes. I sat up and kept my eyes open, and then I lay down on her futon and closed my eyes. I felt nothing dramatic, and since I didn't believe this would do anything, I was confused by my disappointment. Kathy perceives me as robust, intelligent, and healthy, so we are focusing on where my system is overtly broken: sleep. That night I slept with two Temazepam and two Benadryl and had one awakening. I slept 7 1/2 hours and then felt wide awake, much more so than usual, ever really, and ready to go, but the headache I'd been having built into a migraine. Despite the deep pinching pain in my right eye and the nausea, I pulled on my winter coat and drove back for more training. I knew that C4 was the right spot. Even with my enhanced alertness and concentration, I had no sense of how I was manipulating the wave. When I lay down, the Theta wave got higher. I could see that, but I didn't feel it. In the first session, it was difficult for me to do what was asked, which was to lower the Theta wave while increasing the SMR wave with my eyes closed, but by the second or third round, I was able to do it. Theta went up when I opened my eyes, but I was able to reverse this.

In the morning, I trained for one hour straight through, lying down. Initially, my Theta was high, the highest she'd seen. Very quickly, though, I was able to control how much Theta my brain produced. It became easier, almost routine, to meet the parameters for inhibits and rewards that Kathy set.

The migraine intensified, and so did mood lability.

On my drive home, even within the deep and painful cramp of migraine that was spreading, I felt lucid. Oncoming headlights penetrated to the back of my eyes, and I flashed mine on high, more as revenge than as a reminder. That night I slept well. I awaken, wide awake at six.

I left Kathy after lunch on Sunday and drove to Northampton because I wanted to catch a movie highly recommended to me, Antonia's Line. My brain felt different, it has less weight; less shadow. I experienced some lightheadedness at the edge of dizziness at the movie theater.

I had, without noticing it, developed a high tolerance for violence on screen. No one had mentioned the rape and the pitchfork—they have the same tolerance. I had to leave the theater, stumbling in the dark, and almost throwing up at the curb. I considered going back into the small lobby to ask the woman making popcorn why there was no warning posted—I imagined it in block letters, in red—but the sky was darkening, it was cold, and I had a mile to walk to get home. The sky turned indigo, brilliant, and lights blinked on, like stars, as I walked through the neighborhood, dizzy, head aching, clear, lucid, weak, vulnerable in my joints, vulnerable throughout, exquisitely, appropriately, vulnerable.

On Monday, in a rapid press of words, I told Kathy. "I am living in a different brain than I had on Friday."

"Now, I'm getting scared."

"I understand, but don't be. I sound manic, and I am in a way, but I'm not." I told her what had happened at the movie, most of which I never saw and how I'd seen the sky.

"They have a name for that," she said. "It's called 'the clean windshield effect.' When your brain changes, things get clearer." I was glad this was known and had a name, but it was deeper, more brilliant than that.

I had not responded to Neurofeedback as she would have predicted. I felt a profound sense of equanimity, a lucidity, and a sense that the shadow over me was gone. That shadow was the presentation of myself that I sent out before me. At another moment, it felt as if the shadow of the antisocial was disbursed. I could not, at first, even imagine organizing around these aspects of me, those aspects so preferred for so long. Now I can imagine it, but more in memory than as forecast. I have no desire to, no rumbling even of potential desire.

By that Tuesday, I was even more wired. I was also on Percodan for a level nine migraine. My brain felt lucid and both untouched and overtaken by pain.

I moved very quickly, talking to Arles, trying to put this profound experience into words. The pain of being alive, the rod around which I grew, the core element of my interior being, seems to have moved to the edges of my skin, the fear now is a fraying of the skin. I needed him to provide cover for me, to contain the rupturing skin. This has been the troubling physical reality of the past several weeks: eruptions all over my skin of small pimples that itch fiercely at night and when I scratch, open like pox. The scars are only beginning to fade after six weeks, and there are still strange things going on. I scratched my belly and apparently broke many blood vessels. It itches around my ankles. Sam said that whatever it was was on its way out. My liver had been inflamed, and that was better, lymph also, adrenals still up and spleen still enlarged. I have systemic yeast, my mouth is burning, and the diet to ease it leaves me hungry and slightly panicky. I feel as if I'm speaking and writing in a different voice. I don't know who this is. It is disconcerting to feel so suddenly new. I feel pure in a way, but then it also feels as if nothing about me has changed, just that all experience is now sitting on a different ground. I don't know this voice, this character drained of drama, shining.

Mom is in the hospital with her second pneumonia.

Last night, Arles asked me if I liked what was happening. I hesitated because I doubted the simplicity of my response.

"Yes." Then, a little anxiously, "Do you?"

"Yes."

"But haven't you always…?" I asked. The question ached.

"Yes, of course."

I am puzzled. "I have been so engaged in the struggle with my mind, it is part of who I am. It seems necessary."

"Necessary for whom?"

"For you," I answered. "It is not only what I am attached to but how I've been attached."

"Having no mother to attach to, you have attached to your own psyche." Again, it is the metaphor of autism. But it is also more. It is Charlie Boren. It is the necessity of survival, it is the drive toward what could be real, it is a vital energy, it is life force. Arles had said about meditation that attention was not enough, that intention was needed, an intention of goodness. I was interested in goodness, but not motivated by it. I was motivated by truth. I wondered about the threads, about the continuity of the sense of self. What has happened to the antisocial? To the terror?

I have twice been overtaken by fear. The first time I saw myself and saw only Arles' boots. I did not hear him speak to me. There is something monochromatic about this. It has an orange tint to it, like the early stereopticon. An old photograph, trembling, little shots of fear in my body. No thoughts, no content, no memory. It was, I said, as if the experience did not drag a story along with it. It is as if in this being I have cut the line to the story, and the boat is drifting away from its mooring.

"How is that for you?"

"It feels fine; the water is calm—it's very clearly a lake, not the ocean, there are shorelines in the image, there are boundaries—the sky is blue. It's fine." It was only later that I realized that I wasn't frightened because the boat is the story; I am the mooring. I am confused. I feel no need for a past. I am the one who has been so afraid that my terrible memory and the sparse narrative attenuated my very being. I am in a state of pure Now. And then there was the sudden crackling, and I again flipped into some wordless, imageless, throat-binding terror. I cling to him and cry and say, "No No No" and then, following his quiet voice, I finally open my eyes, see the air conditioner, and it's over.

"You know, this really has nothing to do with me, Eva." We were talking about these radical shifts.

"It has everything to do with you! You have been working toward this your whole life. This is the dharma. What can explain this?" I knew that she was right. I'd said to Kathy, "If we didn't have the language of the dharma, we would have to make it up." I have been a dharma student for almost six years and in this therapy for four. I was helping to form the conditions. And I still knew that I was right. This was not me. It was not my psyche. "My brain," I told her, "has a mind of its own."

"My brain," I said to Kathy, "is the other inhabitant."

"This is very special," Arles said quietly. I had cried for 40 minutes about my mother. I told him of the multiple times I have prepared for a death and then my brother or sister did not die, and I would feel undercut and then relieved, only to once again, in their relapses, forgo any hope. I talked more about Kevy dying of aplastic anemia in the University Hospital. She had a patch on her eye. She was dying from this one in a million side effect of Indocin.

"Did you cry?"

I had to think.

"I think I did, but in brief spurts, viciously interrupted, stomped out." I looked down. "I need to be taken care of when my mother dies (*I wrote 'cries'*)."

"You will need that, and you will need that for quite a while."

This is quite something. I continue to experience this change in the ground. Everything is calmed down, but less different, maybe 'less' altogether. I saw a purse left in the doctor's waiting room and thought, without impulse, to steal it, and tonight the profile in the window across the street immediately becomes a target for the imagined high-powered rifle. These thoughts come and go without charge, and so lightly they are only important because they are that shadow, thinner now, almost pale. I told Arles yesterday that I saw it moving toward me, arching over the right side of my consciousness, but just at the periphery. I am not frightened by it, nor does its return seem inevitable. It is there. Perhaps it is just a reflex toward dramatic contention, toward getting into it with Arles. I have been feeling deeply connected to him, the need intermittently strong but without desperation. I smothered my face in the smell on his scarf and folded it carefully to keep it. It feeds a hunger. I am episodically much more aware of smell. I could hardly stand the odors in the kitchen on Sunday following the training. It smelled bad and strong. Blake could not smell anything. When one of my patients moved, I could smell her body, neither perfume nor body odor, in the bursts of her motion. On Monday, after I returned from New Orleans and walked up the stairs to his office, I smelled his vanilla scent powerfully in the stairwell but not at all in his office or on him. I could not identify or feel the need for him. I couldn't smell him. There was a smell of absence, an institutional laundered smell and, oddly, texture, and the dream that I had that was only smell.

On Thursday, I saw Sabelle and Merrit back-to-back, and Merrit left very angry at me. I was shaken by Sabelle's terrible story, by my mistake and Merrit's hate. My sense of ground was gone. I walked to my session with Arles. I needed the company of him. I was not safe, but I was scared of that too, not of him but of the association now with the air conditioner.

"Describe the state you're in, Sebern."

"I don't know what I do, what triggered this." I was working so hard not to get upset. Something happened, and there I was standing up. He stood immediately, took me by the shoulders, and tried to calm me. Very quickly, I started to flip. I remember saying, maybe yelling, "Don't let me go into this, please, I can't." He asked me to open my eyes, to look at him. It was hard, as if my brain were being sucked away from inside my skull and my eyes were pulled with it. I heard him say, "Look at me," and I pushed through this almost magnetic barrier, broke through to him, and it was over.

When I was finally able, I asked him to tell me where he was going. He will be at a monastery for Easter. I asked him about why it was called Good Friday. He wandered away into his contemplations on Good Friday and the Saturday night vigil, but it was him, and there he was, like a miracle, sitting in his chair.

Another session with Kathy. I am righted.

"Do you feel connected to what you were saying?"

"Yes, don't you think so?"

"You seem like someone on Prozac, a kind of matter-of-fact 'OKness' as if nothing could touch you."

I was like that. Everything seemed gray and graceless, but I am not sad or scared.

"Everything seems Soviet," I told him. I was feeling deep feelings without feeling their depth. Feelings about the paralysis, the rack my mother keeps me on, not forgiving me for wanting her alive, not forgiving me for wanting her dead and I was struck by grief perhaps for the first time, over being the one to end my brother's life. It was my decision. It was a clear but awful one. I don't want to make it again. I want my mom to drift away. I want her not to suffer. I am exhausted by death. I cried, a strange pitch, but it was not false. Then the "Prozac reaction," the full amplitude of these feelings is gone, truncated at the bottom range. The feeling is taken out of the feeling.

"It is as if you are brain-injured." Neither of us is thinking about the four concussions. I feel the absence of the other self, the presented self, the part that I push ahead of me that casts the shadow. But things are strange. Tonight, his office looked different. There seemed to be more space between everything, the way your place can look after it's been freshly painted. My connection with patients is more precise, which he feels is because I am less impacted. If that is true, it would cut both ways. Arles is making sense of all of this from within what we think is known. He cannot be in this with me. This is unknown.

Crying made me feel much less exhausted. This is highly unusual and unpredictable. It's mostly my mom. How do I help her?

"I might recover from whatever has happened to me," I said as I was leaving the office. He smiled.

"Yes, I think you could."

I couldn't tell if I was experiencing the same problem, feelings cut off at their depth. I wanted to see the photographs. My reaction was stark. It felt as if something inside me was staring back at this child, just like her;

not a mirror, not a twin, her. I could feel nothing. When there was noise in the hall, my body organized to meet it—it was pre-programmed—but I didn't feel scared. I told Arles that I would kill anyone who came in here, and I said it simply, with a cold resolve. I wasn't mean or angry. I was self-reliant, unafraid, but in this, as post-traumatic as I am when I'm overtaken by fear.

I started to call it 'ambient fear.' Before that weekend, I just lived with it, moment to moment, in my life as a daughter, as a mother, as a wife, as a professional, at full pitch as a patient. It was a beast curled in my belly. It shared the same blood supply.

It is complicated knowing what's what. What is generated from the feedback experience, what from all else I am called to experience. What of my exhaustion was a collapse into the face of that baby that was me? What some errant protocol? What, my inability to weep?

Yesterday afternoon, my handwriting changed to a back slant. I'd seen this shift come on suddenly in my nearly illegible case notes. Last night I began to feel tired, maybe even a bit sleepy, which is rare for me. I dreamt. Slept until 7:15, waking only once. My muscles were very heavy, including those in my chest, which I didn't recognize until I stood up. These things could scare someone. Maybe they should scare me, but it seems like my brain is trying to work something out.

I am distracted tonight. I try to see the obvious beauty of spring awakening, to find solace in it. I walked down to the small pond near the dirt road, raucous with peepers and studied the reflection of the bare maple saplings and white birch. The peepers all ducked away and went silent until I heard their echo in the reeds at the far edge. They could not resist their own song. This is an orgy of competition, of the desperate drive to declare the species forward into another year. I passed a beech with leaves white as ghosts, dead except when the wind blew. The sky is darkening early. I don't trust the energy that hurls me down the road to the Jambs. I know I am not about prayer tonight or rapture or calm. An old tree has fallen across the trail, and I sat on it pressing my palms into the bark, because I am, I can feel it slipping away. I need the information from my palms to turn back toward home. Each time a car approached me, I would pray they would not know me or stop to chat. I was scared of it and simultaneously preparing to be gracious. As it has been all day, I have feet in a boundless terror, but within this containment, still thinking I should call, then thinking that I must learn to trust the container. I can hear screaming. I went to sit on the rock with the peepers to drown them out, but I drowned them out instead.

Last night in the training, I saw myself (I think) dangling over a banister, a patent leather shoe, and a party dress. My chest went rigid like plasterboard. It was hard to breathe. I didn't tell Kathy, ashamed and afraid of any intrusion or even any kindness, afraid that a dam would burst and I would be rent like the trees that used to stand along her road before the tornado. The stench, the background noise, the moaning in my head—it is a drunken black rage, and I am sick with the taunt of it.

I'd never forgotten the time when Hugh did this to Kevy. I was paralyzed on the landing, Kevy was half over the railing, and Hugh, in a murderous rage, was barely holding on to her by her legs. He wasn't listening to me. Kevy was screaming. Our new maid, Evelyn, finally came in the midst of screams and threats and pulled her back. She quit that day. My mother said she was lonely for her family in the city. She said we were old enough now, we didn't need a caretaker.

This is a different memory, a different staircase, a smaller child. I concentrated, I worked to contain my breathlessness. Kathy asked me regularly if I was OK. I whispered to her to note the time. Then, as suddenly as it came, it went. There was only the aftermath.

We looked at the data—I knew exactly where to look—there were wild spikes of alpha and theta, and she thought delta as well. The pattern was irregular and sharp. She wondered if this spiking, mostly right at the boundary between alpha and theta, came first or if the event produced it. It seemed to me that they had to be co-rising. She asked me if I thought this was a real memory. It was real.

Yesterday, I pushed down on the Mentadent dispenser in the bathroom, dripping toothpaste into my hand. My back aches from minor labor and too much time in the car. I bought pansies, raked the lawn, and pruned the raspberries, came inside and collapsed on the couch.

The false-self shadow is still gone, even though I am swamped with moods. I keep being amazed at this as if looking at a new discovery, as if scrubbed of dead skin.

"I have not, you know, believed most of what I have told you, or felt or dreamed. I believe this. This is not a concretization of my mother's absence. This is something else."

"Yes," he said, "this is something else."

The knock at the door cracked the space. I hid my face between the pillows and whimpered. He talked with me softly. "It's UPS, Sebern. You are safe here. No one will hurt you." He found my hand beneath the rubble of blankets and pillows and took it in his.

"I don't want this, Arles, I don't want this at all."

"I know that, Sebern. You won't be in it alone."

I lay covered by soapy water. I do not think that suffering is redemptive. It just *is,* a mundane then suddenly terrifying fact. I am entirely alone, acutely vulnerable without the protection of multiple constructions. I have no layers; there is nothing to get past, I am not false, I am not constructed. I am elemental.

I worked at home on Monday. Girls were chattering on Elizabeth Street on their way back from school. I wrote my report, and then I lay in my bed in the gabled attic room. I felt deeply safe, profoundly at home, cradled, secure, held—an acquired, uninterrupted state of gratitude, of unexcited grace. I was at ease. I have never had such an experience before. Arles asked me if I thought that I deserved to feel like this. I answered without pause, surprising myself.

"No one more than me."

"Yes, Sebern, no one more than you."

That night, I dreamt in the olive drab color of war. *I was waiting for Arles to come to my house on Elizabeth Street. It was nighttime, and I was picking up, straightening so it would look its best. I kept the door to my downstairs bedroom closed, didn't want to, but had to. I heard his car outside and looked out. It was a silver four-door squared off car. He didn't come in for a long time, and I kept picking up, waiting for him to like and appreciate what he saw. He came in the door with several men, all of the same height, all except Arles wearing raincoats. I said, "But Arles, we were supposed to have a session." He said, "All I had was a beer." But I could tell he was under the influence and much more attentive to his buddies than to me. I showed him the house, and without my permission, he went upstairs. He and the men were on a balcony leading to my room, and I said firmly without fear "No you cannot go into my private space." He was oblivious to me, and I suddenly saw that if I did not get his attention and get him to stop, our relationship would be destroyed. I said again without fear, "You cannot go into my sacred space." I didn't know if he would listen to me, so I woke up.* I hated the dream. And it was a first, the first time I had ever dreamed of being in my home.

Arles kept my focus on him, determined to find fear of his oblivion and his abandonment, his inability to protect me from the onslaught. He is standing aside, a mindless facilitator. My mind is in a draw, as tense as two wrestlers evenly matched in that eerie stillness before one gets the advantage and throws the other over his head. In the dream, I see him as a hapless intruder. In my psyche, he is ever-present, pervasive, intracellular, and he is nowhere. I am in a state of transcendent being, of no being, of pre-being. It is non-relational. He is not a factor. Yet I find myself searching for him everywhere, and when I think I see him—even the slightest resemblance—I feel joyful anticipation. He has been so tender with me. He is unafraid and protective. But when I am unable to find the present tense, it feels as if I begin to fire, one neurologic storm setting off the next.

Not all that long ago, I realized that my mother was no longer the problem. She's old and insubstantial. My problem is her, in me. I shared this with Molly to help her with hers. When Molly accused her grandmother's boyfriend of molesting her, her mother lost the father she'd hoped for all her life and banished her daughter. After the hospital, Molly ended up in foster care, and her mother bought tropical fish from Black Mollies. They all died.

I could smell the fog even before I saw it, like day-old coffee. thickening the night over the canal. It is almost Mother's Day, and I have come to be with my mom. She says that since the pneumonia, she feels like an old lady, really, for the first time. She chatted with me, asked after Johnny, and told me of her friend's prostate cancer and his wife's optimism. She wanted me to know where her papers were—her funeral is paid for, the plot information is in the file, and important papers are in the left-hand drawer. All matter of fact, not heartless but without emotion. After talking this way with her, easily, habitually, out of nowhere, my eyes filled up.

"It is important that we have these conversations. I want to have them, but I have to say, I can't imagine living without you." My grief filled all the voids like tidal pools. "I love you so much." Fully and easily felt, without anguish but with the desperate urgency that wrung this out of me as a child. I looked up at her, stole a look really, and she had turned away, looking into the wall, not seeing anything but her own diffuse gray fear.

"Well, it is something we all have to face," she said to the wall. I felt the absence of her comfort, not shock really, but no hand on my head, no soothing words, no embrace. I miss it now. Her response is unnatural, constricted, and devoid. I do not exist in it. She needed to go to bed. I held her tenderly, wholly, and she received it.

"I'm glad you are here."

"I am too, Mom."

She asked me to write her obituary.

❧

"I am a single-celled organism."

"Tell me what that feels like."

I described first the cell wall, then its motility, then its watery and independent existence. There were no other cells. This image of my internal reality overtakes the physical reality. I do not feel lonely.

"What happened to the fragmentation? Is it gone?"

"It seems gone, or it seems skipped over, like this is a pre-fragmented state. It is as if it is time to begin my construction through history." This presents itself clearly; the rest seems to be a process of details, of his curiosity, of helping me discover pieces. "I am," I said, "engaged in authenticating myself." It is as if the doubt was lodged in the false persona, that the doubt has disappeared with the shadow, a flimsy construction I assembled to manage the mother/no mother that I had, to incorporate and embody her, to manifest her certainty and her lie, her predictable but always unpredicted contradiction. When I cried for her, I allowed it. I wanted to cry, to reassure her that I do not want her dead, that I love her. She acts as if she has no fear of being unloved and uncared for, but I know she does. It was a terrible discovery when I found that in her, wrapped in her mother-of-pearl shell. It was worse than finding it in myself.

I walked on Nauset and watched the ocean fall out of the fog. The beach was clear, even sunny. Light seemed sponged up by the crawl of the wave and beneath it as it flowed back into itself— the sand, its rose-purple lip. An intrepid four-year-old dashed in and chased the wave back up, wanting secretly to be caught. The thrill is getting your feet wet; the courage is diving in.

This morning, I woke up sad and a little anxious. I cannot find the source. Maybe it's mom. I can fail to calculate how she makes me feel.

Mother's Day

Once it is not just one thing, it is everything, at once. To me, that single-celled organism is a hard-won simpleness; the absence of affect is the absence of past and future; it is being so deeply attached that it is unattached; unafraid. It is the truth of aloneness floating in love and potential. Elementally vulnerable.

The single cell is the me in his mind and body. It is the me before me. I asked him to hold it not in his hands but to let it float in the space that he is. It is the egg yearning for its penetration to begin life, to find form.

The whole in each cell that only becomes whole in its union with another. I am deeply related, just untouchable. How could anyone tolerate this?

I knew, walking in to see him last night, that this image of the single cell was also one of reduction, of becoming impossible to see with the naked eye. It was an image that achieved life and oblivion at once. I told him I wanted to be as thin as an old dime, that I wanted to slip in between the pages of his book and then be put on the shelf. Oblivion is the habitat between death and knowing, a place to survive. He asked me if I had noticed my swagger, and I said that I had—this walk that I thought I'd willed away, just appeared, like muscle memory, like a signal from a drowning person.

"Don't be angry, Arles." He was ready to be.

"Do you want me to agree to your oblivion, to your death?"

"I am in a time before you. You and I are not able to inhabit the same time." I wanted to say that ever since I acknowledged the reality of trauma, he had in some significant way disappeared.

He sat next to me and took the glasses off my steamy face. I leaned against him and cried. I came close to throwing up. I was feeling so ashamed that I could not bear to acknowledge his presence.

When I could talk, I talked of the plane crash in Florida, a plane with 109 people, no sign of it, buried in the swamp, mouths clogged with mud—they suffocated—; they were buried alive. Somehow, I imagine no impact, more like a hot knife through butter, settling softly into the mud, the screams that descend after them, then just silence.

"The news said the swamp was 'infested' with snakes and alligators. For Christ sake, they don't infest it, they live there!" I've been riveted to photographs of the site—one small bit of debris, and it could have been litter. The whole scene, as if it did not happen.

I was following behind a station wagon, and there was a beautiful baby girl asleep in a car crib. She became agitated and twisted around, revealing another baby, but then it was clear this was a two-headed baby. I said that to the woman I was with. I was not myself, and the woman I was with looked similar to me, but that is not me. They were matronly sisters, with shirt-waist dresses and sensible shoes—handsome women. The face of the other baby was more serene, perhaps even too much so, given the distress of her sister. I exclaimed, "Look, it is a two-headed baby!" We entered a hospital where we'd been going to participate in something, and ahead of us was someone carrying the baby/ babies. I said, "Yes, they are conjoined twins." The doctor took a pair of shears and, more by feel than by sight, began to cut them apart. Then each of the sisters was going to have one of them fused to her. The procedure the babies were going through was rough, primitive—no anesthetic, no preparation. One doctor was holding them in the entryway. Fusion with the adults was temporary to save their lives when separated. Later, I was in a hospital room. Instead of the two sisters, there were four, as if that had always been true. They were in beds all next to each other. Two had name tags, two didn't. All looked happy, and I wondered where their babies were, but realized quickly that after such an ordeal, they must be recovering. The women looked like British matrons, mindlessly content with their situation.

All day, I have worked with and against an extravagant mood. A sadness or sorrow like quicksand—perhaps it was depression. It was not despair. I barely wanted to move. It had me until I went to the river and lay there with Eva next to the torrent of amber water. I considered stopping this quest many times today; it seems common sense. I am afraid of the catacombs, nobody comes here. I am playing with the devil. There is perversion, destruction, and evil here. I cannot rid myself of this. I remember then that it is in my mind, it is no longer my reality. There are friends to call, perennial gardens, and children to nurse to health; sorting books, pinching fresh lettuce, and walks to the Jams. Eva is right here. I breathe into this and know there is nothing else to do but feel it and to soothe it, to ease the cortex, to find a way to smile and hold onto Arles. Otherwise, I am tumbled in shame and terror moment to moment; opening to dread, then closing up, saving me one more time. What am I asking of my patients?

I have begun my lessons on learning to sleep again. I am not a good student. The first night I fell asleep the way I imagined people do and woke three hours later from a dream with this thought: "there is a hole in me as big as my mother's sadness." It was 1:30, and the last sleep I had that night. I trained for twenty minutes at C3 and thirty minutes at C4. I was assaulted by the hallucinations of approaching sleep; the images of sleep were never attained. This morning, I felt a hum in me, not really an agitation but a high electrical thrumming. It's just this side of not bearable, perhaps just beneath agitation. But yesterday I imagined the unimaginable. I think that were Arles to die, I would not be destroyed. Perhaps I would be open to some other journey, a path foreclosed by the necessary containment in this one. It is both comforting and distressing. My liberation is through this relationship, in this relationship, not because of it; it is not dispensable. It is not a skin that I will outgrow and shed. But perhaps like a skin, I will not always perceive it as containing me; it would just be the natural, flexible, ever-present surround, a part of me. There is a vision of a future, even if he should die. I would not fragment or dissolve or go mad. All would not come undone. I would not be left, just standing dazed, motionless, as mute and agonized as stone.

Marsha and my mother called, both with stories of torment. My mother was savagely treated by a stranger in the parking lot outside her pharmacy. He accused her of scraping his car, which she says, sounding a little confused, she is sure she did not do. When she came out after getting her medication, there were grass clippings all over her car. She asked him to take them off, and he said something about her insurance. She was frightened of him and, by her telling, should have been. He was cruel, mocking her, making her afraid. I wanted to kill him. Immediately, I am seized with fear that I will be killed or will somehow put her life at risk. Holocaust images intrude like darting figures in a black and white film, and I am left horrified, once again, in that underlying abiding state of terror. It passes. It took me a long time to notice that she had never called me like this. If I hear at all, I hear months later, when an event works its way into an accusation against me. I called Marsha back. There are moments when she can no longer bear her loneliness. It's often then that she calls.

It occurs to me, when I can pause, that this training is destabilizing me. I have become more labile, more caught in darkness, more foreclosed. I recognized this when I saw a man across the street, out on his porch, gently strumming a guitar. I said to myself, "It is raining, that is all." It is not the end of summer, or the end of hope, or the end of anything. It is just a mood, a momentary eclipse that the primitive in me reads as the end of the world.

I sat with my keys wrapped around my hand, pushed under my leg. He insisted on them.

"You don't need your keys. You are not a warden. Give them to me." He paused as he turned to put them on the table next to him. "But perhaps it is that you feel the need to be locked in." I nodded, this was as true as the need for a weapon. I don't think it is ever to be used against him. I just became so wide open, so essentially defenseless. He is going away, and I have no persona to take over for me.

"I don't know what you're dealing with, but you're worn down, aren't you? Are you afraid?" I answered so he wouldn't have to. "You don't seem to be afraid."

He didn't respond, but he didn't lean away.

"I wish there was something I could do to help you, Arles."

"I know you want to help me in some material way, Sebern, but all that is needed is your recognition. That's what helps."

Sleeplessness is like a water torture, the dark minutes each one glancing off the open eye. He forgot to leave me the sleeping pills. I am hurt by this. His forgetting feels like a deep empathic rupture. The painter, working late, witnessed my betrayal when I punched my hand into the empty mailbox. I hate this melodrama. I don't want to twist into myself like this. I don't want to harbor this raw, unforgiving rage. It is a mistake, not hatred; it is one night. I am the one filled with hatred. What is there to rail against? It is. Where are you, Arles? Why do you leave me?

He forgot me. I imagined this: my presence in his consciousness getting smaller and smaller in retraction, like the iris of the eye, gradually until it is so contracted that it disappears. How do I dare risk my fragile being to his capacity to remember? Last night it seemed clear, there is no other choice.

I spent the night awake. At first light, I was on the porch listening to the birds waking up. It was 4 AM, and I had been awake for 22 hours. My panic was also about the pills. It was the kind of disaster a toddler feels when her Teddy has disappeared. I could not console myself.

Billie and I have been working together for three years, devoted mostly to keeping her from driving off the bridge between here and her home. She could not, she said today, experience the reality of me. I have no impact without my "being feisty," being one step ahead, being demanding. When I get this, one wonders how I could not, and when I act on it, she relaxes. She can't quite account for her sense of my absence, but she feels a quiet but deep despair that comes to the surface as meaninglessness and hopelessness. I try to trace my internal timeline to see how my state has affected hers. She is aware of my fatigue, and she sees this as a factor, but all of this began to surface most at the time of my flashback. She asked shyly if she could look at my hands. She turned them over in hers, amazed, as she might look at an opal or the pink muzzle of her horse. She is looking for the brown nipple of my finger, and yearns to hold it in her mouth, in her memory, for one long week or two, like me.

I closed my car door quietly, not to startle the swallowtail resting on the midnight Iris. I am learning to garden. I am surprised, in general, to realize how little I know. I just could not pay attention to anything other than the din between my ears.

I search wildly for Arles until I remember, in a terrible stroke, that he is in New Mexico. Then I see the bureau in his office and the baby pictures, and I can gather the scattered calm when, now, I don't feel forgotten. I am tired of this, the unsketched, hazy terror that catches me up like a lost piece of newsprint, first stepped on, then blown down the dark street, yesterday's news, oddly compelling, lonely, and rapidly meaningless. Trash, really, no mystery in it, just the sadness of the city night and the tenor sax. I want to fall asleep easily, as I imagine he does after hours of prayer and work. I hope the abbot there sees him well enough to send him out of doors, into the garden or out to mend the fence. I hope that, in between the cracks of this practice, he rests, lush and soft on moss.

"You are opening your heart to orphans, Merrit." I had just learned that she had bought kites for the four little boys in the welfare hotel.

"I think I am opening my heart to everyone. I am filling up on Tess, and it is spilling out, reflecting, a lot like summer sunlight."

Hannah read me two poems for my anniversary today, and I thought when I hung up that hearing a good poem is like finding a piece of pearl in the sand and recognizing it as such, since all that sand is, really, pieces of pearl, before the oyster.

A blue heron greeted me and flew a foot above the pond to a new resting place in the laurel. I found my water body again today. I entered, my belly like a five-year-old, pouting out in delight as I walked cautiously deeper. At first, I refused to swim. I made excuses. I turned back. But lying on the beach, my hunger for the water grew until it could not be resisted. I swam easily out to the rock, and on the way in, I saw the sun on every ripple, my arm turning brown as it stroked the water, my bracelet as gold as the sun, as fluid as the water. Out of the side of my eye, I saw a flash of silver, not the glint of a blade but the dance of a fish. A deer fly chased me into my car, and I went to the solace of the Flat Rocks. I was considering the nature of evil and the impossibility of God without godlessness; there can be no light without dark. I surrendered my body to the density of stone; I surrendered my vigilance. Almost. The stones on the path down to the river are wet. Were I to fall and injure myself, would that be the sudden intrusion of demonic force or the patterned willingness to injure myself? Perhaps neither; it would be the lack of mindfulness. The rock is slippery because it rained. All of this, all of these, are conditions of God.

As soon as I left his office, closed the door and breathed the night air, I was calm. I was OK. I erupted when he told me that he would no longer be seeing me in the evening. I am still torn asunder, and I am woven together of the finest cloth. Until not long ago, he was God, the universe, every morsel of sustenance. Then he became mother, then father. Now, perhaps father and therapist, and simply a man on his own deep journey, paralleling mine, leading mine, following mine. He, too, must have air and time and solitude and care. I must provide for the provider. Today, I must be attentive and tender with my fear.

There is something new, an agility perhaps.

I dreamt that I was on a landing preparing to go scuba diving. Although I was not confident that I remembered how to put everything together, the BC and the tanks, I was not afraid or apprehensive, as I usually am before my first dive. It was Christmas day in the north, but sunny and warm. I realized when I saw someone else getting into his that I would need a wetsuit, and that the water would be cold. Arlen, the dive master, took me to a locker, just a bit impatient that I hadn't considered this sooner, because I would be holding up the others. He pulled several out, all of which were made out of cotton baby blankets. I picked one, white cotton with yellow piping and put it on the bottom, and the top snapped on, and then I pulled some over my feet, expecting to cover all of my body, until I recognized they were booties. I didn't know why mine weren't rubber and rationalized that this would keep me warm because of the nature of the fabric, knowing all the while they probably wouldn't, but it was the best of anything I could've chosen. He was instructing us on the use of the tanks—which I never saw evidence of—as he took the high-speed boat out of the dock. It was a machine which I now recognize was a heart-lung machine. I was worried he wasn't paying enough attention to the course, which was filled with obstacles, particularly at the speed he was going. I wondered again about how it was that this was the way I was spending Christmas. The course was first through a suburban neighborhood and then a large section of water that was a cemetery. He had to steer his boat through headstones to get to the open sea.

When I think of neurofeedback, I will always think of Julie's dream. She was the first person I trained. She'd insisted on it, and with trepidation, I used the protocol for depression that I had learned just two weeks before. She was pale, she'd been crying, she could not meet her classes, she was afraid she would slip into this "chemical depression" and not recover, like her sister, who had taken her own life. I watched with awe as she trained. Her head came up, her back straightened, her color returned, her voice got stronger. After the standard 30 minutes of beta reward, she declared the depression over. That night, her dream was just a voice saying to her, "*The path to the enigma is now clear.*"

I am back late tonight from my third Alpha-Theta training. A couple of days after last weekend's two-hour session, I recognized that my startle response had disappeared. In the last day or two, it has returned, but I still believe that these treatments will continue to positively and often profoundly affect me. There is still no return of the false self. My whole neurology, already deeply affected by Arles, has quieted even more. I am excited about it. Excited enough, hopeful enough to travel through torrential rains in the dark to get a training. We'll see. Arles recognizes the difference.

I just realized that this latest training has disrupted a habit, the habit that, in part, is attention to detail, like reaching for the toilet paper in a place it hasn't been for years or going to hang up the phone on the refrigerator. It feels like a part of my mind is living in a different house, and that if I could catch all these small mistakes and piece them together, I would know which house it was.

The startle response is coming back, but today it was only on the left side of my body; the right side stayed unaffected, unstartled. During the training, I feel simultaneously relaxed, rather deeply so, and alert. This is not so clearly hemispheric, but it seems that the relaxed part is more on the left, the alert on the right. The electrode is on the left, on the back of my head. I recognize the disruption in the ease that habits provide. On a practical, functional level, I am disorganized and often chagrined.

This morning, I drove to the Cape with Sabelle. We ate a processed cheese food and mustard sandwich in the room she is sharing at the Best Inn with Cory and Tess. After they got as settled as seriously disturbed adolescents can, Tess, Mike, Miriam, and I took Ilya, June, Darlene, Cory, and Sabelle to Coast Guard Beach. I played with them for a while in the gentle waves and then just sat on the low-slung chair and watched, admiring their capacity to leave it behind, momentarily, and to be truly happy. The day was hot and blue, and the beach was festooned with color—almost a parody of the perfect childhood—rainbow umbrellas, sandcastles, pails and frisbee. A little burnt, drenched and coated with sand, we turned into the beach for the modest but empty motel swimming pool. I played chicken with the kids, riding high on Mike's shoulders. I was quickly outflanked and spilled into the water. I helped Ilya learn to swim. I promised Sabelle that I would teach her to dive, but she was, ultimately, too scared to enter the water headfirst. I let June dunk me, and I swam underwater with Cory. These are the girls we'd chosen to be in the Dialectical Behavior Therapy group that Tess and I ran together. We'd started the first DBT-based residential treatment program in the country, and these kids were the first members. They had to learn to greet us, to pause before they tumbled forward into the room and took their seats around the table. They ate their raisins (after their snacks), poked each other under the table, and swore. Tess told me after our first two weeks at this that it was her training in musical comedy that made it possible for her to lead this group. Sabelle dubbed them all "Zenies."

We changed clothes and tracked down Cape or up Cape—whoever knows—to Ocean Ridge Resort, which is, I think, a bit of a stretch given that the ocean is 6 miles away across several major and minor roadways. Marsha greeted us and was, as usual, quite wonderful with these kids. She is funny, direct, and acute, particularly with Darlene. She said later, "I could see her neckline get lower and her shorts shorter as she sat there." The kids were a little shy, but Marsha talked enough to keep them going. They'd written her a card thanking her for the therapy, for giving them a chance at a different life. I knew it touched her. She said, "This is very nice."

I miss them when they leave. It's strange to me that I do.

Marsha and I had our typical conversation, secure one really only when we are talking about her and when I can stave off discussion of our differences. We reminisce about my letter to her, our meeting up again, about the Institute and the April swim across the Connecticut River.

"Sebern, what happened after we got back to the Institute?"

"We were separated in the river, remember? I was scared that you might have drowned. It was probably Charlie who told me that you were back and were sent down. Do you remember any of that?"

"I remember being pulled out. I remember the ambulance... No, I don't remember. When I thought back, though, it seemed strange that I was discharged from a locked unit."

"Actually, it might have been Kinnery who told me that you were Ok." I watched her face as it came back to her. Kinnery was the no-nonsense Irish head nurse, who took the same four of us back up to the most secure unit in the place after Shelly picked the lock and, not knowing what else to do with this sudden freedom, we'd shown up at her office at midnight.

"So, what happened to you? Were you sent down, too?"

"I was, but not a locked unit. Charlie sent me down as punishment. I guess he had to do something. He was furious."

I stood, frozen at his doorway. "Shut the door and sit your ass down!" He barely paused. "What the hell were you thinking? Do you have any idea how dangerous this was!" He didn't wait for me to answer. "Marsha nearly drowned. You would've never been able to live with that. I can't believe"... he seemed to look around for what to say next and then bore down on me... "The sheer stupidity!"

"It was hot, Dr. Boren. I'm a good swimmer. Marsha said she was, too. I didn't want to walk back through that foul muck!" He cut me off.

"Think, god dammit! Everything that is in that 'muck' is in that river. There is sewage, garbage and gasoline. It's damn polluted. It's got the fastest current in the East. It's April for Chrissake, there's still ice melt in it. It's probably 50 degrees. What the hell were you thinking?!"

"What more can I say? I didn't know." I was as stubborn as I was scared. "We're not dead."

He stopped yelling, looked at me, and slammed his hands down on his desk. I jumped. "I tell you, Sebern, the only thing that gives me any pleasure about any of this is thinking about how many shots you're gonna get." He stood up. "You're being transferred tonight." I started to protest. "I wouldn't go there if I were you. This is unfortunately all I can do today. I might think of more by tomorrow."

She loves these stories as one does the happy stories from childhood.

Then we had dinner with my mother at Albici's. They like each other.

"I am not a complex person," my mother says to her and, turning to me, she says, "Am I?"

"You are more complex than you know."

"I am an open book." Marsha agrees with her. We eat fish, and I search for topics that will keep us all safe. When we were alone, I told Marsha that she'd been invalidating, and she agrees, but it seems useless to discuss the impact this has had. It ends as it always does, somehow with me loving her. I took Marsha to her car at the Sheraton, and as I drove back to my mother's, I fell into a deep well of loneliness. Is this Marsha's or mine? Or mine provoked by Marsha or by my mother. They are not so different.

The next morning, we sat on her side porch with coffee.

"We are going to go to Weston this Christmas. We can come here on Christmas day or you can come with us."

"I'll just have to see what I'm capable of doing."

"Mom, what I did last year was very important for me."

"Did you ever think that there might be someone else in this world besides yourself?" I checked in. I wasn't bracing, just talking.

"Mom, I spend my life taking care of others." She rolls her eyes at this. "That is how I live my life."

"All I'm saying, Sebern, is that I have never felt more hurt in my life than last Christmas."

"I know it hurt you. I knew it would, and it was the hard part of my decision. This is very important to me."

"Christmas is a time for families to be together. Our family has been ripped apart. The least you could do is..." I didn't hear the rest.

"I do understand. I have always been here, but for seven years, I have wanted to find the spiritual importance of Christmas. It is pressing." She was looking away from me. "What would you do if you were in my place and searching for something so important?"

She paused and looked at me. "Well, I guess," she said, "I'd go for it."

I thought, "This is the most she can do, and it is a lot." I'd asked her not to call me self-centered and selfish, and she didn't I think recognize that she had done just that. I leaned over my knees, toward her.

"There is no one I love more than you."

"I loved having John and Blake here, but," she started to cry, "it was you I wanted."

"I know. I love you more than I love anyone," I repeated.

After a moment of reflection, she said, "I believe that. And there is no one I love more than I love you." Then she added, "Well, you are on a par with Blake, Wendy and Gwen."

I have no idea how this is left in her, or I guess, in me. But something real happened—it was not scary, it did not make me crazy or angry. I no longer need her to be anyone else for me. She may still leave me broken-hearted. I never knew before I was off the Cape.

❧

I want to put the neurological changes into words tonight. The first change is now thinking about these shifts as neurological. The ambient fear is turned down but is still playing. I am not in it or invested in it. My mind, now, keeps saying "I don't want to know, I don't want to know." I don't know what it's talking about, but I believe it. The startle response, although still possible, is quite different. It happens, but it doesn't take me over, and it feels one-sided, only on the left. I jump more physically, but it feels like an exaggeration, almost a parody. It happened once in his office, and Arles questioned it.

"That was pretty slow."

"I know," I said, "it's very weird. But it's real, just strangely delayed."

"You are afraid that knowing will drive you mad. But it is the refusal to know that creates madness."

I thought I wanted him to know and tell me, in part because that would mean that he was alright, unharmed, and able to contain it. There is some threat to him. I gasped, recognizing this.

"What are you experiencing right now?"

I shook my head and tucked myself in close to him.

Thursday and Friday, I did Alpha-Theta training with Kathy. Thursday night, I drove home at midnight feeling as if I had just sat through a two-week retreat—light, fluid, buttery. I swallowed the pills (that I again, as I did a long time ago, referred to fleetingly as birth control pills) about 15 minutes before I got home, and in 10 minutes at home and in bed, I was asleep.

Friday's training went for an hour and a half. My experience of time is altered. Whatever time Kathy tells me has passed surprises me. I have no reference except my body. My sacrum keeps track of time. I experienced a sweep of terror. Just before, I'd thought I should be breathing, that this was, after all, a meditation. It was as if some consciousness (from the left) rose to meet the brainwave, and in the clash, there was terror. There were no images, no words, no warning. Then small tears. Then a slow but even return to the training. I don't feel good; I feel shaken, tremulous, off to the side of myself. I am increasingly more available to myself, simpler but still in some pre-verbal turmoil, a state that is very difficult to validate or receive validation for. Billie calls to tell me that she has Hepatitis B, and I am strangely calm, not disinterested but not distressed about my exposure. I woke up this morning, again with a sensation that I was pinned down on my back all night, unable to move. I was uneasy. I tried to find the source in the news. That was not it. His vacation? No. Molly? No. The school? No. No present-day situation. I felt unable to move and remembered that in the night, I woke up with my hands freezing cold. I hadn't pulled them in under the covers and, even somewhat awake, had to think out what to do. After two hours, I got up. After three hours, I drove to the store for a bagel and coffee and for the company. I read the paper. I could not change the mood. I went to the river, but I wasn't there, so I went home to bring in laundry, stack wood, and make the beds. Everything was an attempt to bring time into the present.

"I always know when you're having a hard time because you tell me a long string of stories of catastrophe," Eva said as we sat together on the long flat rock, our legs stretching into the water. I haven't been aware of doing this. "You remind me of a child in a nightmare. I don't think anyone ever came and turned on the light and calmed you." It is as if, in some echo around her voice, I am hearing a Grimm's fairytale. I am embarrassed by the fear in me and the humiliation. She was talking about her work, and as she talked, I felt a shift in time. It was a slow and smooth reorientation. This is Eva, this is the river, this is now. I began to smell the water and feel the air move over me. I saw the brilliant sun-lit treetops and the flash of a Scarlet Tanager.

"It is really something to begin to come alive." I doubt she can grasp how true the emergence is for me. It is a slow thaw, and a finger wiggles free, and the whole world feels new. I am desperate to find her, to have her understand. She put her hand on my head and my arm to comfort me. I wanted to kiss her knee. I turned and felt the tears running down my neck.

"I love you, Eva."

I am looking forward to my time with Arles. I have missed him. I am filled up. Standing at the river yesterday, I recognized that beneath my contentment, not out of reach and not sought, there was a state of bliss, before that or in that, joy. This contentment seems deeper than happiness and happier than equanimity, but all applied. It all feels miraculous and ordinary. Like Sabelle at the Cape, I "feel so happy, I feel stupid."

I was taken aback by a brief and strange interaction with my boss. An hour before, Sabelle doubled over, crying in my office. It is rare for her to cry, and she trembled. She told me that the principal and several other staff continued to mock her for being dissociative as she switched wildly to manage the humiliation. They were pushing her to the edge of her madness. This could erupt in her system in the night, and she would be back in the hospital. We anticipated this together, and she knew I understood her peril and what was provoking it. She knew I was on her side. She got a little calmer, but after she was gone, I could barely contain my rage. I talked to myself, trying to quiet down as I pushed the papers on my desk into piles. I ran into Paul in the parking lot and, without a thought, turned and confronted him. I was angrier than I'd ever felt. It was an oddly contained fury that arose in me full-throated, in the moment, still rational, not attacking and then immediately released. I warned him of the dire nature of Sabelle's situation in the school. "I don't understand how you don't see this! It's so clear that the school has become a dangerous place. You get other reports. I don't want a fight. I love you and mostly don't want another battle where you and I would be on opposite sides. But there is a crisis brewing, and there are concerns about our accreditation raised by all of this." He was physically taken aback but said nothing and left without comment to go into the Center. I sat in my car. I felt the rage drain out of me. It was a state. It was over. I looked ahead into myself over the rest of the day, and I knew, in me, there would be no aftermath. It was so complete that I expected this would also be true for Paul.

This morning, he called me into his office, and I expected some consideration, some concern about me, perhaps, about my patient. Instead, he was formal, a little anxious, and he informed me that there was "a process," that I should follow it, and that I should put my concerns in writing. My sense was not one of collegial respect or concern for good process. It was entrapment. I agreed, knowing I would never do this. Then he said that when he got back, he would be giving me a written warning. I was shocked, but not shaken.

"For what?"

"For threatening the agency."

"There was no threat, there was a warning."

"Maybe I misunderstood, but we will talk about it when I get back next week."

Of course, even if he had not misunderstood, what he was saying was "use the process," JCAHO, the process I'd just said was corrupted. I can hardly recognize myself. None of this is scaring me. This is not possible. It's left me shaking my head and saying to myself, "This is the world. It kills people like me, whether or not we are afraid." His allegiance to the school is motivated by money, and it will never be discussed for what it is. I don't get it. He acknowledged my earlier concerns about the leadership there, but that didn't make a difference. There would be a written warning. They want to silence me, not engage with me. Why? And the answer comes to me in some exasperated male voice, "This is the real world!" I don't feel the disillusionment I expect to; this does not echo down into caverns in my belly, as it would have, and I am not angry. I will be cautious, and I will try to practice right speech. My outrage in the past was fueled by an illusion that "right" mattered, that good guys win, that the world is not, in the end, too big and too stupid. It is. I don't even get that there are sides; differences, yes, but somehow, I feel I'm being put on a side that doesn't exist. I keep checking in for the interior report, the sonic boom. I can't believe it's not there.

From the time I wake up, I am troubled. Tuesday, Wednesday, and Thursday were days as clear and clean as the West Branch. I felt contentment and clarity, and from this, strength as deep and fruitful as marrow. I was present during those days, and they were happening at that time. But this morning I am beginning to slide. I feel the front edge of the time warp, like weather, like atmosphere. This becomes the only air I have to breathe.

My heart races. It is throbbing in my neck. When I finally get inside his dark office, I ask him to lock the door and when he does...

"It's worse, what comes from the inside."

"Yes," he said. "It is."

"I need to get more under something."

"Use the blanket, Sebern." I lay down and pulled it over me.

"I know if I could just figure out how to do it, I could make a leap out of the time I am in, into our shared time." I handed him my watch. "No, give it back! That was the wrong thing to do."

"Why?"

"With your watch on and mine not, you have all the power over time. You play the time cards." As soon as I strapped it back on, it became impossible for him to reach me. I finally took it off and slapped it down on the arm of the couch.

"Now, time is between us," he said.

"Yes, yes, that's right," and then, like a discovery, "Now you can't come here."

"Is that a line I need to cross, that timeline?"

"Yes, I hope so."

I cannot arrive in the present time.

❧

I dropped everything, pulled on my wet bathing suit, and got back to the river. I first tried the shock of quick immersion. It helped, and I stretched out my body and swam along the curves of rock and along the floor of sand that looks like gold dust, over the leaves that are coins. There are familiar, reassuring nibbles on my feet, the hatchling trout that are raised on food the color of my toes. I slid off the smooth rock and sat with my back into the rapids to get a pounding. I needed my face under. Nothing bad has happened to me in the water ever, even the lionfish and the shark. I am safe there.

On Friday, I felt like I was suspending Arles, making it physically impossible for him to move toward or to stay apart. I didn't want this, but it felt, to him, quite powerful. Both of us spent the entire time trying to find a way for him to breach the barrier, to enter my time. He told me in detail where he would be, what he would be doing and when. "I am OK," I said as I left. "I'm just not fully returned." I have to trust that my psyche will choose its time wisely and that Arles and I will become more skilled at, as it were, the ins and outs of time.

I remember only this fragment. Some guy, a young blonde redneck sort, is being obnoxious and aggressive to someone, and I intervene. I know I've made him mad. I am on the phone already trying to reach the emergency number when I hear the door creaking, and I call out fearfully, "Who's there? Did someone come in?" There is no answer. I am holding the phone and walking to the foyer. He is there, smiling sadistically. I called 911. He is leering and threatening and undeterred by the fact that I am calling the police. I can see the policeman, leaning back in his chair, his feet on the desk, talking to me. He won't come because there has not been a crime. I am confused and frightened because it is clear that I will have to be assaulted, tortured or killed before they will come, even though he is standing right in my house and threatening me. Then I realize the reason that no one will help me—it's because it's New Orleans.

It is Alpha-Theta training that is playing havoc with my sense of time, below and beyond how it is distorted in the outbreaks I have. Sequence is difficult, linear time feels like gravity, a pull with only the illusion of direction. Placing events in time seems elusive, but I know absolutely that I am living in time.

Yesterday, I felt the beginning of this process that becomes runaway terror. I refuse it. I experience it as something grabbing my mind. Once it gets me, I have to try many things to get free—rapid eye movements, cold water immersion, twisting the skin on my wrist, banging my head lightly, pounding my fists on my sternum, cold seltzer, and a eucalyptus inhaler. I listen to the sound of the water over the rocks, but the sound is actually very hard to get to. It is more than I know it could be comforting. This is also not new. It's just more discrete or more discernible; more dystonic; more real.

I am becoming aware of how I imagine Arles. This is new. When I look for him, what I see is his dark office. I don't see him, but I know he is there, absorbed into the dark light. He is not distinct or separate from the room. He has become part of it.

After seeing two patients and forgetting a dentist appointment, I took Merrit and Sabelle out to pick blueberries at the farm with 5 acres of bushes. It was close to 90 degrees. They were awkward and eager with each other, Merrit a little hyper in her peer mode and Sabelle, more obviously anxious. Both were more at ease once they were in the pond, two very bright, very dissociative young women trying to play. I returned to work not entirely housed in my own psyche. Then to Great Barrington for neurofeedback. This last round has left me feeling that I can handle anything. Not grandiose really, just not anxious.

On Sunday night, two days shy of the full moon, a clear, open night, I went to the river. I wanted the freedom of it, so I overrode the undercurrents of fear, slipped off my sweats and went to the little beach at the swimming hole. I was not afraid of any external threat. It wasn't that the murderer could not appear—I am an attractor—just that I could handle it were he to come there. The water was cold, my body gilded silver. I was wary of movement, careful of rocks and the immeasurable depths. I did not experience the freedom I'd imagined, but I did embrace the beauty of it all and the remarkable experience of no fear.

I gardened today, and instead of tearing up my hands again, I used gloves. I was suddenly and oddly aware of a kind of joy that my hands were protected. Zoe came to be stroked, and I felt the sensation of my palm running over her fur and the punctuation of her cold nose. Delight. I am learning about delight.

In this Alpha-Theta state, time is stretched out, slower. There is more of it. I have a child's sense, an abundance of time.

I took Sabelle and Merrit to a steep rocky section of the river with its small pools, and they talked together and left me to stretch out on a large flat rock, looking up at the cavernous stone and pines and a lacey young beech overhead. I thought of Arles and what he has provided. It's too small a word, "provided," for all that has come, but I can't think of another. From the first moment, the rocking, soft tones of his voice, the "fetal fish," he created the universe. When I think about going to see him, it is less now to curl into his body than it is to curl into his universe. It is, probably, not really different from what they mean by a holding environment—if anyone really knows what they mean by this—but this vocabulary of the universe is right, in origin and in scope. It seems the reality of this infant, now abstracted from his arms, made as large and as complete as the universe. This universe has rules to maintain it as a closed and negotiable system. The rules include the tone of his voice and the centrality of me, and they are beginning now to include him.

Arles used a phrase to describe his countertransference. "Maternal... and I cannot remember so I fill it in—'degradation,' 'deprecation,' 'disinterest,' 'disturbance,' 'despair,' 'desolation'..." It was 'dejection,' maternal dejection. He was being replaced by neurofeedback.

"It used to be that I would see myself as a small child running up to you, and you would pick me up. It is as if I have stepped out of the metaphor."

"This is not a metaphor! Hegel says, 'words kill the thing.' Making this a metaphor kills it. I am here, and I will pick you up."

I have been experiencing him as missing, as already and permanently gone. I have him, and he is gone. I see him, I see him in the office, but somehow, he is missing. I want him back. And it's OK. When I returned from the Cape, I turned to the machine for regulation, not to him.

"I am so casually annihilated by my mother, I will not risk it with you."

"You have never said this before, that you feared that I would annihilate you!"

"I thought it's all I've been saying, nothing else, in the running toward and running away, being torn to shreds by my own movements." He is absolutely with me—I am not alone—and he is not with me, and I am not alone. I cried. I wept over missing my mother. This is, well, unimaginable.

I awake with the first part of the dream fading away from me, something about a lot of people, refugees maybe, and rooms I didn't know were on the second floor of this house, old, ramshackled, no insulation. I looked down at my leg, and there was a spot on it, then I realized my whole body was covered with them. They are oval and the color of café au lait, and it frightens me. Someone says it comes from dirty sheets. I started to cry when I told him the dream because I thought it was about being unable to change my spots, like the wild cat. And then the image came that I called "the internal fact." I am wary. I am a child jumping on his chest. I am crying out with rage, "Stop being dead!"

The dramatic infrastructure of my history is gone. This is like a sudden true maturity. Tomorrow, I go to LA for qEEG, a brain map, then to get trained in how to provide neurofeedback.

❧

After two near collisions, I got out of Santa Barbara and found my way to and through Los Angeles. The brain mapping was straightforward and simple, and I have finished day two of the training. A good deal of Siegfried's lecture on the first day soared over my head. "Timing; hertz; frequencies; the laws of physics; the rules of timing." I ate lunch by the pool. The others passed by me on their way to lunch, deeply engaged in a conversation about the lecture. I have no need to join them.

I am struck the most by my own state. I am here now. I have no wish to be elsewhere, almost as if I have no sense left of anticipation. I have become aware of many moments that, before all this, would have sent me into the boundary land of dissociation, and they don't. The system, though, is significantly perturbed – there is a sense that there is information there, but I am not mobilized, no flight, no fight. It disturbs me; I notice, I will talk with Arles. That's it.

I had two sessions of neurofeedback. The first was standard SMR, and it gave me a headache. I moved on to Alpha-Theta training, and during this, I felt a sudden, hard pressure on the top of my head. During the second one with Bill Scott, I had even more of this and a sense of a kinesthetic memory of the dive. Pain shot into my ear, my neck hurt, and I began to whimper. I could hear it, more than I could feel it. I know if I were home with Arles, I would grieve this, but I am able to contain it without corrupting it. It is not suppressed.

Some of the same strange disorientation or orientation to another time. Tonight, it happened when I was looking for a towel hanging on the back of the door, but that was not here, nor in Elizabeth Street, nor in Plainfield.

I dart along the landscape of the present to find a clue. Arles is away; Eva is not returning the call; Merrit and Sabelle are both in the hospital, but my anxiety doesn't seem to be at any of these sites. Each adds volume to the flooding stream, but the stream already flows full and deep. It would be different if Arles were close, or Eva were predictably accessible, or the girls were OK. It would be easier, but it would still be.

What is it to know something? It is always a function of memory, and when it is something to be known of one's own history, it is your memory confirmed by the memory of another? How will that ever be for me?

I drove into town for what turned out to be a 2 ½ hour session with Merrit, who was first a three or four-year-old tantruming little girl named Bitch. She picked the shark to play with, one of the puppets we'd bought at the Conference on Trauma and Dissociation. Tess worked with her seamlessly, and I mostly just watched as she helped this little girl to comply. She made a list of favorite activities, including learning to ride a bike, sledding, and sitting in Tess' lap when she is cross-legged. Merrit came back after much cajoling of Bitch and was a little disoriented at being there. She asked to speak with me, and we discussed her situation. She believes that ghosts have inhabited her, and one of them, an older man, believes that he can throw her out the window and walk away from it. She's afraid to let us meet him, but she finally agreed to let him out for five minutes. For five minutes, he was uncontrollable, and when he went back in on the cue—I had threatened to call the police—he began to threaten her. "He" tried to flee through a window that he broke, but he did not try to attack us. He'd threatened to kill her cat. Tess and I are vigilant, and I am numb.

I have kept track of where Arles is every day, which means I placed him in time and space.

I have stopped caring whether he returns.

I want to see him.

I don't care if I see him.

I love him.

He is nowhere in me.

He is part of my cellular makeup.

I know what he looks like.

I'm glad he is back.

The girls have both been admitted to the 5th floor. I am tired, and I'm just coming down from hyper alert.

My conversations are about the turbulent Now. The staff at the hospital has made allegations about me. There were outright lies that only the kids could refute, and my administration refused to talk with them. The psychiatrist there had told me that multiple personality disorder was very rare, and asked sarcastically what the odds were that I'd be seeing two kids with this. I am not allowed to see either of my patients. I am glad they have each other, but of course, one is not able to quiet the other. They escalate. I coach. "They will separate you if you raise the stakes. Don't do it!" But they are a long way from my voice, and they are overwhelmed by many of their own, in a place with people who essentially don't believe that they or their experience exist. When I shared my despair about the way they were being treated, Vicki got concerned. She has put me on forced leave until I am evaluated for stress. Tess works with Sabelle and tells her what's happened. She, as usual, accepts it too readily. Merrit calls me several times a day and, of course, we speak. Randy, the new administrator here whose position in the hierarchy is still unclear, came to tell me that they are removing me from her case for "overinvolvement." This came down to two issues for them: "you see her three times a week" and "you push and fight for your patients." I reminded him of ethical guidelines around patient abandonment. He said he's making an administrative, not a clinical, decision. I understood his position—new here and in the crosshairs—, but I said that he can't fairly or ethically alleviate his stress by passing it to Merrit and to me. He ended the conversation when I said, "No one is ever going to say that they are abandoning a patient—there will always be a rationale. Merrit meets none of the criteria for termination of care."

I am exhausted with interrupted crying, with too many assaults on me and on the interior space of my relationship with Arles. I sat in his chair, and after a few minutes of shared silence, he said,

"How do we get back here?"

"Actually, that's what I'm trying to do." He knew. "What I have lost are structures. When I asked the question, 'Where did that part go?' I was thinking of it as a structure, the sociopathic persona. The structure of the persona is gone, but I can still call forth the function. When I perceive abandonment, I perceive the residue of the structure as a voice, not as an impulse or as a wish. I talk to myself. This morning, the voice said, 'Don't go there,' 'dress in red.' I don't go into the structure; I don't even act on the voice. I'm not irresistibly drawn in any longer." Quietly, as if not to startle me, he asked me to move to the couch, and there was no question.

"No."

"Why?" he asked gently. My response was frozen in me. He waited a few moments, then he stood up, took my glasses, took my hand, helped me take off my jacket, and when I sat down on the couch, he sat next to me.

"Everything you said is important. It is profound. But it is not relevant. You are not in it, and I want you here."

"I hate all these people who take up my time, who act like I don't exist!" Then, an eruption. "I hate you for letting it happen!" He contained me quickly and soothed me with his quiet "Yes." I fought just like I used to, but quickly realized that all the circumstances around Merrit and Sabelle had deepened my anguish over separation. I stopped.

"What are you feeling, Sebern?"

"Humiliated." I thought he said, "So what."

I was crying, and he couldn't help but laugh when I asked, "Did you say, 'so what'?"

"No," and then, after pausing, "But now that you mention it..." We fed each other laughter, me crying and laughing and angry, like a kid being teased out of her position, not wanting to give it up easily, feeling bad, and it was funny.

"These people don't know the damage they are doing to these girls. The lie is indelible, and I was forced to participate in it. It's a fucking re-creation of the betrayal, violence, lies and abandonment they have lived. Perversion, corruption, protectors turning into persecutors, everyone impotent, unable or unwilling to help, blaming the victim, mind-fucking, raging at them and at me, willing to injure, willing to degrade, and defame, willing to make others crazy..." I am heading toward explosion or collapse, and I could feel him preparing for both.

"Yes," he said, calmly, "It is exactly that."

"Merrit asked to see me, but the therapist at the hospital denied the visit. She wanted to go to the human rights officer, but she was scared. She was being punished, made to bandage her own cuts, status kept loose, and made to do her own room search. The staff is mocking her." I stopped. I looked around. "Something is set off in me, Arles, working with Merrit and Sabelle. And the way they are being treated." I paused and asked, "Am I exaggerating what happened to me?"

"No." He said "No" as if it were a fact. "I think it was much different but psychologically just as devastating." As I began to say, "We don't know yet how different it was," someone opened a door, and I flipped into another time.

He talked so close to my ear that I could feel his breath. He had me look at him.

"This is me, here.

"No one is coming.

"No one will hurt you.

"No one will come in here from the outside world. That is noise in the outside world.

"Look at me."

I looked up and opened my eyes as deep down as I could open them.

"Good. Look around now, find the walls you know, the chairs, the couch we are on here, now, and see if you can let this move through you." I followed his voice and again moved out of the grip of something I know and have no memory of.

❧

There are snow flurries, and the day is the dull amber of November. Merrit was transferred to a special unit for dissociative patients at McLean's in Belmont. Yesterday, Eva said, "No one knows. Who can put names and dates? Merrit doesn't know either." I wonder what that means, except that in memory there is no fact; there is only memory.

I spoke at length with Sue and with Siegfried late this afternoon. Sue took me through the brain map and concluded by saying, almost offhandedly, "This is dissociation, most likely."

"You can see that in a Q?" I asked, surprised and exposed.

"Yes. We'll look at this together when I see you next, and I'll take you through it." I felt the reality of my situation: a beleaguered, abused woman, integrity and sanity still intact, but feeling as low and dark as the early night and seeking the sanctuary of their warm afternoon sunshine.

The ninth circle of hell is for those who betray. One of my colleagues went to the hospital with heart pain; my boss has been out sick for a week. How does Randy manage his shame? Barry is exhausted. The clinicians are under siege and seem desperate for my return. I won't go back until after Thanksgiving, and then I will plan to leave. It is not a place I can work any longer. It is a frenzied, heartless system that crushes its patients and grinds their caretakers into dust. I will find a way not to live in it.

I lost Arles. They have pushed past him, or gotten around him and then got to me. There was no protection. He said it seemed as if Hitler had entered my life. He was right. I was the pathetic, naked Jew, small, speechless, hopeless, betrayed, and ridiculed. He was destroyed. He did not exist—perhaps this is how I explained it. Perhaps I made him disappear to protect him because they'd gotten me already. It didn't matter. No one could have known how shattering all this was. He insisted on the third appointment on Wednesday. All I remember is filling up and spilling over with grief. I saw my lawyer and became reacquainted with the realities of law. There's no recourse there. I met the psychiatrist at Eastspoke, and he put me at ease. Unlike the clinical people at Cooley Dickinson, he was not ashamed to see Sabelle's torment as, in other circumstances, no different than his own. He talked about Margaret Little and Sabelle with respect and empathy. It was this meeting more than anything else that allowed a shift. Even more than Tess saying, "If I'd been through what you are going through, I would've driven my truck off a cliff," or Vicki, one of the perpetrators saying, "You have handled all of this with grace," or my lawyer saying "You have a case" and hugging me before running off to get his daughter. The events overtaking me got relocated in the nastiness and disturbance of the people on the fifth floor of Cooley Dickinson. It was no longer my private holocaust. I will not be understood; the system will get worse, and children will die. But I won't let this happen to me. I recognized that although there was a lot of crazy—making intent a particularly vicious form of deception—I could decide not to be vulnerable to it. This would not have happened to me several years ago; a new vulnerability in me drew this rage. I was so overtaken by the willingness of these people at CDH to savage my patients and me that I hardly noticed this. It is new.

In the midst, Marsha called. I was crying as I told her what was happening. She was appalled. She went off on a brief tangent about the psychodynamic concept of "over-involved" becoming a "reality," but she was genuinely worried and at a loss. My voice trembled.

"I am re-traumatized."

"Get untraumatized! They can't do this to you!"

"I don't know how to do that, or I would. And, unfortunately, they can and are doing this to me."

Arles and I talked about all this and the brain map. He was astonished that I needed to see this on a graph.

"You were changing states here constantly."

I don't believe these very real phenomena. This is a disorder, at its most basic, of self-negation; no sense of self that continues reliably over time. One sense of self is often violently overtaken by another, or softly sucked up by another. I am suggestible. There is nothing to trust except the validation of graphs. I told him I spent most of yesterday post-migraine and in bed, leveled and dazed, in lag time. With this kind of attention, the migraine did in fact seem like a slow seizure. He was going to get milk.

"Please, don't go." I heard my plaintive voice. I heard him come back and sit in the chair and put his keys down. I don't know what happened; the cue was internal, but it was sudden and vicious. I am at no remove from all this. I see nothing—it's almost as if I go blind. He talked me through it. I saw the rug, and then I knew where I was in time. It's a problem of time and space.

Tess and I drove to McLeans' for a three-hour visit with Merrit, who has seven stitches in her arm and the message "I will kill her" carved into her belly. She says this time at McLeans is very different. She has friends, and she goes to a group.

Her therapist joins us, and we are suspicious of each other's shoes, hers black velveteen pumps cut away at the sides and mine, Dutch walkers.

"They should be ashamed of what they are doing to you. If they are not ashamed, they will never learn. They are lost." Eva's voice brings me toward her, away from the abyss in time.

I have cycled in and out of an irrepressible trembling and a swath of dread. I work to remind myself that I have another mind, not this track alone. When I visited Sabelle today, she said that I was different, that I was anxious. She sat on the floor of the seclusion room, her arm bandaged to her elbow, asking to go to McLean's. "You will be no safer anywhere else. You have to find a way to talk and not reenact." I am steadfast in this. I asked if she would feel invalidated if she were not to get shut away. She answered me, quietly, "No." She is subject to so many dramas and cross currents that she's hard to read, and in a grotesque way, hard to believe. Grotesque because I completely believe the slaughter she was subjected to.

How do you think one should react to the destruction of care for the most helpless of all people, if not to get angry, to cry, to lay one's head down in despair? They have been attacked, slandered, removed from my care, lied to, betrayed, abandoned, mistreated, humiliated and asked to endure it all without recognition of the harm, without outrage over what was done. So have I, without someone in power rising to protect my patients and me. Vicki is frightened of emotion, and she mistakes suppression of feelings for stress management. I never hear anything from either of my bosses and, oddly, don't see them. They must hide out. No one will apologize.

I will take three more weeks off, except to see Sabelle. I worry about the stress this is on the others, but there is nothing else for me to do. I need time to see if I will recover from this enough to make an orderly withdrawal from The Center. I brought Sabelle a copy of Catch-22. She sat on the floor of seclusion and read it. When she finished it, she was deemed ready for discharge.

It is unrelenting. In answer to my question about what the school is doing to Sabelle, Paul said, "Sebern, we are not going to fight back." He went on to say that he fully supports the program director's decision to terminate Merrit. "Why?" I asked him, "She's in the hospital."

"It's his call," he said.

"Paul, what are we doing here?" He answered too quickly.

"We are moving kids through the system." I was angry and nauseous. But the ground, as barren as it is, is clear. I ran into Randy going into the agency. He looked uncomfortable—as well he should—and muttered, "Have a good day." I didn't respond at first, then said, "I don't want to be rude, but I don't know what to say to you." He said he understood. These men are pathetic to me. I returned to a call from the psychiatrist treating Merrit at McLean. She, too, has decided that I am overinvolved and she prohibits me from seeing Merrit. My jeans and Dutch walkers? Bringing her chocolate milk? There is an aura of punishment in that unit and a willingness to scapegoat. Three days later, I received another certified letter banning me once again from the program. I was under investigation for overinvolvement.

"This is shingles," my doctor said. He paused, considering what he was about to ask, "What's going on at your agency!?" It was clear others had come too, felled in this disaster.

The mental health system is falling into a ruin of disgrace. Friends of mine are either numb to it or complicit or both. I've just begun to fight this. It is indecent. I spoke with a woman at the Department of Mental Health, and I've left messages at the Center for Public Representation. I will file against the program.

Thanksgiving is cold and gray. I didn't go out. I lay in my room by the fire and spent time with the inexhaustible four-year-old, Sammy, who has come to live next door. Eva and John cooked. At the table, we talked of the five years ahead, and my mother said, "I'll be dead in 5 years. I don't want to live." Eva spoke into the awkward silence. "Well then, we hope you will at least come to haunt us."

Arles just found a space in his monastery in Big Sur, and he leaves tomorrow for a sudden, unplanned recovery. Only a small place in me feels the shock of abandonment. He has no abandonment intent. I kinda feel wrapped up in a woven bundle and carried along. He has placed a spongy earth beneath me. I still fall, but not far and not convincingly. I remember him. He gave me his number, and I carry that card with me.

"It's just better," I said, "when you're here. Better for me." I stopped and then said, "I hate to be one of the people that you must leave to recover."

"I do not need to leave you, Sebern."

A week ago, Paul read the bill of particulars: the letter threatening my job, in fact, my life's work and completely unexpectedly, I felt the gifts of my own recovery. "It was," I said, "like being beaten to death by pillows." Paul began the meeting, "It goes without saying how deeply I respect and value you." "No, it doesn't," I said softly. He acted as though he didn't hear this, then proceeded with mostly bogus concerns, all of which could be said without threatening me. He had produced a memo that would quickly restructure the clinical team, demoting Barry, and me. They spoke of the need to investigate two cases, both mine, Merrit and Sabelle. I cannot fathom their conscious intent.

"The queen," Arles said, "is only one moment away from becoming the scapegoat." They are trying to silence me, discredit me, wrestle the power of my creativity away and somehow retain me in an "as if" state, as if they had done nothing. I scanned myself for hate or retribution, a wish for harm to come to them or to the agency. I cannot find any. The perversion of all this is unspeakable, but they are not perverts. They are fearful and unconscious. I will not contend with them nor appeal to them, and they hate me for this and attack me more viciously. I will leave them to contend with themselves.

The day that I got the written warning, I also got confirmation of the loan for the EEG Spectrum equipment. Many friends want to try this. It will occupy me, perhaps distract me, while Arles is away.

I feel his absence, but it has no catastrophe in it, no bottomless despair. I have, though, become less able to concentrate and a little disorganized.

The Neurofeedback system arrived yesterday. John came, and we both trained. He did a half-hour Beta session after which he said he felt like he does after meditation, a general sense of well-being. I thought there was more color in his cheeks or face as a whole. He made abundant Alpha when he tried the Alpha-Theta protocol. I did two SMR trainings, each for half an hour, with a bipolar placement at C3-C4. This is an easier placement, with less likelihood of headache. During my Alpha-Theta sessions, the power went out twice.

"I can't grieve. It annoys me when you say it. Talking isn't helping. I want to try the machine." One of my patients had objected to the system being in the office, and she was right. It was a powerful third, an intruder in my small office. It was beckoning Billie from the waiting room. We did the training I was taught for high arousal, even though I was confused by its effects on me. It was as astonishing for her as it had been for Julie. Billie could cross the bridge without any pull to drive off it. She smiled. She could think. She needed me to talk with, no longer to govern. But it wasn't over. There was her father.

I began training today with Merrit. I was not allowed to see her before they terminated her, against her wish and my advice, but now they have no say. They continue to investigate my "overinvolvement." Tess brings her here to my office on Elizabeth Street, which is also my home, and I am seeing her without charge, and they would use this as "proof." She noted no problems and no gains with training. I'll look for both.

I am learning this system slowly, and there is a lot to learn. I did 40 minutes of Alpha-Theta two days ago and another 35 minutes tonight. I begin to feel anxious when the Theta band and the Alpha band touch momentarily before the Alpha sprints up with the sudden thought, "I don't want to be here." And yet the sense that I can handle anything is returning. I seem unafraid of the people at work. This probably relates to the training, too, but it also comes from sitting and flooding my brain with compassion in meditation. It's inextricable. Alpha-Theta deepens my meditation.

I told him of my dream images. *I was connected to the machine. Someone walked toward me and touched me with so much static it hurt my brain. In another case, a former patient returned for treatment. She said her name was Fear, but I didn't understand her or recognize her until she became impatient and reminded me that she'd changed her name. It used to be Lucia.*

"Lucia," he said, "is the name of the town that the monastery is in." We both let that settle into the space between us, and then he changed the subject. "I am worried about the weight you are losing."

My weight loss seems inevitable in the present and necessary to the past. I am a waif in the sphere I find myself in. It is as if I can disappear my own body as a way to survive in it. I have no appetite. It's the background terror we seem to visit at every session. Stress around my patients and my position at the Center gained momentum again two days after training. I am being hunted, in the day and in the night.

There was another meeting at the agency. I was not mentioned by name, and my position was eliminated. The consultant for the JCAHO audit asked me to lunch. "The best way to fight back is not to fight back," she advised. Barry said, "You have been preparing for this for years, and if you can just hold on to yourself, you will emerge stronger, clearer and even more powerful." He spoke of my courage. I don't, except very rarely, experience this as courage. I have no other way to live. I have said I did nothing wrong. I will begin to say that what I have done is right. I am bowing to superior power, power to humiliate and destroy. They terrorize. They are in a frenzied momentum. I told Vicki, "If it would help my patients for me not to love them, then I would not love them." She turned away muttering. "But Vicki, the proof is in the pudding. My patients do better."

She sputtered, "The proof is not in the pudding!" And I laughed a little and raised my hands, palms up, almost in supplication.

"I don't know what more to say."

Paul and Vicki left this meeting stooped over, in the hush of my silence. Their only redemption is in that posture, their only acknowledgment of shame.

I am trying to find my position in all this. What have I contributed? Is my confidence experienced as arrogance? Am I arrogant? Have I humiliated others? How do I speak about all that has been done without becoming the victim?

I took Merrit and Sabelle out to the Depot. It is decorated for Christmas, and when I asked, they gave us the table near the fireplace. Taking them to lunch, once just an act of simple pleasure, is now a death-defying rebellion. When I took her back to the program, Sabelle said that she was just happy and that she was beginning to get glimpses of what her life could be.

It is the winter solstice.

Chapter 7

John tells me that Johnny is coming, and I'm glad. He has bought himself a crucifix for Christmas.

All positions in which I argue with my tormentors or identify them as tormentors or insist they see what they are doing, or that others do, or that I am in any way an undeserving victim turns sour in my stomach. And it torments me. It singles me out, out of the flow of human history, outside of the banal reality, outside of the safety of faith. I cannot be other than misunderstood. It is OK. It is about doing what is right and being met with fear and hatred. At the risk of illness, I have taken the Eucharist each day here on retreat at Weston. There is a lot of flu. I've taken it, I think, to bond with this Christ, to find my experience in his, his in mine, without arrogance or self-importance, as a reminder. Those who know not what they do cannot know what they do. I cannot expect that or condemn them for not knowing. I will learn to find harbor in the way it is.

I am trying to untie a knot. The more I perseverate on injustice and blindness, the tighter it gets. It begins to relax in me, to unravel when I recognize "it just is." There is nothing in what they are doing that is new or hard to believe. It is commonplace.

Johnny didn't come. We got his Christmas call. He was drunk and telling me things like how it made his skin crawl when I had asked him if he wanted to sit between John and me; that he cannot come here because no one here understands him; that it was a scene that held only bad memories; that Hugh was his only respite, someone who gave him understanding and a sexual outlet—I went into high alert—and he quickly said that Hugh did not exploit him then lapsed back into his rant, laced with alcohol and therapy cliches. He was inhabiting a different voice last night, and it was eerie. It occurred to me to be hurt, and there were flecks of it, but I wasn't. I do keep looking in the background of my mind for feelings that would have been there. Their absence leaves little blanks, little question marks. My mother said that Johnny must have lived in his own world of torment. I was astonished and relieved. She wasn't shaming him. There were moments last night and today where I see her just as she is, stooped, eyes going, her elegance giving way to soft, almost goofy sweetness. Her will and anger now just serve a hopeless battle for control of the thermostat, or the quality of the asparagus or her determination to be left alone and to die. She talks each time I see her of dying, and I hope what she hopes, that willing yourself dead predicts a quick end. I surrender, to the Center, to Johnny, to my mother, to what I still must learn, but I do so like one who is getting electric shocks and cannot escape.

The child they brought to me, who has cerebral palsy and who turns away and bites, is changing dramatically. Her mother reports that it is like "night and day." She is calm and easy to be with, cooperative and turning toward her parents. "Last night," her mother told me, "She finished her dinner, folded her napkin, and asked, "May I be excused?" If that's all that neurofeedback ever did, that would be a miracle." Three sessions. Brains are organized to be pro-social. Something has to go very wrong for a brain to turn against its own company and the company of others.

I think I should be asking questions like 'why me?' or 'why is this happening?' They don't arise. I am not raging against my fate. But when Arles asked me why I thought this was happening, I cringed, ready to hear the accusation. Others see a defilement in me that justifies this cruelty.

Monday, I received a call from the JCAHO consultant. She said she wanted to ask me a question as part of the Merrit and Sabelle investigation, a question related to "boundaries."

I saw Nieves, and she greeted me outside Sylvester's with a hundred-year hug. All of her health is in that connection, in that "boundary violation." I met with my clinical colleagues at Paul and Elizabeth's for lunch, and then Tess and I went to the office to do the DBT group. On the drive home, I experienced a profound shift. All of my protests had arisen in part from believing that I had done something wrong. It is not true. There is no shared ground, no shared vocabulary. Nothing I said or did could reach them. Nothing will change, except that it can all get worse. It was over. This was not cognitive or emotional. The landscape before me that was littered with wreckage was now clear, open, and beautiful. Dread, shame and anger were all gone. It was a wise mind, a kind of clairvoyance without object. I wrote my letter. I erased every line that began with an accusation. Finally, it was simple.

"Dear Hal,

"Sadly, I am writing to inform you that I am resigning from The Center effective March 14th. I have loved working at this agency, with many exceptional people and these very special children. The events of the past few months, however, have made it clear that my vision and values are no longer consonant with those of the agency. I ask to continue to see the patients I am now seeing until they leave the agency. I wish you only good fortune in your attempts to navigate these terrible times."

I handed it in with copies to Vicki, Paul, and Barry. I called Tess to let her know. I couldn't read the letter without crying. I felt safe for the first time in months. I was beyond their reach. Tess was stunned when I told her, saying she found it hard to imagine working there without me, that I was the one who distinguished the place. Barry looked deeply distressed and said, holding the letter, "I'd hoped we could get through all this without losing everything." Vicki closed herself in her office. I heard nothing from anyone who received the letter. I had moments of fearing that they would figure out some further outrage, but these were thin, even wispy, fears.

Vicki had said, almost wistfully with only a trace of accusation, "You are different from everyone else here." I repeated this to Arles, and he asked me in what ways that was true.

"I think it's because whenever I am made to choose between my patient and the system or the agency or another staff person, even my own reputation, I choose the patient. I cannot abandon them." He was listening, and I continued.

"My allegiance is unwavering. It's never been understood, really, but it's been episodically appreciated or at least well tolerated. These kids are unconsciously or not so unconsciously degraded by many who care for them, one of the therapists described her patient as 'white trash!' for Christ sake, and a DMH supervisor told me the runaway would be 'roadkill.' I was tolerated like they were tolerated, as long as they brought in money. It used to be that these kids at least contributed to the system's welfare. Now they don't. The more disturbed they are, the more they take of shrinking mental health resources, and the more they represent a threat to the survival of the agency that is functioning to serve them. There are more administrators to write and administer the grants than there are residents, and then the grants never cover the actual costs. The administrators feel themselves on the rack. They manage this by scapegoating, and they chose me because I was the patient and because I chose the patient." He nodded several brief acknowledgements.

"I brought Sabelle the Simple sneakers that don't fit me right. She left her ratty ones under my chair. This is the evidence against me, and I offer it."

I had a glimpse that perhaps, with him, I could return and become small again, under the wing. But it seems impossible.

I told him of the dream of *many people coming to sleep in my room, being invited in by someone other than me and my fear or annoyance at this, my belief in the dream that the inclusion of them would make it impossible to sleep.* It suddenly occurred to me that these dreams were about integration. There is pressure in me now, integration pressure, that was in its way as intense as the pressure that brought fragmentation. I resist this collection of selves in the dream—I want to be left alone so that I can sleep. There is an inevitability, a knowing that I cannot change the circumstances and that someone other than me is inviting and/or forcing this arrangement. The second dream was one of the ubiquitous *large house with multiple rooms, and everyone was coming into my room to sleep.* Two nights ago, *I dreamt of two rooms and many children, all of whom needed Arles. He kept trying to come to the room I was in, but he was always interrupted.*

There was another event on Friday. I felt my head turn towards the left, pulled from the inside and turned from the outside. The hands were large, with clean fingernails, pink, and the skin was a dark, chocolate color. I am resisting. It did not seem to frighten me. I narrated this to him. "My internal state is a little dazed and on automatic, but still I'm not afraid." Then all the doubts take over. Without terror and without the opioid numbness, what do I make of these flashes? Arles remains abstinent. I am not tired of these happenings. I am tired of being tired of it and of being afraid. I don't know what there is to know, I don't want to know; I want to know.

"Vicki doesn't feel very good about herself," Sabelle said, looking up at me from under her long lashes, seeing if it was ok to go on. "I know from the way she walks. I walk like that when I don't feel good about myself." I brought them to my home office. I listened to Sabelle and Merrit talking with each other, and I felt moments of deep happiness in the normalcy of it, these two beautiful young women, survivors of unspeakable horror, chatting in the sunny kitchen, drawing, all very regular until—of course—I looked at their pictures. They are of small children and a Hitler-like man from Merrit and a grotesque naked woman from Sabelle.

My skin sensitivity has gone down, and the mental fog is fading. I slept fitfully after one hit of strong marijuana. I have an increased sensitivity to drugs as they predict with neurofeedback. The brain needs less to feel whatever it is. Except for sleep medication. There has so far been no change.

This week will be hard. I will fight to continue to see Sabelle and to provide her with neurofeedback. Then I must tell her, the others, and the staff that I am leaving.

I have been living out the Christ metaphor. I want to live by the Buddha metaphor.

Tonight, as I was leaving his office, I said, "I can't imagine anyone more committed to attaining wholeness than I am."

He put his hand on my shoulder and said softly, "I think that's true, Sebern, I think that's true."

I caught this this morning. My brain felt excited just beneath and just above the bridge of my nose as I came close to jumping the time track and ending up back there. I asked Arles to put his thumb at that point in the corner of my right eye at the bridge of my nose, in energy medicine, a survival point. Too much and it just hurt, but firm pressure organized me and kept me in the foreground, in the present. He experimented with it. When he lightened the pressure, it felt as if my eyes were focused on a place in a picture. I couldn't remember the term until Arles said it, "the vanishing point." When he took his thumb away completely, for a moment, my visual field was washed out in white light. I was in nothingness, and I felt physically disorganized. Like a frantic calf searching for the lost teat, I moved my head to find a point of pressure. He had to hold my head to help me stay with the incipient disorganization and white out, to stay in the exploration. The organism refused. I would not willingly succumb. He insisted I put this into words. Then he put his thumb back. I organized and was no longer at risk of switching time. He tried this on himself, but there was no effect. He may not be disorganized beneath the bridge of his nose, and it was his own hand, not his mother's.

"Part of the shock you're experiencing is that you are emerging from within your own head into a reality that has been mostly inferential. It is separate. It is Other."

I am a very small being with the carapace of a psyche. The end is torn off, and I have my first view of the world deconstructed. The carapace is gray and floating, like an abandoned hornet's nest, and the scene is the flat rocks—the scene of a dramatic episode of time travel, sitting with Eva and rising through layers of time until I broke the surface and was sitting there in the present. The exhausting miracle of forever being born.

The next journal has disappeared. For now, it is just my memory.

First, I told Terry. She was going to graduate next month.

"I hate this fucking place," she said, tears rolling down her cheeks.

"I am angry too, Terry, but don't let this get in your way." She asked for a hug, and I held her until the sobs began to quiet. "I trust you to do this well, kiddo. Let that be our heritage." And then Sabelle. I saw the familiar change in her eyes. "Don't descend, Sabelle. There's nothing there for you. Stay on this plane, and we will work together when you get out."

I prepared with Arles on how to tell the staff that I was leaving. He said, "Don't leave them motherless." He didn't intend this as a koan, but it was. And then the kids. One challenged me before I had a chance to tell the lie she expected. "...and don't tell us you're leaving to spend more time with your family!" I told them that I had the staff, but I lacked faith in the administration. How could I not leave them motherless?

The next day, when I came into work, the magnet with my name on it on the IN/OUT board was gone. When I asked about it in the office, everyone scurried and finally someone said it was a mistake. The next day, I was escorted out of my office. I'd been instructed not to tell the kids or the staff why I was leaving. Paul or Vicki or both had told me to make something up. I couldn't do that. Telling the truth about these kids and to them was the crucible. It was JCAHO procedure to have me escorted, like a perp walk, down the long hall, Barry, at my side. He talked softly to me all the way to my car.

I visited my mother on the Cape for her birthday. For the past nine months, since beginning neurofeedback, I have looked forward to seeing her and have come every month. She'd cut her hair something like mine. She told her friends that I was her best friend. We shared Stouffer's at her kitchen table. She'd become urgent about learning Tai Chi and had arranged for a class to be held during the day so she could drive herself there. It was her form of Eastern practice. She asked me if I'd like to see her "forms." Of course. The pride she took. It makes me cry.

My mother died as she had wished to die, of a painless or at least an unregistered heart failure. She had wanted to die as her mother had, at 81 in her sleep. That morning, she and her friend Steve had gone to the rehab center in Hyannis to visit their friend, who was failing to recover from a hip fracture. They visited together and then drove back to his place in Barnstable. In the car, she'd told him that she didn't want it to end that way for her. She'd already had two major surgeries for cancer and a heart attack, and weeks in the hospital at Tufts. She'd told him what she'd told me, "I don't want to leave my little house." They settled down in Steve's home theater in his basement, and she chose the film. She decided on GoodFellas. When the movie was over, and he turned on the lights, she was dead. It was April 12th. She'd turned 81 on April 1. She wrote her own death. I was at the movies too that afternoon, with Eva. We went to see Kolya, about an orphaned 5-year-old boy in occupied Czechoslovakia, taken in by a reluctant 'father'. John was there, as he always is, to give me the news. I don't remember how I took it. I do remember Arles saying, alarmed and unforgiving, "Sebern, this is your mother!"

My second grandson, Luke, was born with an anoxic brain injury.

Molly is holding her baby, with tears in her eyes. She never cries. "I don't know what to do. He only sleeps for an hour at a stretch, and he screams when I try to give him to anyone else. He startles for no reason. I'm exhausted; I'm worried." She paused. "Do you think neurofeedback could help him?" Luke was five months old. He was born hypervigilant. That's what can happen when you nearly die at birth. After three sessions, he slept five hours between feedings, and the startle went away. He could rest in the arms of others. Molly could sleep.

Billie began Alpha-Theta after she felt stabilized with eyes-open training. She dropped deep into the waves of theta. She was looking for something long denied by her family, and this is what she found: "I am on the ceiling looking down. I'm in a crib and my father," she stopped to check back in from outside of this state, "My father is fondling me." She did not look away from this. "I know this happened, Sebern." I listened. "Both of them said it didn't, it couldn't have, but it happened." There was an outside threat to remembering and to being believed, coming from the False Memory people. "You know what else?" she said, still in, then out, of what had just happened, "There were other things about him and about my mother that I have believed and somehow in this session I knew they weren't true." I asked her how this left her. She shook her head slightly. "I don't know. I don't get it, really. I don't feel bad. I'm not angry with him."

Reggie came up the stairs. A professional woman, conservatively dressed —white shirt and pantsuit (but hiking boots)—, a referral from Sam. She has come to consult with me about neurofeedback for her husband, who has been hitting her in his sleep. But after she talked with me, she and he decided that Reggie would become my patient. She wanted to address her "attention deficit disorder." At her third session, she arrived in a see-through blouse with sequins, in red heels, a bold dash of red lipstick and no apparent recognition of this difference in her. Over the months, there were others who came in during Reggie's hour: a young and utterly helpless teenage girl; a redneck man, overweight; this crudely seductive one with lipstick on her tooth, and a very competent nine-year-old who'd made soup for the family since she was five. And there was Reggie, too. There are, I would come to say, many reasons that a person has trouble "paying attention."

I woke up with the image of Uncle Theo's 1997 holiday letter. I read it three times. He made no mention of my mother's death. She was obliterated. How could he do this to her? She had no protection. Someone wrote about walking in graveyards, hearing the whisper, everywhere, "Remember me, remember me." She is not in an unmarked grave covered over by snow. She is safely tucked into her warm death. She cannot be hurt except by being forgotten. What is this madness?

Two trainings since I got the equipment back, and yesterday, I talked with Arles about my new state. The images were from the ride to IMS, looking down at Turners Falls, seeing the light glint away from the river as the sky turns silver.

"I felt serene and quiet but not deep. And the images have ice all through them."

"What do you mean, not deep?" he asked.

I answered by describing ice diving, which I have never done. "I am tethered to someone above the ice. The sun is out; it's a clear sky. I'm swimming in these clear ice blue waters, turning over and looking up at the ice from underneath. The ice suffuses the sunlight. It is as if this layer, the deepest layer of ice, has drawn in and holds all the sun."

"It sounds like Alpha-Theta," he said, and I feel, again, my relief that he has done at least some of this training.

"Maybe, but it is the sense that I can't access that particular richness that my images are about. But there is nothing superficial or unimportant about this quiescence." I paused as I thought this out. "Soon, I won't need therapy."

"When you don't need therapy, then you can want therapy." I mistook what I heard.

"Can I want the baby?" I asked. Then I caught up to what he'd said, and I continued. "It is actually the same thing."

"Yes, that's right. Do you feel a loss at not needing?" I couldn't answer. I feel too new, every cell feels new. I feel detached, maybe more than unattached, as if there is a large space around me, a space filled with light, but I am alone. *And* I am alone. I feel no opposition to it, no dread or loneliness. Nothing bad or good; just a fact. But I still live within the context of my history. Do I? These issues of attachment, and attachment failure, of ice and surfaces are still within me.

Marsha will not hear about this training, and she will not see her own resistance, even when I pointed out that I've been talking about this for two years and she has not pursued it. That recognition silenced her for almost a minute, and she may have thought about it.

"I never pressed you like this about Zen," she said after that moment passed.

"You didn't have to."

There was another pause on the phone, and then she said, "Actually, that's true," once again redeeming herself.

She does not recognize how deeply she has internalized her invalidating mother and how systematically and offhandedly she shames others. She will end up alone. I want to edge her into this for herself even more than for her patients, but tonight I doubt it will ever happen.

Chapter 8

The holidays are over, and the emptiness and sadness of Christmas have ebbed away. I have a red protection cord around my neck with two knots— one for commitment to practice and joy, and one for the observation of the precepts. I am back from the New Year retreat with Jack Kornfield. At one point during a sit, I looked up, wondering, 'What is this about; what am I doing here?' It was not a pragmatic question, and it was not triggered by fear or confusion. Many times, in the night, it felt as if my brain was shifting in my head and it could leave me in a kind of silence I have never experienced before—three or four-dimensional, dense, and physical. The people there looked lost, driven into meditation, looking for peace, looking for wisdom. What does it matter if you shave your head when it is crowded with nightmares? The meditation hall can be just a more formal way to become attached to. There is no truth in the zabuton; no truth even in the practice. When I got home, I described my practice as follows. Nothing happened except these shifts in my brain from ear to ear. This is neurofeedback, and I have no preference.

I feel as if I inhabit a field, now, that is flooded with warm light. I can see the edges of it, and it is as if some 'me' arrives from outside the field, from the right, actually, an airy being. I can see opaquely through the body, and it is coming into the field, naked, unashamed, translucent, tiptoeing. This being has entered the me that inhabits the field. It has snuck into me, and it enlivens me.

"What happens if this therapy is about the future distinct from the past?" he asked me. I had the image of a mother anticipating the birth of a child, of the mother walking toward the image of her baby, and that being entirely about the future. It would not be, then, particularly about repairing the past or reconfiguring it or resolving it. It would be about taking my brand—newness at face value as a real state of being, as a new being who needs to be nurtured so that she may be brought fully into life. What would that therapy actually be?

I, though, still have to face a chorus of ridicule to feel anything but disdain or disgust when I look at the photos. I would have to come to a place where this new being incorporates this baby. I thought that before I could do that, Arles had to; that he had to open entirely to that baby, then, in his wake, I could follow.

I could not separate myself from The Center until I felt a glimmer that I could survive without it. This is a common dilemma, and it is spoken of most frequently in reference to economic survival, to money. But for me, a larger and earlier dilemma contextualized it all – I could not leave the nexus of my survival, no matter how bad it was, without some sense of my own continuity. This is not as straightforward or as seemingly time-bound as separation, although it is; I am sure what makes separation possible. It is the experience of a continuous other, a predictable presence that allows the child to slowly gather around her a sense of self that persists back in time and forward into time. This sense of continuity is embryonic, but it does exist.

Marsha called. We got talking about my neck. She had forgotten my telling her that I had broken it in the dive. She felt bad about it.

"You were not responsible, Marsha, you were the inspiration." I reminded her that she protected me on Thompson Two.

"If you get paralyzed, I hope it happens after I'm dead." We talked about the layoffs at the Center and about my pleas to deaf ears, that none of them were safe. There were three paid therapists, 10 to 12 people salaried in the business office and numerous middle managers. Everyone there is miserable. They are walking around like Lilliputians in the decomposing corpse of the mental health system. Once they gave up the vision of taking care of kids, and it became a place to secure jobs, all was lost, including jobs.

I find myself thinking about the transference cure and its taboos. I brought my motherlessness to Arles not to be understood, to be mothered. My transference was rich and troubled and demanding. Somewhere in history, someone believed that all that was needed for a 'cure' was an accurate and timely interpretation. I don't think Freud or Jung really believed this, but this is what therapists in-training are, not exactly taught, but left to believe. 'Transference cure' is all but dead, and when alive, limp, and ghostly—in name only. Yet all the taboos, structures, and rules around it go on strong, a mindless life of their own, strangling all innovation, spontaneity and honest relationships for litigious protection. This is what I am accused of. "Overinvolvement" is breaking some vestigial sense of what, really? Marsha has no truck with transference, and she detests the concept of boundaries. In DBT, she has replaced boundary with "personal limit." There's pushback, though, from a profession so deeply intimate that it cannot trust itself.

Rosen

For Christmas, Peggy gave me a gift certificate for a session with Lee, a woman who practices the Rosen Method in Great Barrington. I thought it was a massage until Lee took my frozen wing into her hands and said softly, "This shoulder will take a lot of work."

Soon enough, I felt comfortable enough with her to say, "Please press deeper, Lee."

She was hesitant as she did. "How can you tolerate such deep pressure?"

"I know you are there, but I can hardly feel it." She may, in fact, have gone too deep. It is as if this bruise is held in the subtle body, the body between the surface and its history.

Reggie is doing better, she has me back. When I do left-side training for myself, her experience of me becomes stark. I become suddenly unavailable to her, and she is devastated. I become cold and punitive. It's subtle to me, but she's right. I am gone, I resent her, I drive her out. This is what Arles sees in the swagger. During my holiday crisis, my answering machine broke, and she arrived quivering at my back door. I turned her away, angry, frustrated, overwhelmed. It makes me sick to remember it. I was cruel. I could not do the simple, decent thing and just wrap her up. Her need seemed endless, and I could not forgive it.

"I understand Theodore Kasinsky better than I do the men who molested me. I identify with him. I picture his victims as powerful white men in suits, Westchester country club men."

"Are they people?" he asked me.

"No! They did terrible things, they will never be punished, they should be blown up!"

"Yes, yes," as if coaxing a child out of a nightmare, "They should be blown up."

"Why?" he asked a few moments later, "Do you think that 'memory' is more important than intuition?"

"Don't you?" He didn't respond. "I don't know. Memory is more privileged by everyone." I told him of the mind that I live in now, the default mind, that steps into the shower with appreciation for the great comfort of hot water and, at the window, feels near rapture for the cardinal. He said the other mind is the one that either takes for granted or wants more.

"Intuition stands apart. It looks on. It has nothing to do with the eruption of fear and grief that comes unbidden in some code, organized and understood only deep in my brain." I paused to notice how important his question was before I responded with mine. "Where would my memory come from? That vacant baby, how could she remember? And then there's the hole burned through the cortex, the white-hot needle of current. Then the denial of its harm, the eradication of memory, as if the loss of this most singular, precious capacity of the human mind is a mere side effect. The multiple head injuries, the bashing of my head that was itself, like the red queen talking, a manifestation of memory. I want stepping stones that will lead me from then to now and memories to set down across the path already cleared. I want to step from one memory to another through time. My continuity over time and space rests in your memory and your witness, your participation and determination to provide a past and a future. Without reconstruction of memory, I really have neither. I have an endless present that is claimed by the past. I don't live in the river of time and space. I am held away from it and dare not move. Nor breathe. I am inanimate. I have the fact of a life lived, but it is as if I did not live it. I want what was true and actual. I want the markers of time to organize a sense of myself over time." I stopped and remembered. "I used to love 'connect the dots' games as a kid, to see the hidden form emerge. This is what I hope for from Alpha-Theta, just enough dots."

I tried to describe the mind I needed him to be. Finally, I got it. "Like a dream catcher."

"Not open," he said, "that you could slip through."

"Yes, broad, but netting is not enough. I need a containment wall."

CEREAL KILLER

Why is it that discovering the realm of the sociopath seems different from the discovery of the unconscious? I was unaware of that substrata in me, an entire landscape of organization of self. It was a revelation of a buried infrastructure. It was not a revelation of yearning. I knew that. I presented that, performed it, disguised it, costumed it, paraded it by him – yearning as obvious as a Macy's Day balloon, a four-story head severed from its body—a show of yearning so as not to yearn. It had become hollow; desperate but hollow.

Perhaps it is accurate to assume that every baby has the capacity for an unconscious, and that the unconscious, like memory, is a relational development. Carl is unaware of 99% of his psychic reality. He said once, "It's just beginning to dawn on me that when you give me something you're not trying to hurt me," this after 6 years of devoted treatment with me and in the residence. What was that dawning? The very beginning of relational potential? It was not the dawning of an unconscious. He lives in the predawn dark, not in the unconscious. He never gained me.

On Monday, my feet went out from under me, and I fell on my back down four stairs. It felt accidental. In today's context, it was. On Mondays, perhaps it was not. It's strange how that could be true—not just the observation of therapeutic convention but the ellipsis of fact. It's not just that the fall should not be addressed today, but that in the consciousness of today, that fall was an accident. In the consciousness that may still be afraid to leave, it would be anything but an accident.

This morning, I felt the frozen infant state and a state of fundamental, adult security simultaneously. There were only small spikes of fear.

I brought oil for the hinges of his door that squealed, and heard him say as I walked into town, "the squeaky hinge gets the oil." Here I am, no longer that, no longer wanting to be that, but instead the bearer of the oil. Everything in me is quiet—a quiet of hopelessness, a quiet of serenity and infinite capacity, perhaps even the quiet of breathless terror.

Sabelle graduates. I have been forbidden from attending.

Alpha-Theta dream

I fell back to sleep at 4:30, and the dream started. *I am driving with Sue up a mountain road somewhere in the developing world. We are going to the conference called Future Health. She is driving, and the road is made of large stones, orange and smoothed over the years, with cement or sand between the stones. It should have been a very rough ride, but Sue was so skillful that it was as if we were driving on pavement. I commented on this. Suddenly, there was a huge boulder, three or four stories high and wide, rolling down the road directly at us. We were going to die, to be crushed. I yelled over the rumble of it, "Don't let it hit us, don't drive over the cliff!" Then I was gone, wrapped in dissociation. I felt the impact of the boulder against the back of the car, but it was muted by my state. The car was stopped. I couldn't see. "Sue, are you alright?" "Yes," she said, "You must get out of the car now!" I didn't immediately understand, and she repeated herself emphatically. "Get out of the car now!" She was already out and afraid that it would either explode or fall over the cliff. I got out mostly blind and inched along the side of the car on a narrow lip of land. What had seemed to be a cliff was now a gentle slope with trees. The light was shimmering. I got to the road. I asked again if she was all right, and she said "Yes. I have a different history than you," she was steady. We walked down the road to a small beach. There was no evidence of the boulder—no scars on trees, no trees run down. There were three kids playing there, but oddly diminished in size, as if I were seeing them from a long way away when they were right there. At the edge of the water, we could see a double line of mountains beneath the ocean surface, but there was no path in the sand and no boulder. An old man who was up to my left says, "There used to be a gap in the mountain range, and now it is filled in. This must be where the boulder ended up. Submerged under the water." I could see, and I was confident, but I was also dazed. Not only was there no sign of damage done, but there was no sign of the reality of the boulder, except the witness or merely the hypothesis of the old man. Maybe there was damage to the side of the car, but having walked past it, I did not turn back to see.*

I came awake very slowly, falling back into the vivid reality of this dream repeatedly, unwillingly. I knew I was in a room, and it was dark, but I didn't recognize it. The boulder part of the dream had been in three dimensions. *The boulder was granite, different from the rest of the landscape. It was going to crush us.* I could not get awake. I called Eva. I remember the light on the dial, and by this time, I knew I was in my room. This was only a fact, not a comfort. It did not really compute. I could not reorient. Eva's voice on her machine pierced the state for a second, then it took over again. I told the machine what was happening; I tried to get out of bed, but I was too weak, and my body hurt. I felt like I'd had a concussion, there was a painful pressure in my head. I felt like I'd been run over. I could do nothing but lie in bed and keep the alarm going in snooze cycles. Between the alarms, I would be dragged back into the dream/nightmare/neurological event. I finally had to get up to pee. I had regained some muscle, went down to make some tea, and came back to bed. The rest was waiting for help; the kind of waiting that you do in a hospital bed, helpless and weak, with patience forced on you. Eva called. I was able to tell her all of this and hear her soothing voice. This is unlike anything I've ever experienced, and nothing she has experienced either. I struggle, but I cannot get free until she tells me of a boy named Franklin who is as happy as he looks. He described to her a sudden biochemical change a few years back, which left him with daily periods of exuberance. This story changed my state. The impossibility of the day dissolved into possibility. My body still hurt, but the shock and terror of the dream disappeared.

Tonight, I have had glimpses, surges really, remembering how awful that dream felt. And now, like the boulder, the dream has gone to rest at the bottom of the sea. It is covered over, and without this account, all it represents would be unremembered.

"This was a near-death experience," Arles said. "It is beyond all meaning in your history, inclusive of it, but not *It*. It was not a dream 'about,' a dream projected on a two-dimensional screen. It was a dream from the space beyond the third dimension, nonspecific and archetypal."

He asked me to describe the mountain ranges. I looked back into the dream.

"They are parallel to each other." I paused, looking away from him and down over the mountain tops under the water. "This seems strange, but they are running next to each other and," I stopped again to confirm this impression, "And they look like the double helix."

"Yes," he said, quietly, "Cellular memory."

Sam felt trauma, both old and chronic and acute. Old in the way it felt; new in the way it yielded. My body ached. I felt concussed. More so today than yesterday, but I got up like a shot, shocking my body that is used to a gentle morning ritual. Last night I tried to get worked up over Johnny, and I couldn't. It was just hollow and habitual and finally just foregone. Big flakes fly outside Sam's window, and as he moves the bones back in place around my head, my whole body goes as still as snow. I realized, driving back to town, that I had nothing to say. I stopped and got a pillow and brought my journals into Arles. I lay down on my pillow. He tucked the blankets in around me, brought his chair up next to my head and read my journal. He capped my tousled hair with his hand. At some point, the exhaustion began to ebb away, and my body opened up.

"I think I saw God, Arles. I am still trembling. It's been going on for three days." I felt the depth of his attention. "I don't need to remember anything anymore. Every event was in the boulder that is resting at the bottom of the sea. The gap is filled."

"And remember the quality of the light." The light was vast. It shimmered. Arles was asking me to look at what he saw as the dream's overarching goodness.

My heart broke open in my love for him. Love and gratitude. And for all of them: for Blake and Chelsea on the beach; for my mom, for John finding his way; for Johnny, whose heart is building capacity and flexibility; for Molly, whose patience seems endless and who is gracious and generous with herself; for Eva, who is turning in circles too small for her but just big enough for me. I feel rich with people and free of sorrow.

Before I left, I told him about being with the fragments of Reggie. She and I pictured her picking up the neon orange salamander, her two fingers around its little belly, an animal at that moment in terror, and stroking its head, its throat, and finally able to turn it over to stroke its belly, the slightest brush of the fingertip and the whole universe of this being changed from terror to bliss.

"This is your lizard brain, and this is what we are doing." Then there is the part that yells at her, telling her that all of this is a lie. I asked her what she did.

"I say back, 'That is not true!'"

"When you lived in Boston, did you ever come across a man on a box preaching, exhorting, condemning?"

"Yes."

"Would you argue with him?"

"No! Of course not."

"Why not?"

"Because it wouldn't make sense to."

"Right, you just let it go by, not particularly attending to it, right?"

"Yes."

"Could you do the same with this part of you? Perhaps contending with it is not as useful as letting it pass by and treating the ranter with compassion."

"This came from a wise place in you, Sebern," Arles said in his quiet, soft voice. "Thank you for telling me."

HYPERBARIC OXYGEN 1

Everything is ordinary. Driving in LA, living in this hotel. On the way here, waiting patiently for the plane in O'Hare, I saw the pilot making preparations, I saw that the waiting room was empty, and I made nothing of this. I did not hear the boarding call, and in the absence of this, I made nothing of the other data. It was as if I had lost signal anxiety, as if I am, at base, so without anxiety that even when I should be, I am unable. I will have to adjust to this. Here is the difference between equanimity and mindfulness. They called my name, there was nothing lost. I was surprised by my initial inner protest at my seat assignment which was way in the back near the galley, surprised when preferences and judgments are still so strong, surprised that it doesn't disappear immediately once I see it, surprised at how quickly it does give way and how superficial it is—all of this at yet another level as surfaces deep within me smooth out.

Yesterday I went to the factory near the fashion or, more truly, the sweatshop district. It was one of the few places I could find in the country to try hyperbaric oxygen therapy. Jamie, my friend and neurofeedback colleague, recommended it to me, if only to kill the parasite that I'd picked up swimming beneath the waterfall in the river in Belize. This parasite has been provoking the yeast that has a hold of my system.

I'd come to promote neurogenesis. Flooding the brain with oxygen under pressure, I am told, does this. I'd come on trust and intuition.

I parked on a side street in the neighborhood I've been warned about, staying aware but not anxious—another new capacity. I did not feel menaced. Belle, my technician, is a thin French redhead with a southern sweetness in her voice and demeanor. I walked into the receiving door through a section of the factory where there were three chambers in partial assembly. There were two large oxygen canisters and a few odd chairs, two gurneys and the chamber that the patient leaving described as a snub-nosed submarine. There are two bubble windows on each side and another in the door that seals the chamber. You cannot, once the door is closed, get yourself out. It was raining and raw outside and gloomy inside the factory, but in me, everything was fine. I took off my shoes on the Kmart Persian rug at the entrance to the chamber, pulled on my sweater, grabbed my pillow, and climbed in. I was cold. After covering me with as many sheets as she could find—ones they used to cover their projects at night—Belle closed the hatch, and I spent the next hour and a half going down to 33 feet, adjusting pressure in my ears, thinking about meditation, monitoring my state. It was unremarkable, just cold.

High winds, pounding rain, streets flooding over the sidewalks, and I make my way back and forth to the unwelcoming steel of the hyperbaric. My body adjusts quickly now to 45 feet of pressure, and I begin to relate to the tanks more as a healing force than as a potential death trap. Belle takes me down in the morning, and Dennis in the afternoon. More sheets appear each time, and today, a tablecloth. I wrap up and breathe. I asked the parasites to let go. I visualize them releasing their hooks in my intestines and being carried out by oxygen—I wish even these parasites a peaceful death. All else is staying dry and settling down. Just settling down.

I sat for a long time in the tiled hot tub at the hotel, watching sparrows, thinking about the pigeon who hopped on one foot, the other seemingly congenitally deformed, and noticing my reaction to the people I saw. One Black man, dirty, ragged, and schizophrenic, and almost immediately I saw him as a little boy, bewildered. The plump elderly maid;

another old Black man, well-dressed but harried; two Hispanic women trailing two little girls, many people and all of them I look at, and I wonder what their lives are for them. Who are they? Who have they been? When I drive along Pico in the rain, Mexican migrants stand draped and dripping in garbage bags waiting for work. I am taking these people in.

Today I read a bumper sticker three times: "There is no rescue from domestic abuse." It was only after a few minutes that I realized that it didn't make bumper sticker sense. I read it more consciously. "There is no excuse for domestic abuse." Sometimes my mind goes like this.

Palm Springs: Future Health

I tried the new 1 - 40 frontal squash protocol, for 5 to 7 minutes without any apparent effect, this afternoon and woke up at 1:02 AM clear, focused externally and completely unable to sleep. There was no need to sleep. Even though I have never formally studied physics, I knew I could take a physics exam then and pass it. I asked the developer the next day what he did when there were untoward consequences, and his answer was that there were none. I told him mine. And then I got it: the big problems here with this whole field are very high development costs, fragile egos, and mysterious phenomena. I am going to have trouble tonight. It is familiar. I cannot move from an external to an internal shift that helps me sleep. This used to be a problem with hypervigilance, but right now it is hyperfocus. This executive function is more like the workaholic CEO function. I felt extremely bright and scientifically capable, intuitive, creative, though not very in my body or emotionally present. Linguistically fluid. Some restless legs tonight. Appetite is even less. This will pass, but not it seems without migraine. Siegfried chastised me as if this should be obvious to me. "You can't go around and sample at these booths, Sebern, not with your brain."

I went to Carol Schneider's talk on the orbital frontal lobe. Injury to any part of the brain can eventuate in injury here, injuries that abrade the cortex and leave it torn. I have moments of seeing how serious my situation is.

When the conference ended, I felt a tinge of sadness. This gathering is perhaps one of the most practically revolutionary of any in history, an event marked by compassion and brilliance, humor, and grasping. Siegfried and Sue took me to the living desert, Siegfried with his video and tripod, Sue full of botanical notions and a warm detachment. Siegfried burns brighter, and his smile, sudden and full, delights me. We ate last night with Len Ochs and Mary Lee Estes. After the hyperfocus in the middle of the night, I'd become unable to organize notes. My receptivity, both emotional and intellectual, felt occluded, my handwriting fell apart, and I was getting a migraine. Len decided not to train my brain. "He recognizes a swamp full of alligators when he sees it," Sue said. Standing at his booth, he gave me a deep shoulder and neck massage to ease the pain. "Wow," he said, "Your left shoulder is burning hot and then ice cold." Stuart Donaldson came by with a bevy of learners around him and, pointing at me as a specimen, said something about how I hold my shoulders forward because of trauma. Len smiled and whispered to me, "Duh."

I have no ambition. I have no other place to be. Right here, right now is fine.

❧

I could feel grief in every cell. I couldn't find the route until I sat down with Arles and I saw an image of my mom in her apron standing in her kitchen, little, cute, exquisitely vulnerable, and my heart tore open, and I wept. I wanted only to protect her, to hold her, keep her safe from all harm. We are inseparable in my grief, in her numb and inchoate suffering. I am a stunned baby. So is she. My route to grief was through the sudden, awful knowing of what had happened to her. He just held me. I do not yet truly know that she just couldn't do it.

I miss my mother. I discover myself leaning toward the Cape, mentally, physically, as if she were still there and missing me. She got to that place toward the end. She was able to miss me; she was able to wish I would not go, which made my going poignant and finally possible. Before that, leaving was a minor geographical rearrangement beneath which I felt an unspeakable loneliness. Until the last nine months, I was most alone when I was with her. I had been desperate to get up the short staircase, then to sink into the deep tub. Her skin was soft and fragrant with Nivea cream, I loved the smell of her. Slowly, in the last year, she learned to receive my kisses as they became robust in me, unambivalent, unafraid. My mother was scared. She was confident in her beauty and in her business and scared nonetheless. She feared, I think, that she would be humiliated in conversation with others, with me. I hear her in me, in the habit of control. I carry her wallet. I remember her face, her fear of suffering, her wish for a sudden peaceful end.

"When I was a kid, I scooped up her face cream on two fingers and, well, I ate it."

"Yes," he said, nodding slightly, "Yes. I see this."

❧

"I think you talk too much and with too much certainty about neurofeedback," Peggy told me after we ordered appetizers. "I want to hear about you, not neurofeedback."

Without much defensiveness (surprising), I agreed. "I don't know what to do. It's like I've just discovered the existence of sulfa drugs and no one on the TB ward will listen to me."

Last night, Arles stayed with me as I tried to understand the anger that is so immense when I would say how hard this Friday cancellation was, and he would do nothing to make it right. This was dissociation time, and I couldn't. I was cuing for an explosion, but there was none, not only no will to explode, but also no capacity. I was enraged at him for canceling. It made no sense in 99% of my being, but this one percent held sway. I couldn't get out of it.

At the EMDR conference, I wanted to remember. I thought that if I remember, I will have events in which he can intervene. I can bring him into a scene, and he can extricate me; we can rewrite the psyche's history. Suddenly, I realized he's already doing that. Depending on where I position him, I disable or enable him. I can keep him, withdrawn, at the periphery, or I can see that he has been intervening constantly, that he has been rewriting my history.

Lee laid her hands gently on my lower back. My sacrum was bowed. My breath, she said, was careful, as if I wanted to move as little as possible. As she worked, it was as if memory parted.

"Lee, I always thought the sacral pain was from the car accident. It wasn't. I was kicked." I could see the color of the boot—a light mustard color—, and I could see my position on the floor. The room is dark. Lee's hand felt 10° warmer on my sacrum than on my upper back.

"You must have been a terrified child."

"Actually, I don't think so. I was numb." But this, of course, is just a layer above.

What does it mean to believe this happened? I don't want that. None of this. It is not interesting. It is not important. I needed to know why I lost my mind. I know. It is enough. It is more than enough. No one loses their mind without reason. It is not a congenital defect. I don't want to be hurt anymore, not on the street, not in my mind. I don't want this. I feel a new empathy for Johnny. Who can stand knowing? Who can stand not knowing? There is a rope around my neck, high under my chin. I am pulled here, then there, slowly, delicately strangled.

"I don't know what to write." I flatten the seam of this journal with the heel of my hand. "It feels as if I am straddling two moving walkways 'trauma time' hurtling me into a nauseating warp and 'now time' that is as clear and promising as early spring. I was torn into pieces by an unnameable terror, and I'm all right, upright, not tumbling at all… Both are fully simultaneously lived. There is no observer. Somehow, this should not be possible. It is the difference between memory and present fact, between remembering and being tormented. I know I am 'in' something, but I am neither detached from it nor judging it. My desperation is encapsulated in the other time that I momentarily inhabit on the other walkway."

"Don't let them get me!" I am breathless. It is always "them." I don't see anyone. Just the color of the boot. He quiets me.

Forgotten. Absence. Neglect. There is not enough in these words. From them alone, no one would understand that there has to be another word.

"Maybe there is a word in French," I said. He smiled. His smiles are empathic moments. His laughter and often his "uh-huh" and his sighs. His anger too—loud so I can hear it, demanding so I have to, quick to take me by surprise—is empathic.

But there is also something that can tighten in his chest, and he turns away.

This is Reggie's complaint. This is what I do. She wants this to flow freely from me, as if it were mine to give. I speak with him about a kind of flexibility that can meet ruthless desire. It is only a baby asking, for better or worse.

It feels as if I have tread every inch of a small territory so repetitively, so necessarily, but so unendingly that nothing grows now on that patch of earth. It is gray clay, hardened by my constant footfalls, compressed and barren. At times, it is my mother's body. I don't want to walk on her. I want to lift her up, breathe air into her, round her out. I want to so deeply forgive her that the thought of forgiving her is gone. I want the truth of her, but I do not want her body and psyche to be reduced to the platform of my suffering. I want to know and say what is true without demeaning her, without stealing from her, without flattening her. We were mute in our own distinctive ways. She refused to talk to me, her stoic crushing silence, and I was afraid to talk to her. The patch of earth is the square beneath my unrelenting feet, unable to leave, unable to stay still.

I am quiet. "Arles, what happens when something keeps imploding, getting more and more dense? What happens in physics? Does it explode then?"

"Is that what you're feeling now?"

"No. I cannot explode. I was just trying to understand what happened, all the exploding that I did. This is beneath it." He waited for me. "How could I have loved this illness, dramatized and romanced it?" He waited, still. "I did it as the ultimate defense. It kept everybody's attention on the presentation and off of me."

"That is very insightful and important to know."

"I've become aware that this was inevitable. Once I was born to my mother, there was nothing else I could do. It had to happen this way." We were looking at the photograph of the baby propped up against the pillow.

"That's right. It was unavoidable." His voice is quiet, even gentle, as if he is also talking to a baby.

"Someday," I said to Arles, "I'm going to be a little bodhisattva. I will know all varieties of human suffering. I will embrace it. It will pass through me, and it will not find a home."

"Yes," he said, "you will."

"You too," I said. "I don't want to be alone, so you have to." He laughed, but he did not affirm. He doesn't know yet that this is possible. I will find ways to clear the energy in my home office. It is, as he said, an electromagnetic field that builds up. "Don't underestimate the impact."

"I am the whaler walking inside the still bloody body of his prey, up to my waist in blood; swimming in trauma."

"Is that your mother?" It was to me so clearly about trauma that his question disoriented me. Later, I answered,

"My mother is dead, and she has left me with all this bloody body."

He nodded and sighed.

"I am tired. It is Alpha-Theta exhaustion. I can feel it inside my brain. It is where I ended. It is where I became a bombed-out building with window eyes, charred inside, the top of my skull blown off."

"Who is looking out?" His question puzzled me.

"No one."

"Who is looking in?" I shook my head.

"This is what keeps me from moving into Theta. It interferes with my meditation and my training. I cannot, in that moment, feel anything other than shattering. I don't believe I will shatter. It is not about prediction or future; not about the past either, really. It is just the reality, and it cannot be." My brain vibrated with it. Arles sat with me as I tried to feel for it: "Yea, though I walk through the valley of the shadow of death, I shall fear no evil for thou art with me." The big bang: the moment of destruction and creation in one. What was created in that implosion? It was a riveting discovery of something that was not new.

"Who is 'Thou?'" I'd asked myself the same question. The answer then just came.

"It is you, you as you are and you, infinitely expanded."

I can feel the cramped quarters I live in. I cannot stretch out my arms. The air is stale. I have no freedom, no range of motion. I can point to exactly where the toe of the boot landed. It has become isolated. It is no longer diffuse but sharp and deep. One hard kick. There seems to be no relief from the sacral pain. Chronic pain is memory.

"I just don't want it!" Tears are streaming down, "I refuse." And then I am still, only a little scared, lighting the lights, changing the sheets, listening to the rain.

Tomorrow is Good Friday. Arles will tell me why it is called that.

I am here at the Cape. I miss her. I miss her doing her needlepoint with the sun coming in over her shoulder. I miss our laughter, finally genuine, over the crossword puzzle. I grieve for the very hard life she had and for the nearly impossible lives she gave her children. I don't want to ever leave her. I don't want to give this place over to strangers. I know today again that she is dead. It isn't about being mothered; that is not what is lost or what I feel lost about. It is about the absence on this plane of the body/psyche in which I once lived. Where is her pelvis? How can I still be alive and she not be?

I need to sit here until the sun goes down. Instead, I will go to the lawyer and settle her estate.

I dropped back into a traumatized state. I canceled with Sam—something I've never done—believing that he might hurt me. Too exhausted to fight this, I crumpled back into my poorly used bed. I considered canceling with Arles, too. Every interaction had to be carefully managed. I finally got up and walked slowly into town in the warm gray mist, like walking in a kitten's breath. I knew I had to cry. Arles was impatient, maybe, like me, disappointed that this technology delivers better on deep than on smooth. It has been a terribly rough course for both Reggie and me. He denied being angry, but he was—this has been a long course of misery. He swallows his discouragement, knowing that everything is indeed changing profoundly. He pushed me to know what I was feeling; I didn't.

"Once I was no one to my mother, I positioned myself as an object for the rest of the world. Every abuse, every injury, every accident were manifestations of this original broken arrangement. I did not exist to my mother. I did not exist to myself. My body, my psyche, my spirit were all someone else's indulgence. I knew nothing else."

"I know how you feel. I really do," he said. I knew he did. We sat together in silence.

"Look at those flowers," he said, nodding at the spider mums on the table. "They just keep going... like you. They don't have to keep going, but they do."

My brain will be like that rich yellow mum, holding and spreading the sun to everyone who sees it—one day, one day, just not this one.

I am still thrown by these cyclones. I land in a heap. Someday, in a heap of spider mums and forget-me-nots.

Suddenly, shockingly, he made me aware of my hatred. I didn't know what he was talking about.

"You have been telling me that I am not helping you." He was right...

"I have, but it isn't true," I said, confused. It only becomes true if he believes it. In this unrelenting state, I have been unrelenting. He is a bystander. He watches my torment. I slip, saying, "You tor..." stopped, but it was said. He is not only a helpless bystander but an active torturer. This has been my accusation for weeks, "You are not helping me. You are torturing me."

"When I am saying over and over, 'I don't want to do this,' I am saying 'don't do this to me.' I am telling you something is being done to me."

"Yes, I thought this too."

"I am absolutely helpless; no one will help me. They are all bystanders."

"Describe the bystander."

"It was sex..." it escaped my mouth, and it clamped shut, my hand flew to cover it. "No, no, no, I wasn't supposed to say that!" I turned away from him.

"What will happen, Sebern?"

"I don't know. I was never supposed to say that. Ever."

"Look at me. No, not away, Sebern, toward." It hurt my eyes.

"This state is a state without you."

"How can I let you know I am here?"

I closed my eyes and shook my head, but whispered, "Press me."

The chickadee just lives out her nature. I want to stretch and yawn and smile. I want to invite the opening of life, not turn my shoulder against it. I am guarded, vigilant and turned inward, forced to feel what should never be felt or to live with a transcendent lie.

"I don't want to do this!" I repeat this in multiple chords of agony, almost in accusation.

"Can you accept that you cannot accept this?"

I am imagining a compromise, a way around this core reality of no other. Or a way to live with it, only partially exposed. Like the shell from World War II, uncovered in a random excavation. Roped off, gawked at for a while, then hardly noticed. Commerce grows up around it. A pastry shop and a mobile store. We memorialize the unexploded relic. Plaques are engraved, flags on scrawny sticks are pushed into the spongy ground at the corners of the rope. Is this a live bomb or a dummy? It landed here without exploding the first time, just at the end of the war; why do we suspect it now? The town meeting addresses this: we can't take the chance now, there is the pastry shop and town pride. Who will come here? We have no other attraction. No one comes for the peaceful grazing of the black and white cows. How would we thrive without the bomb? And think of the lives at risk; the shattering of bone and psyche. It must be left alone, this decrepit metaphor, this potential crater where life had been, filling with cold rain, turning into a jewel of ice. Ice that no longer has any relation to water. Ice that is stone.

Neither implosion nor explosion—a steady state—the baby left motherless in the presence of her mother; in the absence of her mother.

I told Arles that I needed a squeeze machine. What I wanted was his hands up underneath my skull, cradling my brain.

"Short of that, what can I do...?" For a breathless moment, I felt the terror that my sense of him was true: he could not help me; would not help me. That was the faintest hope, the hope that the shadow memory of his presence was gone. Short of the impossible... Didn't he use to do the impossible? Didn't he routinely reach inside the bones of my head? Didn't he once ease me into sleep? I cannot find him in my nostrils or my belly. I don't miss him, he is everywhere. Everywhere and obliterated.

He is my therapist. In the truest sense, I am alive because of him, and just now the memory of the smell of his office, of him, made me smile. I cherish him. I don't need him. There is no place for him in the place of no other. He asked me what he could do, and my hopelessness flares and burns out.

"There is nothing you can do. We both must tolerate that. I am in the land of fire and ice." I tried to look up at him across from me in his therapist chair. "I hardly exist. I am safe enough to experience this terrible epic. I can only hope it is a passage."

I left him a message. "The terrible belief in these states is that nothing can touch them, but today it was not true. You changed everything."

I woke up still listening to a dream, someone talking about me: "Her mother needs help to die."

Tuesday night I smoked, and I saw myself as a dark-haired woman slinking about, dressed in dark brown, hag-like, cold, killing. I was actually several women, identical, in a crowd, all of this underground. As I said it, I realized there was a yellow star pinned to my chest.

"I am vermin, Arles. I only feel hate. I have been so debased that I have no capacity for love. I am recruited for the resistance. I will become an assassin. I am beneath the ground, maybe in sewers." Is this a metaphor or a memory? Arles said nothing. I was restless, but there was no better embrace of all that I was stumbling toward than to be receptive, receptive and still. I became grateful for it.

On TV that night, a physicist said that if you were the right distance away, you could see the birth of the Earth. The closer you could see the span of all life. Closer still, you could see the history of all humanity. You would only need to change the position in the slightest bit to see the Buddha, Christ, Hitler and you and me. From a certain distance, it would all happen as if simultaneously, which is, of course, simultaneity. Isn't this then the entry into parallel universes? Once you dispense with the notion of linear time, or try to, it actually seems a likely possibility. And what then is the barrier between these universes if not primarily our belief in linear time?

My patient Godwin said about himself that having no passion, no love, was like having no central nervous system.

How is it that training the right side of the brain the right way allows us to feel safer? My own training seems to have dropped me down into an even steadier, less perturbable plane. My speech is a little impaired, forming too slowly, and my syntax is a little rocky. But I feel safe. I experience myself living in the present, and time moves at an expected pace. I have no desperation about Arles' absence. He remains important and constant but no longer central. I do not organize around anyone or anything external to me or internal or intrinsic—no other, no ambition; no preoccupation. I am fluid, moving with time and space, one with time and space. This is not a mystical experience; it is a practical one.

❧

Mother's Day 1998. One year, one month. Cold and rainy like the day she died and the one she was buried. Pink petals cover the lawn, the car and the neighbor's roof. This and the cardinal song had begun to annoy my mother. She called it "mess and racket." She was becoming tired of living. She could've said that, though in a sudden twist of mood at any time. Any time I knew her. Until the last nine months, she became easily and bitterly annoyed. I held my breath around her, unable to know for certain what would trigger an assault; just to know that suddenly I would, or some past injury, stored like doomsday goods in her dark and angry larder.

As I became unafraid, she also became unafraid. She took her finger off the trigger. She forgot there was a war. She danced Tai Chi. No longer angry or bitter, she welcomed me, and I welcomed that. My elusive mother, the one who turned her face from me, who would not touch me, who could not cry for me, asked me if I wanted to see her forms. I couldn't hold back, openly crying in gratitude for her sudden willing vulnerability. Many times, she granted me relief with her generosity. This time it was a gift of joy. She was proud of herself, and I was proud of her—but not for her forms—for the first time ever trusting me enough.

Mother's Day: the span between her birth and her death is brief. I have, in that interim, recognized her in me. It is as if I can feel the line of her nose beneath the ridge of mine; her temper animates mine. She seems to be in my joints. This is not a foreign presence, although it feels very new. It is disquieting. Her body lies beneath my bones, the covert structure. I do not see her when I look in the mirror. She isn't there. I don't really yet see my own eyes, they go blank before each other, refusing entry.

I have the sense again that I am seated, my brain is held calmly between my ears. It rests in my body. It is not, this morning, anything as dense as gray matter or white. It is more like John's description of a molecule, the nucleus and the swirl of potential. The movement is organized and, to accommodate the slope of my head and brain and the telemetry of planets, it is circular. It is dense with potential, more dense and more electric, but perhaps like dust in the light. There is no center to it except what shape and motion imply. And I feel seated in time as well. I am participating in Now. I am at this moment as accomplished as an old monk.

This organism, which is, in some way, myself, has abruptly and calmly experienced the absence of my mother. Her death is real, and the fact of her absence does not grip me. Maybe this is my increasing sense of her in me, in the way I turn my head, or write a sentence, the literal flow of ink; I feel her in me. This is new and at first unsettling. I am suspicious of these aspects that are suddenly in me. I experience myself as she might have experienced herself were she self-aware. I seem ready to allow her to create herself within me.

I am having some speech difficulties, almost stuttering, some word reversal, some footwork clumsiness and an inability to grasp scientific concepts. I cannot get them into any place that I can visualize. John is a patient teacher. I told him that if I could find a way to intuit volts, amps, current and frequency, I could remember this stuff.

I started to have all kinds of difficult associations as I anticipated the blood draw. The last one had been botched. I felt an aversion to giving blood, but I went. The same solicitous text, the same chair, every prompt for physiological arousal, including anxiety, but my blood pressure was 110/64, and my pulse was 57. It felt as if the feedback loop that would convince me that I was going to be hurt was broken. The body part of the loop was refusing to be aroused by the mind part.

Arles and I are preparing to part for the month. He asked me how I evaluated training and therapy in terms of importance.

"I have no doubt. Neurofeedback is the single most important breakthrough in medicine since the discovery of DNA. Not just medicine, but the expansion of our understanding of being human. No theory of consciousness is complete that does not include the understanding that we can change its course through feedback to the brain." I looked at him, but I couldn't tell if I was hurting him. "But 'therapy' and 'You' are not the same. Very few therapists would have done what you have done for me. Your presence has changed me. I don't know what neurofeedback would be for me without the surroundings of you. Slowly, slowly, it has made you more real to me, more than your presence alone could have done."

I must have looked away or set up the screen of white noise. I don't know what he felt about this.

Before I left, I said, a little confused that none of the old constructions of catastrophe formed up in me anymore, "It would be terrible if something happened to you. It would not destroy me."

Before the ten-day retreat at St. Michael's, we had a day of mindfulness for members of the Order of Interbeing at Maple Forest monastery. Thầy said, "You have a right to suffer. You do not have a right not to practice."

The pressure here for "as if" mindfulness is not entirely bad; it is the beginning of mindfulness. First, adopt the behaviors. One of the members said that Thầy had been skillful, and I said Thầy had been present. So, I too am trying to be present, just present, just honest, just kind.

A few days ago, I reached over to my bedside stand in a moment of impatience and habit and thumbed a small ant. The part of its body that I missed struggled to escape, fought to live, and I was suddenly deeply stricken by what I had done. I ended its suffering with a tissue. It was a terrible episode of enlightenment, I saw it all clearly. It was life. I had ended life. I had created suffering, fear and pain. I have vowed to protect life. I have been tolerant of ants, but more as an idea than as a reality. I didn't see this creature or value it; it was a prop for my mindfulness play. That ended suddenly. Now I have a more challenging practice. When I took my shower, I saw that someone had killed a mosquito dragon. I wrapped it and asked forgiveness for our casual killing of these beings that bring us life and who cherish life in themselves.

THE VIRUS

I interrupt the meditation silence with deep spasms of coughing. There is a virus pooling in the dark of my lungs. My throat and my ears are sore, and yesterday I began to get a headache. I am waking in time for morning meditation, but my lungs can't support my going. There are times when it feels as if I will cough them up. Grieving? Of course, that is it. On my way to Plum Village, I had ended up in Notre Dame and could sit there only for a few minutes. The realm of no mother, the ocean realm, that is what fills my lungs. I've become susceptible to this disease when I become confused and have to learn again that grieving left undone stops you from breathing.

A private sanitarium somewhere in Europe, between World War I and World War II. TB, I think. I am a person of privilege, the daughter of wealth, but I cannot breathe. So I am in the mountains, quarantined to my own room, left to write, to reflect and to grow quiet. I came here restless and angry, filled with pity for my illness. But everyone here has it; some must even be wrapped in white blankets and taken about in those elegant wicker vehicles. Everyone walks slowly. Their lungs can support nothing else, and there is no place to go. No place to be. I must ease my struggle for breath.

The discharge sheet at the little clinic said viral pneumonia.

The sun rises under the leaves of this beautiful tree. "The first green is gold." Up today at 5:15, I had a peaceful private shower in a bathroom filled with sun. The images of the sanatorium are vivid again. All white tiles. I can almost smell the place, enough to know it is not familiar, not American and not the present time.

We were caught in a sudden downpour. Thầy was out in front, followed by three tiny nuns, one of whom tried to shield him with an umbrella. They were all rescued in short order by someone in a new white Volvo. I just walk. It's not about Thầy anymore; none of this is about Thầy anymore except that I love him. His teaching soaks into me like a gentle rain into desert soil, first only in the outermost level, then in deeper and deeper until the flowers that have lived only as potential begin to grow. Dharma rain.

As the monks and nuns chant this morning with Thầy as the bell master, I thought of Charlie. He is 64 today. I liked the way I was celebrating his birthday. He will never do any of this in any form.

I arrived back here from the retreat expecting solitude and met Johnny in the kitchen. We shocked one another. The porch was being painted, and the kitchen was filled with porch furniture. We stared at each other over this tumble of chairs caught in mutual suspicion and hatred. Just in time, I remembered that this was a mentally ill young man, and I took care of him. On the way to the country, I asked him what he needed that he wasn't getting. He paused, "I need some acknowledgment that when I wake up in the morning..." "Oh, yes, Johnny, I know that's true."

I canceled my patients and spent the day in bed. I drifted, rocked in a boat, in a sheltered cove in the Aegean; walking over tawny bricks in unrelenting sunshine, seeing the play of light on a three-story gray house, the shadow of a tree... I was in no time, no place. It was transcendent; the illness, a surprising gift.

Years ago, when Blake was about ten and out with her dad at the movies, I had an encounter with a young Holocaust victim who I knew had committed suicide. She was in my room, inviting herself to take refuge in my body. I thought at first that I should allow this, I should save her. She was coming into me through my feet, then my calves, my knees, my thighs. I would be a righteous gentile. But I was not her harbor; she wanted to become me. I abruptly told her she had to leave, and I felt her jarred but willing to go. After she withdrew, I saw scenes as negatives. Between coughing spells, I realized that this was the same as looking at the family album – we are faintly etched in white, emerging ghostly out of the slippery blackness. Not quite a skeleton. And inside me, I keep coming up against the negative, the blinding black hole in which there is no memory, only haunting. And then there's the picture of my friend Mary as if she didn't die that year, hands filled with Amytal, the Beatles on repeat on her stereo. Kevy is in the picture too, but she is eternally young, not dead and motherless. And my mother too, the one that ultimately only I, by sheer perseverance, could claim. Sheer perseverance and failure to die.

The phones are off, and I am silent. I hardly know the time or day. When I move, phlegm moves in my lungs, and I explode into a spasm of coughing all to harvest one small gray-yellow marble rolling around in the deep pocket of my lungs.

Swimming in endless pools of Theta and sweat.

Tiny sugar ants land in my glass of water, and they are not easily discouraged. I have lived with them as I have lived with this cough, almost constantly.

Ginger pack, then tiger balm, then magnets, then Benadryl, then meditation, then the horrid Chinese tea.

Back in bed, coughing. I am riding this horse and returning to real time, quietly.

On Saturday, I walked slowly into town, aware of almost every footfall. I was ambushed by neon advertisements and kids screaming, laughing, 'fuck, fuck that', and there is no pause, no thought, no stillness. Everyone seems angry or fogged over by despair. There is no light in their eyes. They smoke cigarettes and use the ATM and exclaim over shoes in the window. There was no comfort to be found on the streets. No one looks up. The same ones who used to just hang out on the streets now peddle them as beggars.

"The trouble of today is much worse than the trouble in the Buddha's time. An entirely different order," Thầy reminded us. I am not blind to it. It moves like a river after a flood, and it frightens me. The only refuge is a stable mind. I try to discern the wall of cough syrups. A kind woman arrives just in time, the pharmacist makes his recommendation and steers me confidently toward the store brand. And then two bottles of chocolate milk.

All day today, the door clicked open then shut. John, Johnny, Blake, Chelsea, and I listened for them from the tree hut that my bed has become. I wander down in the same flannel nightgown that the night before was drenched in sweat. Everything in me and around me is limp with this disease. It feels like a debt accumulation, a dense gathering of unshed tears. My weakness has always been in my lungs. My silent breath suddenly rises up in a spasm, grabbing me inside the throat, pulling me upright in bed, gasping, choking and tearing up, staggering almost sightless to the bathroom, coughing, choking, gasping until the marble is exhumed and lying in the tissue or the sink. And then I return lightly to the troubled sheets, swallow water in tiny sips to keep the spasms from starting up again, then a little juice, then cough syrup. "Try to lie down, easy, keep your head elevated on the third pillow, on his chest."

Silence today, interrupted by the definitive clicks of the lock. Thunderstorms, blessed downpours and this maple, like the one at Saint Michael's, sheltering me.

Johnny is stumbling out of the wilderness of psychosis, bloated with terror and fatigue. He is not yet completely with us, and it is very difficult to discern if he actually remembers the prior states. He was unable to read or drive when he arrived; a week later, with training, he is doing both.

Do you notice how, even more surely than cats, ants always land on their feet? The persistence of ants, pastries of phlegm, Fugitive Pieces, the pillow that is the possibility of his chest; the epoch of bronchitis. I am worn down by illness, and in the silence yesterday, I wondered what I did that discouraged care. How would it be that I was so sick and no one called to see? I was more curious than lonely, but today I noticed a slight seepage—then moments of suicidal despair—as old as my mother, as old as her mother. I have spent much of the past week in some other time and often in some other place, patient or, if not exactly patient, feeling no need or ability to be impatient.

I am still sick. 20 days. I am as motherless as a loon's cry. I am three or four, told after the birth of my sister that I am too heavy to carry. My whole body yearns upward. Just to be picked up, under the arms and tucked into the corner of his body. I settle back on my heels, my feet bewildered that they are still on the ground when all I need is one moment to be swung free of sorrow's gravity. There is no one above me. They're all dead.

I began antibiotics today, drifting and timeless, wishing for rain. I was crying at my doctor's office. Some belief in my own resilient health has been shattered. He prescribes antibiotics.

I felt the entire weight of my body cradled in the arms and belly of this bed. I surrendered. Flowers are everywhere, on my comforter, on the box of Kleenex, on the tray from Reggie. I am not restless. I am not afraid now. I am sick. I meditate on the release of these pathogens. In the vast realm of human suffering, this is a speck. Deep within, Arles recedes from me. I throw ropes to haul him back in from the black tide. Yellow ropes. It is futile; I am too small, too weak.

It feels as if my mind is bending. I turn off the air conditioner because it plays the Virginia reel. There seems to be no outside.

I finally reached Arles, sobbing, fearful, "this is an emergency." He answered and said he was just looking up my number. We are finally able to settle that I am having a drug reaction.

"My mind is like a slippery piece of liver, and I am watching it slide away from me. It is horrifyingly familiar."

"It reminds you of the hospital, but I think also of a much earlier time, near your birth: the state that led up to the photographs."

I got dressed, picked up my stuff and tried to free myself from the grip of the state by going outside. It was gray-green, thick air, threatening clouds. It was as if I had walked into the weather of my own interior, and I couldn't get out. Everything was flat, the way you see things when pressed up against glass. I went and bought a book since everything in my room was dripping with madness. I got Under the Tuscan Sun, which is actually quite annoying, but it wasn't about my brain bending and turning into offal. It was part of my climb back into normalcy. I bought two Heath bars while waiting for the new prescription to be filled. I told Paul, my pharmacist, what Bactrim had done to my mind. He looked it up. "Chance of psychosis is rare," he said, "but reported."

It was humbling to be so sick, and it was humiliating and terrifying to be so out of my mind.

"It was a toxic state. You can't give meaning to a toxified brain." I think that's right, but I don't think he's ever experienced psychosis. I know the state. This was not so distinguishable from the theoretically "untoxified" brain in the seclusion room. And really, isn't everything about a toxified brain? There are so many poisons.

Part of it was my encounter with how it must've been for Kevy and Hugh to die without their mother with them. She wouldn't have been here either. How did they bear that? How did she?

I have re-oriented treatment with Reggie, she is enduring it. I am insisting on a midcourse correction. We both have to acknowledge my limits and my collusion in her deep fantasy of a mother with endless resources. She did not deny her greed and her neediness; she saw all she's been asking and all that I've been giving. She feels humiliated by her need and even more by my limits.

Arles's presence has been more ghostly, more not there than there. Oh, the demands on him with his own perilous attachment. It was his not coming; it was not daring to feel what it felt like that he did not come. I am not unloved, but I cannot love him. I dreamt about this. *I came down a long hall and went into his office. He wasn't there, and I said, "Good, this is my time!" The room was white, almost sterile, and there was a double bed with white sheets. I sat on the bed, leaning against the headboard with my legs stretched out, and waited for him. He came through the door, his hair standing out on the sides as it does when it gets too long, partially red, partially gray. He stopped and smiled, glad to see me. I asked him how the retreat was, and he said it was good. Some hard times, but good. I was glad to see him, but detached. He said, sitting now, "Prepare yourself for a spanking. You will feel this." His tone was no-nonsense. I didn't think it would matter. I woke up.*

My love for Arles has become passionless but undiminished. This is biologically difficult to understand. He has been my universe. How do planets stay in orbit without the passion of gravity? But who sees gravity as passion or even as connection? It just is, a force of nature; a bonding that is granted and taken for granted. It does not engage the question of need. Yet need is still deep in me, and deeply disappointed. We are held to each other in orbit, cool as the moon and the earth.

The hopeless body of an infant. Still here. Still yearning. Still refusing to yearn. It is our nature—as sure as migration is to birds—to seek the body of our mother and for her to seek ours. It is as if she had a missing chromosome. She had a missing mother. I have not felt his presence except for the strong hand on my shoulder holding me back as I started to leave. "Remember that I love you." I left happy. "That will be enough," I said to myself, stepping into the vivid colors of the summer morning. But it wasn't.

I have to face the possibility that this primal hunger cannot be fed. As I talked with him, I felt the unspeakable, unbearable pain that precedes the anti-social position. It's not right to call it sociopathic. It is first just a frozen death. Then I become only the glare. I am arching away.

I wondered with Arles yesterday if the intense Alpha-Theta sessions have opened the door for this infection and the secondary growth of yeast that I've been dealing with for the last six weeks. He asks if I think Alpha-Theta done too early could impact the immune system. Maybe it's just a matter of interrupting the stasis as we begin to reorganize the brain. The immune systems of chronically stressed people are suppressed. I have always been confused by this since I rarely get sick, and now, six weeks.

I thought more broadly about dissociation, that it need not be so tightly linked to trauma. For me, the major indication that I am dissociated and the degree of dissociation is measured by how I experience time. I could not find the platform of real time during the pneumonia. Bactrim wiped away any remaining vestiges. A mother not there, and what is time? Without time, without my mother, nothing is quite real.

My experience of the suffering of another has changed. It's quite dramatic. I knew that it should move me, and I would try my best, but some pathway was severed or never developed. It now just comes; it is the natural response. I have noticed it most as Eva tries to find her way through her father's cancer. He is disorientated and near death. My responses are about her. Sabelle is developing empathy, too. She, too, has cared about people, but this, as I am discovering, is something different, not quite the same as empathy.

"I want to know as much of the map of devastation as possible before I can no longer feel it. It is a moral imperative to make this known." I had the image of the explorers' map, like the first crossing of the Rockies. "It's now an irrelevant map, we can see it all from the sky or from space. It will be an artifact in a museum, appreciated but no longer needed because of neurofeedback." As soon as I started talking like this, his absence vanished.

"Personality" may be, in some essential way, the accumulation and reification of mood. There is something that endures in this complex process of neurofeedback while all around it changes.

"You said you didn't really care if you ever saw me again. Do you know what that felt like?" His chin trembled, "All that I have done, how deeply committed..."

I didn't hear any more. I was overtaken by remorse and a shocking recognition that, of course, that would hurt him, and of course, it was still in me, it pervades me even as I try to herd it into the corner of the pen. It is an ugly fact still living out its independent existence.

But I am coming fast into adulthood; this well-organized brain. I am ashamed of the searing residue of childhood. I am forced out of the transference in some ways right on time, and in others, prematurely. I became aware of some ephemeral but persistent fantasy of growing up with him, not just negotiating infancy but all the rest that I have missed. I don't have many images or concrete desires, just the sudden awareness that I missed all the connections with my parents, all of my childhood. "Infancy," I asserted to Arnold Wilson in his class at Smith, "is about ruthless need, met, or unmet. Met it dissolves as ruthless and is just a need. Unmet?" "Klein calls this aggression. This is a terrible distortion of human nature, of the nature of babies and mothers."

I could not think my way clear, but depression ebbs away as I lie on the rock looking across the water at the green-gold apples. It feels as if there is no other response possible to the circumstances of living, perhaps in this case, to the fracture of hope. My furious need will not be met, cannot be; it can go into recession; it may dissolve in the organized brain, but Arles does not have the stamina of the idealized mother any more than I have. He cannot persist forever against this unyielding core. It affects him, and it affects me, and this perhaps more than anything gives rise to deep despair. It was his being 'above it' before that gave me hope that the void in me could not engulf everything.

Sabelle now says "I love you" with love. She looks at me full-face, open-eyed. With this training and my steadfastness, she experiences herself as being born – born into color, into a universe more of sadness than of horror, of insight and exquisite and prolific poetry, of assertion and self-inventory, of clarity and lucidity and genuineness. And what would have happened to her, this precious, terrified child? Now she sees a future through the veil of tears. Godwin told me, "Until three days ago (several trainings in), I had never known what it is like not to live in anxiety. I always sit with my back to the wall in restaurants. It's been hard to tell you that, I am too afraid." These words finally slipped out beneath and around his shame. At the end of his last session, he said, "I have never before in my life felt this relaxed. This is good." He will learn to feel safe. They are all amazing people, my patients. Even Reggie, perhaps the most injured of them all, is beginning to arrive in some clearing outside the transference. At least this is my hope. I am just learning to be there.

Raspberries, river solitude, clean sheets and laundry on the line: I am moving slow. This depression is not about losing Arles—it is about never having had him. I keep looking for my own clearing, and when I get glimpses of it or have moments of really experiencing it, I am awed, and I retreat. I move away. It will go on like this for a while.

I begin to turn my attention toward Alpha-Theta training, feeling increasingly sure-footed in the mysteries of cortical process. I think so much more clearly. I am, for the most part, unafraid. Peace remains elusive, but I know of it. Johnny's brain is finally coming around. And maybe me too, and Reggie, my three toughest cases.

This depression doesn't lift, and it too seems time-locked. I am dragged by a back current and can't quite swim up into it, or lift my head to see the blue sky and fields of flowers or even the shadows on the dirt road. Time must be marked relationally for an infant, or it goes on forever. A mother's predictability is the rhythm of time. She arrives; she defines epochs, that this is over, that this has begun. Her movement toward her baby delineates time – holding the baby stops the endless flow of time. It contains the eternity. If she's predictable, she domesticates time. She quantifies it. She picks the baby up out of the free float that follows the disorganization that follows the anxiety, that follows the unmet, hated need.

I wrote a thank-you note to Mary, who sent me photos. After that weekend at the Cape, I could no longer imagine her as I had. She sucked the breath out of me. She was the hungry, voiceless orphan who played solitaire and took the bus to Atlantic City. I know the fact of her leaving, my giving her mumps, all part of the constructed narrative, but that had nothing to do with Mary as she is and perhaps even as she was. I loved her and still do. I wonder what she was like then. What was the nature of our attachment? What was this like for her? I have no one to ask. If she were the person that she is now, how did she save my life? Mary raised me, and when she left the attic, Maddie and Moses moved in.

I loved many people, just about anyone who would present themselves for it and many who didn't—they only had to be older than me and beckoning. I went from one to another, like Sammy, who lined me up as his next mother when, inevitably, his present foster parents would give up. I always felt that I got something from the coach, my English teacher or Leonard, the pedophile. I learned to make a meal of morsels.

When Arles called to say we would be meeting, my depression dissolved. I was delighted that I would see him and wondered how, given the nature of my nearly perpetual attachment crisis. I was just happy to see him. What of all the rage he'd been feeling? What of my distrust? I still don't understand what's up with him and me, except that he is insisting in angry spurts that I see him, not just the function he fulfills. He sees the arch of my back.

"I have no say in this."

"So, it's structural?" he fired back at me.

"It is inherent. It is the way it is. This is the truth. 'I am tired of this arching' is not. It would be like getting tired of breathing. One could be, but you just aren't. I am tired of its repetitiveness, of my lack of choice. Yet in this position, I would only choose arching." He has left behind a well-intentioned ghost, and I move through him.

Johnny is reorganizing, or more like it, organizing for the first time. He has no complaints about being overwhelmed. He is present behind his eyes. John trained him last night and reports that Johnny had two flashbacks during Alpha-Theta—you can see these in the EEG. We'll see how he manages this. He did not report any awareness.

I am looking at the juncture between mind and brain, a privileged view. It requires a paradigm shift: the meaning of symptoms, the responsibility of the symptomatic person; the position of the therapist, the role of the therapist, transference—still there, but what about it?—stigma, the DSM. We are explorers at the edge, at the opening to inner space. How are you listening? What are you listening for? What questions do you ask to elicit what information? Therapists using neurofeedback must understand what trainees experience; to be part of the experience; to hold the patient through when things get scary, to know it works and the way it works, the obvious and the subtle and the profound. This will inform their listening and their questions. They will encounter attitudes toward the equipment as interloper or savior, as significant other, as inhuman, and neurofeedback as being referred away; all of this and then the question "Where is my therapist!?" Therapists must first train their own brains.

I saw my neighbors across the street sitting down for dinner at their picnic table. Very soon afterwards, it began to rain, and I saw their curved backs as they headed indoors. The abandoned picnic scene felt forlorn, and I realized that my relationship with Arles feels exactly that, like an abandoned picnic, the hope rained out. Forlorn, not tragic.

When I told him of my fear of losing him in this rupture—the telling of which, of course, made me afraid—he said, genuinely and softly, "What can I do to reassure you that it won't happen?" I reminded him of the havoc viruses play on the brain. He did not deny his depression. He listened and, knowing I have reason, asked me not to be afraid.

❧

"It should never have happened."

My statement hung in the air. Sunlight overtook the lamp light, and I knew the day was turning clear.

He echoed me softly, "It should never have happened."

I turned toward my mother, who stood to my left. She was like this at every age—thin, cool, tough and fragile. I see her beauty and the powerlessness of her old age; I see the absence of her alive and the presence of her dead.

"But except for some sense of justice or rightness, that statement has no meaning. I would not be without them, these two parents. Exactly how they were led to my being, it just is, it could be no other way and the fact that they were who they were led to all the other facts. There is no protest left, and there is no refuge in wishes. I cannot fling myself backwards, saying I wish I did... or I wish they... That voice is stilled."

This is what it is. I must grieve until the grief is spent; I must have faith (this is less and less required) that it will be spent, that I can lift my dark body out of my light body, like Kunta Kinte held up to be blessed by the gods, but no longer living in me.

Last night I had a cannabis breakthrough. I suddenly and vividly experienced others as three-dimensional and separate. They were propelled away and suddenly separated, in their own containers of space. Some vague, unrecognized sense of myself as fused tore away, like Velcro skin coming apart.

I asked him if he'd learned anything important or new during the time we have worked together.

"Oh yes, many, many things. I learn something every time we meet."

"It is important to me only because I want to know I have given something back to you."

"Yes," he said. "You have. You do."

My confusion over the nature of my unconscious has returned, and again I have the image of the Mobius strip, the outside becoming the inside but then pooling in time for a nanosecond before it becomes the outside again. I have been raised by therapists. I learned the need for awareness as a second language. I was able to name the secret motives; they were on the tip of my tongue.

"You act as if you have no unconscious," he said, "or it seems as if you have no unconscious." He doubted me, believing, as most do, that there is always an unconscious. But how does this happen? Are we just born with it? I think it requires a mother present enough to grasp the reality of the infant, to lend her the experience of structure, to put her hands on her, to give her shape. No self means no Unconscious. I was taught the form in psychotherapy. I became increasingly self-aware as much for protection from interpretation and shame, as for nothing more, really, than to please. When I say that I have come to understand myself, it is not that my unconscious has been revealed. It is coming to see how, deep within all the shaping of experience, I was still unformed. Hollow suggests structure; that hollowness comes later. It comes after the sudden newness of the relationship, after the insistence of his hands. The moment my mind shattered, my nostrils were filled with my mother's perfume. She was on her way out, and I was gone. So for years I have trodden through discovery, and now at the nub of being, the tender shoot begins to grow, a voice learns to cry, and my mind breaks open like a warm, raw egg spilling over with light into light.

I was talking about the wilderness.

"Did you recognize what you just did with your eyes?" I hadn't. "You looked out the corners, like the cat."

Rilke's panther is caged, in the most pitiful zoo in the Jardin des Plantes, gawked at, sure to be shot if she ever escaped. They throw meat between the bars and hose down the cage and the cat. She is degraded, soiled, caught. I can feel the arch.

The river is low and cold, crisp as a winter apple. I saw the first red maple leaf. It will all change. Who will remember?

Lee was using a light touch on my back, and the storms began. She asked, and I told her what the thought was. "Touch me deeply or don't fucking touch me at all." It feels tantalizing. And alarming. This rage emanates from the dark body, the body that was never touched. I need impact or no touch at all.

Sam's fingers rocked the center bones of my sacrum, "There it is," he said, meaning the site of injury, when my body was still light enough to give way before bone. Exactly, he was right where it feels so bad, where it never stops hurting. I felt, or maybe witnessed, a state shift, more as if I were remembering a dissociative state than being in one. It was quiet there, but I wasn't scared. I didn't even remember being scared.

Arles kept me waiting, and even when he apologized, I could not free myself from anger.

"I am enraged with you."

"Yes," he said, "for not being here; I know." He took my foot in his hand just for a second, reminding me that we knew each other, that we shared a history. He talked me through the fight in my body.

"I can't help it." I went to buck.

"I know it's in your body, and it's strong, but you can help it.... Don't fight, you don't have to." He tightened his hold around me as I pushed against it. "It is blessed to receive, easy to give, blessed to receive. Quiet, quiet, shhh, shhh," he almost whispered, "Take what's being given here and now." It was as if my body figured it out, following the map of his tones, his rhythms, his hands. This is what I have come to learn to trust.

I am thinking more about my emerging unconscious. I have always brought him gifts, often gifts of food. He has always blessedly received them. Wasn't that always an act of the unconscious? But it wasn't. It was the act it was; now it is an act of the unconscious. I have begun to form around the being of another, and this begins the structure of the unconscious. Arles said you can't have an unconscious without structure – and structure comes from "mother-child," "child-mother," "mother-child" over and over, simply and repeatedly repaired. The child is in the presence of the other. My first acts of giving food were the first acts of relatedness. I could not look at him. He was distant and wan. He simply received them. It was a kinesthetic reality test. Oh god what a disaster had he chosen to interpret! And the very first were not really gifts for him. They were symbolic representations of me: Wooden pick-up sticks, each one lacquered and polished. Only later did they give gifts of food to address the sense I had of his ghostly need for nourishment. There was nothing beneath these acts. They were symbolic acts, but they were not acts of the unconscious.

The loving of another has power in it; being loved is powerless. Power is too aggressive a word, but strength isn't right either. "It is," I said to him, "just like a baby. She cannot stop loving her mother; she can try to stop caring whether she is loved."

I don't remember, maybe footfalls upstairs or at the door... "I am holding you; you are safe. I will not let anyone hurt you. Breathe... breathe."

"More than ever, I do not want to know, but it is gaining on me..." And then it did.

In the attic room, my voice and my syntax changed, and I saw Maddie standing on the right against the wall. She looks scared. I can feel fear crawling up under my ribs now as I write, and I was either scared by remembering or remembered being scared. I was not re-traumatized; I did not go blind, I knew the whole time where I was, that I was being held. I could see and recognize the room.

"Arles, I've just gone numb. I've gone dead inside."

"What do you see?" he asked, gently, firmly pushing past the deadness. I had no response, and then my body stretched out trying to get away from being held. He gathered me back, and everything shifted again.

"I know what happened." My voice was small. But I could only stutter. I tried to say, but I couldn't. Then I tried to show him, wanting him to say, but he didn't. I pushed two fingers into the air and then into my mouth. I felt his slow, deliberate breathing. I kept trying to say it, but every attempt was shut down. "I don't even know if I said anything." I felt his arms strengthen around me. I think I was crying, but I remember screaming, "I have to take a bath, I have to take a shower!" I got very cold. Arles pulled a blanket over me. And then not much later, it was over. I picked two black curly hairs off my tongue. I just noticed. I was seeing it all from a distance. Time buffered me. It added layers of thickness to the air through which I saw what I had to, finally, see. When it was over, it didn't seem that I had been through an ordeal. There was no aftermath.

"This is true," I said, quiet and bewildered. "I don't know if it is factual, but it is true."

"Yes," he said, "I was here. I saw it, and I heard it, and it was true."

As I left, I turned back to look at him, "What do I say? There is nothing."

I had trained at FPO2 for a minute. It didn't at the time seem to affect me, but the way I went through this was very different—the fact that it happened and that I could manage it. Several times, I think, I let him know I was all right. This was from the training.

I woke up full of energy and feeling lighter than I remember feeling in my life. I wonder if it's over, I thought, maybe I know all that I need to know.

It is as if I am in a fort. The walls of it separate this terrible experience within me from all the time and self that is outside. Last night, Arles called to ask me to come in for an hour. I knew that we might talk about what happened on Friday. It was as if I believed that, like the boulder, it would leave no trace; that like my mother, he would not remember. And my state validated nothing. After training Sunday night, I felt once again all lightness and grace. Until I started to talk with him about what I had seen, I believed I had no feeling about it. When I started to see it again, I couldn't stop. At some point near the end of the hour, he asked,

"Do you know how important Friday was?" It took me a long time to discern the truth and say it.

"No. I know it only when you say it."

"Friday was critically important." And then it was as if I'd been grabbed, kicked in the head, overtaken, possessed. My skull was the boundary between past and present, unreal and real, a precious container. My mouth contorted, and the voice, "You fucking whore," and my head pulled back. Inside my head, I was in extreme danger. My brain was hitting off the inside of my skull. I was suddenly in an unbidden, strangely familiar force field. It happened again this morning, and it came as a convincing threat that I feel more than hear, that I will be hurt and die. I knew right then the power of this force in Merrit and in Sabelle. It just sounds like a factual statement, a real threat in a male voice, a threat over which, in a different state, a less competent state, I would have no control. These episodes puncture my reality, but they do not overtake it. They will not make me crazy. My startle response is back.

Last night I dreamt that *I was returning home heavily burdened with packages, and the door to my house was blocked by three red tricycles of different sizes tangled together. I had to pull them apart and set them down to be able to get in the door. They were there as a barricade. When I got in the house, it had been overtaken by Sabelle. It was strewn with stuff, drawings, paints, clothes thrown on the floor, and food everywhere. I asked her what she was doing there, and it was as if she lived there and was entitled to create chaos. She had a slightly evil glint in her eye. I had no impact on her. If anything, she enjoyed my distress. There were some other younger kids there. She was impervious and imperious. I got so frustrated with her that I spanked her. But my arm was suddenly weak, and even though I tried to spank her hard so that she would feel it, I couldn't, only fueling her contempt. It seemed, though, that to some degree it still mattered that I had, as it were, taken matters into my own hands.*

There is terrific pressure in my body and head. But this is all. This is the steep ascent. "Don't ask about a person's depths, ask about their path of ascent" I wrote this to myself in my journal in my disheveled script, a paraphrase from Fugitive Pieces.

Finally, I paid attention. On Monday night, I felt the shift into a trance and each time, subsequently, I've seen blocks of sandstone. I couldn't make much out of it, but it didn't go away until I realized that it was a color I associated with Egypt. Egypt didn't make any sense. Moses was dark-skinned... then, "oh Christ, Moses came from Egypt!" I saw my Bible story books. It was proof, like a photograph might be.

My light body suddenly became heavy. My head was slowly pulled back. He had my hair. He grabbed my throat. I could vaguely feel the pressure. It all happened. I couldn't leave it. Arles asked how he could help me. I asked him to lift my head. Once he did, holding it from behind, the heaviness drained away. He worked with me about using my eyes, they were glazed over.

"You mean look around when I get out?"

"Yes," he said, "look around, see the street, the cars, the trees and feel the air."

At some deep place, I lie stunned but not completely. I have known everything, I am just learning. I was unafraid and in the present. I tested it. No conjuring was successful at bringing on fear. I felt free. Another subtle radical shift.

It is Sabelle's 19th birthday, and she looks radiant. She is on her path of ascent. She is learning, emotionally and academically, at an extraordinary rate. She has a long road before her. At times, we will pick our way along in the darkness, but this all has an end, and we both see that.

Lee was working on my tailbone. I was thinking about the easiest route to Tanglewood. Suddenly, I am grabbed by the face, fingers into my eyes, my brain seized. I was lying face down. I didn't move. She asked how I was, and I couldn't answer, but I had to; I didn't want to scare her. "It's difficult to say," was the best I could do after a long stretch of struggling to say anything. Later, she told me that she'd felt two small calcium deposits chip off my tailbone. She'd asked how I was because she felt a sudden, strong sense of disorientation herself.

There is no other place to be. I look to the sides of the experience. I search out exits but as idly as if I were in a movie theater. I wonder if part of this acceptance is also memory. A memory of the shutdown, like just before you know you will die, all becomes calm.

I am in the whole long, terrible and awesome process of learning not to suffer my suffering. Perhaps that is what I mean by stability, what "inhabiting the witness state" means. I have struggled anew with the fact that intense emotion singularly validates intense experience. I only feel that now "within the memory." It is encapsulated, felt deeply within that capsule, but not felt at all outside of it. This is the realm of not suffering.

I watched Sue cut Siegfried's hair. It comes to me as a revelation that this can be done at home, that I could cut John's hair. This was my mother's house. I would give it to them. We had lunch at the corner table overlooking the salt marsh. We puzzle over the tide chart in the Cape Cod Times.

I am not sad to see summer pass. It has been a thug. The long June days were consumed by bronchitis, and the weakness in my lungs and legs persists. And the turmoil of memory: state shifts that deliver me to the attic room and the aftershocks which really aren't shocks at all, but a continuous daze interrupted by sudden trances or sudden clearings. I do feel split down the center, maybe as if the two sides of my brain are not sharing the same geography, even if they share the same time. When I lose time, or have in the past (I think the dissociative epoch is over), all of me is caught in the tidal drag backward. This is different. I remain in the present, in the "now" but not in the "here."

It is too strong to say that I am at the mercy of some other forces, but I control nothing. Everyone else in the supermarket is inhabiting the same world; my presence is in another. I observe, to try to learn the rules. How much I feel this and how alarmed I am by it are significant measures of my state. Coming back from the Cape that morning, walking into town to see Arles, I was safe. No one was better than me, no one had a stronger grip on reality; they were moving through life asleep, many were frankly dejected, or angry or frightened. They weren't better, so I wasn't afraid and ashamed, but they weren't entirely the same as me either.

The next morning, walking to town, I was vigilant. I didn't need to take my keys, but I considered it; my breath flowed differently. I can't really see others for who they are, like I could the day before. Some diffuse threat thickens the air. It is harder to be alive. He sat down next to me, and I huddled against him, pulling out of a trance in which my head bobbed like someone falling asleep, my eyes sunk into my head, fluttering wildly like Clarice's did, the blind girl, in fifth grade...

I have to continue with my article, but resist leaving the quiet of this pen and paper reflection covered by my sky-blue comforter, accompanied when I can hear it by birdsong, to go to the straight back chair and keyboard and the distant report on neurofeedback, the instrument that has made all this possible.

On my way to Lee, I made a left onto South Street and crashed my car into the curb. Arles and I talked about my responsibility now, and I think it is to be aware that this is a dangerous time. I have to be very careful.

"Do you believe this happened to you?" Then, again, I am stuck... "What did you hear me asking you, Sebern?" I repeated what he said, "No, that's not what I asked. I asked if you knew this happened to you."

I realized in the waiting room of Pep Boys' that I wasn't upset about missing my appointment with Lee, and I heard the male voice, "this is just a warning bitch," then a flash of threat like a jolt through my body. My car cost $1000 to fix.

"It is hard to live afraid of what you could do, living out an instruction from over 50 years ago."

"And you must not."

Sabelle is ascending. After a few minutes of Alpha-Theta, Tom arrived. She turned to it. The waves that are Theta are still crashing when she opens her eyes into a torrent of grief and stunned incomprehension at being offered up by her mother as rent payment, of the madness she endured, at the abandonment of her father. She wept without constraint, and as quickly and completely as it arose, it was over.

"This stuff is amazing. I feel stable. I can breathe." She looked at me and asked if I was alright. "You look sad."

"Oh yes," I said, "This makes me very sad."

"I guess if you weren't sad, I'd be worried."

"Exactly, Sabelle." She felt released from something. I had to guide her there; she wanted to distract, but once there, she felt it all, no dissociation, no trance, fully validated and somehow able to bear it.

I mentioned getting food at Whole Foods.

"What are you eating?" he asked.

"This morning I ate granola with a banana, but the milk was almost sour. I ate it anyway."

"What if it made you sick?"

"I'd throw up."

"What would you throw up?"

I pictured it. "Brownish milk, I guess. Why are we talking about this?"

"Whose milk?"

The answer in my head jolted me. I went into the near edge of a trance, not completed because he kept asking...

"Whose milk, Sebern?"

I shook my head, no, no; no, no

"You can tell me of this milk, Sebern."

I looked away. I closed my eyes and started to cough. I covered my mouth.

"It's Ok. It's important to tell me what's caught in your throat."

"Cum milk," I whispered.

"Who's cum milk?" By then, he had my hair in one hand and a knife with a blade against my throat.

"What kind of knife?"

"A big knife." I almost felt it on my skin. "He will cut my throat now", I reported softly, leaving him behind. There was a silence taking over the office.

"Open your eyes." His voice was gentle, but he was giving me a direction, "It's ok, open your eyes. Look at me." I was pulling myself up. "Look around."

"Ok," she said vacantly.

"What color are the walls?" He waited for my answer, "Do you see? ... No one will cut your throat." I felt his weight on the couch. My eyes closed. I felt the wall of his chest. "The knife was in the elevator, Arles. It wasn't Moses, it was the junkie in the elevator. He trapped me there. He was sweating..." I trailed off.

"What happened in the elevator?"

"He wanted money. I'd cashed my paycheck and put a fifty in the deep pocket of my wallet. He was shaking and sweating. As soon as I got it that this was a robbery and not a rape, I just stopped being scared. My wallet opened to a picture of Johnny holding Blake as a baby. He looked at the photo, then at my face. He threw the emergency switch and ran down the stairs."

"It was he who held the knife to your throat?" I nodded.

"It kept happening, things like this. That time, I was so mad that after I called the police, I banged on every apartment door to find out who had buzzed him in. I only stopped when the cop came, towing a Black kid he wanted me to identify. It wasn't him."

"Was there another incident with a knife?"

"I don't think so. The other one was a cigarette. The security guard wanted to touch my pregnant belly. When I said no, he menaced me with his cigarette. He acted like he would burn my stomach if he couldn't touch it." Arles took in a breath, put his hand on my head and sighed.

Yesterday, I put my confusion into words:

"I put you in two places at once. You are 'during the abuse,' and you are 'after the abuse.' All time began with you. I discovered the absolute and infinite horror of no mother, and slowly I took you in so that you could mother me. I felt elemental, as if at the beginning of my own creation. As I began to recover memory, it is not in the context of biological, sequential history, but in the context of being born and alive in my relationship with you." The way these memories come, in these trance-like episodes, compounds the perceptual warp, and then he is present at the edge of the attic. I don't see him there in any of the scenes, but he is co-present in the hypnotic epoch that now includes our whole relationship. He is standing by and letting this happen. There is no innocent bystander.

I want to be delivered to him at the rehab center at the edge of the peaceful ocean. I am four or five when I am brought there. I don't know where I am. I am just the weight transferred from the driver to him. I feel heaped into his arms. He carries me, and I think he has on a white shirt, sleeves rolled up. He is rested, and somehow, I know he wants to take this case on. He is willing and patient. They feed me Pablum and vanilla pudding. I can imagine more steps, a room, a bath. White tiles. I can see the blue sea and the blue sky, somehow on the coast of England, which has nothing blue in reality. It is England, but more like Greece.

I am writing about neurofeedback for presentations I am either making or proposing to make. At times, I pause in my certainty about this process and what it predicts. I am out on a strong limb, the kind kids build tree houses on, to look out at the world from a different angle. Limbs can be sawn off.

It all began to change as I drove to see Lee. The skies got darker, and gusting winds brought on blizzards of leaves.

It is the quality of her presence. I drifted into deepening states. I felt the indentation of large fingers, rounded tips gripping my shoulder, my face pushed down into a mattress or pillow. I panicked that I couldn't breathe and felt a sudden burning sensation at the back of my mouth and down almost to my stomach. I heard an attack on Lee, "Tell the bitch to get her hands off," and I say, "She is not a bitch... She is not! She is not!"

The rain had stopped by the time I started home, but several times I felt like I would drive off the road or that I was driving nearly blind. I stayed steady. Near home, I felt a hypnotic shift begin to pull at me. I got a sudden vice-grip headache. The kitchen light stabbed my eyes. I opened my mail, and the bank says that there were no checks in my deposit envelope.

When I told him, he said, "No, Sebern, it does not scare me."

It would have been absurd to imagine that I would ever talk, even privately, about some force that exists outside the individual traumatized mind. Evil. I don't think it is a force outside of the mind, but it is a force outside of an individual's mind. It is a force of the collective unconscious, a collection of all of the horror and degradation possible. Fear is the conduit, fear and belief in its ability to destroy you. It will not destroy me—that is absolutely clear; I don't quite understand why it has such force in me or what its nature is—, why the headaches? It is as if I am in some kind of fit that I can watch but can't control. It has hold of me; it will not kill me.

Last night, each time I tried to talk, my headache would become so bad I was almost breathless. My body got very heavy. The headache was all on the right side of my head. The left side seemed oddly unaffected.

"He called mommy dirty names."

"What names?"

"White bitch," my chest collapsed, and I wept.

I just watch the waves as they roll in and out below my window. I stay in bed and look at the sea, and I don't talk. I want to feel the weight of someone sitting down at the end of the bed, making no demands, like Arles last night, as I doubled up, as twisted as a girl with polio needing help to breathe. There's nothing else to do. I left last night sobbing as he helped me on with my coat. I smiled and said, "Contrary to appearances, I am alright." The headache was past. I was reoriented in time.

It does not matter the hours I lie through the night, unaware, it is not rest. I take refuge in this rehab by the sea. Everyone is quiet, picking me up gently to change my sheets or dress me in a soft flannel gown. No one asks anything of me. I absorb their belief that I will recover through all of my senses. There are no words. They do not ask me to smile or even to look at them. They find food that is easy for me to swallow, pillows that are soft and white, and comforters. They sense when I need a bottle or hot chocolate or tea, or a soft egg on toast. Even when I can't eat it, they bring it on a tray with a flower or a postcard, and when it's been too long without food, they feed me, and I eat, dazed and robotic, beginning to note not only the all-important texture but the taste and even the color. Their insistence is gentle, for without it I would not move. My capacity for movement, even for thought and speech, is gone.

I described myself as a dumb animal, that this is a dumb animal recovery. Dazed, senseless as a dog, that from then to the end of its life knows only to trust until the motion is too quick or too near its head and then it flinches or cringes or bites. This state, the one in which I do not hate, feels like a betrayal of myself.

"Why animal?"

I saw my dog, Elsa, who bore her suffering moment to moment without complaint. I saw it as noble and dumb, as pure Zen, as no capacity for an attitude or a protest. Less suffering, really much less. But as soon as I glimpsed a four-year-old, I started to cry, not about what happened to her but from her, the round hot tears of a baby.

The states shift, each one different, seeming to offer no access to the other. As I talked with Arles tonight, it became clearer still. I functioned pretty well, I did meaningful work, and I raised my children. When I came here to begin this therapy, this fragmenting psyche was there, beneath the one that took me from day to day. It needed to be excavated, but there it was, the neurological and psychological dispositions. He agreed, quietly, I think, understanding the enormity of this discovery for me; still going very slowly, not pushing me. The story was the container. It had protected me from seeing what the story was about.

Arles' arrivals surprise, frighten and relieve me. He is almost always present enough, but sometimes, in some revolution in his brain, he is fully present. Nothing separates his awareness of me from me. And I come, again, back to life.

"I'm good. I leave Thursday for Tulsa and then the Clinical Interchange Conference."

"No, you aren't 'good'. I don't even have to look at you. I can feel it in your body."

I recognized my return to the default position of cool aloofness, the need again for impact, frantic and enraged. "No, you aren't good" was, for the first time, impact enough.

Slowly, my jaws have clenched tighter, the front of my face hurts, and my brain is sore. I have headaches. I trained twice. This should not be from the training. Body memory? I have been reading about tardive dyskinesia, and this, it suddenly occurs to me, is what it felt like. My legs are numb, too weak at moments to hold me up. The undersides of my toes are numb and prickly. I am not well. My memory is poor. My notes are disorganized. I put things in the wrong places, and I run into doors. I am not sleeping. I feel explosive cellular pressure, but I am not explosive. My brain moves like a wet sandbag. I still cast about like the orphan calf in the snow: brave, stupid and lost.

Arles was gone again, into his frightened, unctuous mode, stepping away, saying he wasn't. I crouched down before him, steadying myself with my hands on his knees, and locked him in my eyes. "Don't leave me." And he started to, and I said it again, striking him on the knee, "Don't leave me!" Before I went over to him, I screamed, "Train your own fucking brain, Arles!" Crouching in front of him, I said, "This is not therapy. This is not a breakthrough, there is no presence that is not mutually felt, you are a limiting factor for me. I am not for you, but you are for me." He would almost smile, almost come out from behind the veil, almost tip his hand to himself, but then he would, like a lazy eye, retreat from the gaze. I hit him. "Don't go away," he said something about my eye contact and about my eyes, "bright, wet, dark, no longer hooded" and I agreed, "But not yours. Your eyes are behind your eyes." I was back on the couch. It was too hard watching him slip away out of reach and deifying his inaccessibility. It is frightening how he gets like this, softly robotic, unhinged, more stupor than stubbornness, but in this state, he would abandon our relationship. He called this, finally, "being inner". It is part of the revolution of his brain, like the Wheel of Fortune, like a revolver. But it is a focus on himself that is disturbed by the other, and he fends off the intrusion of the other psyche, and this is his mother. I did make eye contact, and he could not come to meet it. I took "inner", thanked him for acknowledging it and as I hugged him, hit him hard on the back.

"There was nothing between you and me except you. The call for that kind of presence comes only from absence." It is a miracle, really, that light is not swallowed up by the black hole; that light illuminates it. My presence remains; his absence fades. He knew all of this today. He was with me.

I have suddenly and mysteriously lost the fear of death. I inhabit an endless universe of light. This is not a sweet state. Everything feels limitless, except it isn't, and I know that. I don't feel rage, but I feel true, boundless anger. I am restless and impatient and immediately dismiss, not always out loud, anything false. I am also kind, empathic and generous. I am unbounded. It all feels dangerous. Unfamiliar and only sparsely inhabited. I can't see anyone. Only light. Kicked upstairs. Accidentally transcendent.

Monday night, I talked to Arles about the apartment on the third floor, the lumpy couch with the blanket folded over the arm, the amber lamp light and the two windows facing the cobblestone street. I see the gas-lit street light making a halo of the dark. I can see this place. I told him of a father, my father, an old religious man who was sure of what he was saying, "They cannot kill us." I am the grown daughter there to cook for him, and I say respectfully and factually, "But, father, they are killing us." My rabbinical father. We were hearing the boots. Maybe our last words before the door broke open, and they took us away to the playground to be shot. He is old, and my body becomes his, helpless, even gnarled. Arles does not find this hard to understand, almost as if he expected it.

I have no boundary. My neuronal fibers extend beyond me into outer space. I have no substance. I said to John that I have no idea what this life offers me, it's so oddly ambiguous, and it frightened him momentarily. I have no casing. I am serene. This state is vast. And I feel rudely interrupted. I was just getting to grieve, just beginning to feel the whole experience of being alive in the particular way that I have been, and suddenly I am here, no longer there curled into Arles long body crying; no longer trembling at the unexpected footfall. But I am a disappointing representative for the state. I can feel less quiet. I need protection, but I don't understand why. It is very new. Unfamiliar. In the trance on Monday, I said, "There is no safety. Once you see that, fear drops away, and then you live in a different universe, with different rules of order. Or perhaps it is that when fear drops away, you can bear to see this."

Monday night, I kept the bathroom dark and lay in the bath with a bottle of chocolate milk. My belly felt full of air and light, dynamic and buoyant. Not a body I've known either. After the session on Monday, a session Arles said was "about the father," when my body was old and sunken and male, I started to cry deeply, nonspecifically. I was more the tears than the one crying them. I had walked there in the minced gait of the very old, and I was keening. Maybe I thought when I hit the blessed cold air, my head would clear. I would regain the contours of this time. But not entirely. Everything was familiar but not mine. Not my town or even my experiences.

When I got to the front register of CVS, there was a blind man buying dish detergent and skin cream, with pennies and quarters pulled from his pockets and splayed across the counter. The chubby girl with green hair and glasses counted it all out. He said loudly that tomorrow he needed to buy Tylenol and Ben-Gay, and he started to gasp with seizures of pain. She handed him his bag of purchases, and as I was buying my milk, he sat on the floor, his back against the candy aisle, moaning and mumbling, rubbing his foot. I bought him Ben-Gay and Tylenol. I didn't speak to him when I handed him the small bag. I felt the fear of his wild, crazy, endless need that would find me on the street corner.

He was dogmatic. He said, making the face he does that gives him away, "If this were a pure state, you would have no fear of abandonment."

"Christ feared abandonment."

He stopped and then said, "That was a transitional state."

"This is too." He said, "Uh-huh," slowing a little but not enough to catch himself. He challenged me, saying that I would feel equanimous, not seeing what he would usually see, and that that would be impossible.

"I am making this comparison with trepidation, but what other example is there? Christ is often described as angry and impatient. Unless you decide that his entire life was a transitional state, feelings like these might somehow go along with no fear of death."

"Why would abandonment matter if you're really not afraid of dying?"

"Because I love you." His silence was embarrassed. "Because I love you." And I looked away.

Monday night, I stepped into the crosswalk. A van was bearing down, not stopping. They didn't see me until the last moment. My thought was that it would have felt better than this. It shocked me, but the need for impact had arisen again; the need to feel the physical reality of my body. I sense the satisfaction in it, the need for it, even now in imagining the crash. It is not about death or crushed vertebrae. I felt like I needed to be rolled up in a rug and sat on by someone heavy. My body is wild; neurons don't stop at my skin. My nervous system is on the outside of my body. I am vibration, and that which is not vibrating the same is not me. I wonder today if somehow I arrived in Non Self. I no longer feel reluctant. I am much less angry. Bronxville is a different epoch, and it is closed. I can't be still, but sitting quiets me. I have pressure in my brain and eyes, and my head moves on its own. It aches. I feel extremely alive, but I am not contained. I pound myself on the chest the way apes do to manage my distress. I am hyper-aware, sensitive, patient, and impatient. Baby Luke, my tiny grandson, is quiet in my arms that vibrate.

Beca came here directly to my office three months ago after being checked out of Austin Riggs. She was deemed "untreatable" and they'd finally settled on Bipolar Disorder for her diagnosis. While there, she'd skipped most of her intensive therapy sessions, and no one came looking for her. They finally learned she wasn't there when her car landed in the median divider on the Mass Pike. I have seen her four times a week, and we have trained her orphaned brain twice every week. Her progress has stunned me. She was drinking herself nightly into blackouts and slept with whoever she found herself with. I believed her when she told me that, even so, she was not an alcoholic. She stopped drinking within two weeks. She has enrolled in a community college. She has weaned herself off five medications. She has a steady boyfriend. And now, I think she is describing her own version of this tumult. She is taking five baths a day, and she describes herself as both "uncomfortable" and "OK" at the same time. Her dog, for the first time in their five-year relationship, is sleeping next to her. I have been training her low on the right temporal lobe, and she became dramatically, palpably quieter. I wonder about this. Is it attunement? Well, of course, it is exactly that, the oscillations of our nervous systems.

I follow the breath. I was where I was, in no hurry to be elsewhere. It is easier to be in my body. This morning, I could fall into the weight of my body, into the density and comfort of my bed, into a deep state of rest. No anxiety. A sense of abandon.

Sabelle told me that her last training landed her in her body.

The present moment, before a flicker unknowable in its briefness, is now vast, inclusive of all time before and all time to come.

I took the dead calla lilies out of the vase and held them.

"What part of you is dying, Sebern? What are you mourning?" I shook my head. Then stopped.

"It is I. My Self."

He nodded, "This could be true."

Sitting in the waiting room, I thought, 'this is coming to an end'. Every premise that I knew or only barely knew that brought me to therapy has changed. He agreed.

"I used to think that if my house were to burn down, I would care about saving only the lives within it and my journals. Now I don't care about the journals. None of this is important." As soon as I said it, I thought of Anne Frank and knew I was wrong.

"Yes, that is wrong. Your journals are very important. I can think of no document like it."

I have asked Arles to be my monastery, to provide for me. These states are what monasteries are built to house. It is demanding to participate in the dailiness of life during tectonic shifts. I need someone to make my meals, but a cookbook from Eva suffices. John makes dinner. I feel taken care of. It's just that it has been difficult to attend, to get the bills paid, the food put away, and the trainings planned.

Jamie tells me that EEG Spectrum is now $800,000 in debt. I don't know why, but I am not alarmed. It cannot be destroyed. That is simple. I don't know how to save it, but I know it will be saved. My calm clearly calms her. Last week, when we talked, Sue told me that they'd gotten a bomb threat. She didn't talk about their debt.

"A bomb threat! What the hell! Did you get out?"

"No."

"You didn't, you, why not?" I asked, still alarmed.

"We get them periodically. They're reading EEG as egg. They think we have something to do with abortion."

"Oh, good god, Sue, that is sheer madness. You should still get out and call the police..." She thought I was being alarmist. Whose judgment is wrong here?

I've come back into town to get some work done, to spend the afternoon with Eva and to get free of TV. Johnny still has an institutional air, a day-room kind of aura. Eva and I ate at Haymarket as we talked of many things, most importantly this time, her mother. When we were getting into the car, she asked me if Arles had talked about what I meant to him.

"It must be a one-of-a-kind therapy experience for him."

"I guess. Well, probably." I pulled the door shut and strapped myself into my seatbelt. "Yeah, I guess that must be true."

"I have just been living my life since I saw you last."

"When did you see me last?"

"Last time."

"I greeted you in Thornes. You looked right through me. I know that look-vacant disconnection."

At first, I was just baffled. I had no idea. Sorry, I've done it. Wishing I had seen him. "I don't remember."

"I see that. Is this 'just living your life'?"

"Were you hurt by it?"

"No, but affected," he said. "It was the memory of hundreds of those looks."

"Are you feeling that I have left you?" I started to feel scared as I asked him this, afraid he would wipe out the truth of all that had happened and afraid of the haunt of this uninhabited presence in me, exhausted by it. Many times, I came back to myself after staring out the window. I found myself in the hollowness that is sadness before it becomes sad.

This is what I was trying to tell him. Johnny is deeply injured, and we will always need to care for him. I accepted he might never recover, and I am determined that he will. It was OK. He was OK. This is "just living my life" and the moments when I saw my life as it is, filled with abundance. These are not moments of the antisocial. As we talked about what happened in Thornes, I kept waiting for some structural collapse, but that did not happen. Arles agreed that it could all coexist.

"I feel like a bird taking wing, and you have just caught my foot, and I'm still flapping, believing in my flight. I just don't know the nature of it. How does that baby fly, except away? I don't even know the nature of the bird's foot. Is it webbed or clawed? Am I harbored or trapped?"

I trudged to Arles, hard up against my distress, dense, entangled and unnameable. I fought for descriptions of any kind of any aspect of this. The image arose of the face of Moses, burned beyond recognition in his encounter with God.

"The ecstasy of trauma," he said.

"I can't comprehend what you're saying." I felt obliterated by light, like Nagasaki, only a shadow left; yet dense, and tangled, sickly, confused. I saw only two images: Moses, his face like the English Patient and a child curled in a corner.

"Ecstasy does not mean liking or pleasure. It is nothing like that. It means the tearing of oneself out of oneself."

I cannot take in what Arles said. I cannot take in what happened. Eruption is not too strong a word. I was on the verge of throwing up, coughing, crying, choking, driven by fear, but I was not afraid. Arles weathered it with me. It wasn't post-traumatic; it was nothing familiar.

"Whatever 'me' is left, Arles, it's just fronts moving through. I was not torn apart; I was moved through."

"I don't know how this all goes together, but today feels like the first time I am working on a non-traumatized body. Amazing." I looked up at Lee, tears rolling into my ears and onto her hands.

It feels as if a tide has receded, leaving me enriched for its having been, but no longer awash. There are treasures on the beach. I am not afraid. I am quiet. I am clearer. I am sadder too. When I am sitting, stillness settles in. It has its own weight. Sometimes it flutters through me before resting in the deep bowl of my pelvis.

I am crying a lot, and every time it seems like a new language.

A thud overhead set me bolt upright, eyes wide open, going cold.

"I'm sorry, Arles. I'm sorry."

He wanted to reassure me. "It is only children playing," he said, and I cried out and twisted away.

"No, no, no children playing!"

There is no refuge in time, even when I have not lost it.

❧

I asked Arles about the impact of my suffering on him and of this whole endeavor called psychotherapy. He has never exempted me from concern over this question or over him. He has stayed silent.

"It has had an impact, very much. The question of the right granted in this institution for one to inflict their suffering on another is a profound one. The answer is not simple. It has to find context within the people we are."

"How else would I have ever known you?"

"We will talk more. Next year."

Chapter 9

I dreamt last night that I went to the place where my Christmas tree was, and it was gone. I told someone it had been stolen, and I couldn't understand why someone would do that. Then I realized I was looking at the zendo window, not the window where the tree was, and that was why there was no tree. It had not been stolen at all. There is no reason for despair.

Last night at the candlelight service, I recognized how appealing the idea is of surrender to the other, of worship, of hallelujah, of falling down in awe. I don't think that the Buddhist journey is ultimately low in awe, but there is no other to be in awe of.

I am torn out of myself: "Me" to "No Me." Thầy said that once you've gotten this, you will never lose it. Brother Placid read about not seeking, just being, letting the mind settle, the mind as clear, cold water, as fluid as melting ice. As fluid as melting ice, that is how this is. When I am afraid—so much of the liturgy is about fear—ego limps back, self-conscious and dramatic, and I get discouraged and question what has happened, not the validity, actually, but the thoroughness. And then I hear the teachings, "It will come. Stay on the path." As fear ebbs, so does ego. Perhaps ego is fear, just fear.

This morning, I walked up the hill alone under the Big Dipper, pouring stars into my mouth, each one with the sharp, soft, cold, then warm taste of a snowflake. The chapel is lit only by candles. Services are honest, unperformed. Do they hear each time what they're saying? Do they resonate with their own prayer? Do they yearn for the Other as their prayers do, as I have done; do?

The baby Jesus has been stolen from the creche here. I thought even at my worst, I would not have done this. But that might not actually be true. I was a thief. When I didn't grasp the natural consequences to this, Arles, like any good parent of a three-year-old who runs into traffic, imposed them. My relationship with him has rewritten my moral code. The brain that training has brought me has been organized in his presence.

A lot of today I spent embraced in time, wondering at the predictability of it, stretched out into it, slowing it down, watching the sun rise during vigil and set before Compline. I am, for the most part, free of thought or the constraints of worry. I just am, neither happy nor unhappy, but so ready to laugh that it surprises me.

"Let us be new." That was my prayer in our New Year's Day meditation. Let us be new.

Philip and Lara brought Sammy over, and as they chatted with John, Sammy and I played marbles, my godson, this tiny orphan who has crawled into the lap of my psyche and sits there stunned. We know each other. He repeats my name like a mantra, "Seboin." Neurofeedback is making it possible. When he left, I found the photo of Luke slid under the corner of the rug.

I lay in bed, looking at the fire, then out on the moonscape. I am the most fortunate of beings. Tomorrow, I fly to LA.

I had a brain map today. Sue has become intrigued with them and somewhat with my brain, and wanted one for me. The technician abraded skin on my face and ears, and then used a blunt needle to abrade my scalp. He didn't tell me what he was doing or when it would end. He was warmly apologetic about it but equally rough in cleaning it all up. During hyperventilation, a process I think to induce seizure patterns that risk inducing seizures themselves, my legs became insubstantial, and there was a ribbon of weakness down the center of the back, like the seam of a stocking. It felt something like the beginning of a trance, hints of it. My eyes retract, and there is pressure in my ears, like wax that rings. I trained a group for Sue and Siegfried that afternoon, and my legs were airy columns that would not hold me up. Sitting down only helped because I knew I wouldn't drop to the floor; my legs felt exactly the same. My balance is thrown off when I move my head. My handwriting is terrible. Back in my room, I took Gabapentin, a medicine Siegfried had encouraged me to take until my brain could learn to stabilize itself. He said it would make it easier for it to find its way to regulation. My legs gained muscle as it took hold.

❧

"Since the very beginning of this therapy, I have challenged you; I have asked you to do extraordinary things. It seems to be no different now. Now, all of this is about neurofeedback and my wish that you could enter that stream with me. Not just your toes but your whole body, immersing yourself as deeply as I do. Believing what you have seen, this transformation, becoming skeptical not of me but of your own disavowal."

"How have you transformed?" I am speechless. He is right there, has been, and somehow, he asked this question as if innocent of all that has happened. He heard this in my silence.

"Is it as if I witnessed the crucifixion and then acted as if it hadn't happened at all?"

"Yes," I responded enthusiastically. I know I risk now being dismissed as a "true believer," as a fanatic, but I take that risk. "It is that profound." But this was a strange metaphor, really, for him to suggest and for me to accept. I called later and left the message, "No, it is the resurrection. Witnessing the crucifixion requires no faith, no assumption of miracle. Crucifixion is a common practice. What you are seeing and denying is my resurrection. I want to get this correction on the record before the weekend."

I picked up my messages, a brief one from Sabelle, "I am at the margin. Call me." She never calls me, but my response was fury. Her boyfriend had tormented her relentlessly. She blacked out and woke up with a deep cut on her leg. The cuts were stitched and bandaged. She was regaining her footing as we talked. She felt disappointed and discouraged, both new feelings for her. I didn't do it well at first. I was too mad at her. She could hear my unfortunate impatience, and she began to list off the positives in the situation. She was over it, calmer, and none of it was now throwing her. I got calmer, too.

"How are you going to go about the rest of your day?" She answered me with her plans and then asked, startling me,

"How are you going to be moving into yours?"

An hour or less after training, my brain seemed upright again.

"You are at the far end of a telescope."

"What do you think this is?"

"I am going along, going along, exploring one depth, one transformation after another and suddenly comes 'manic defense' or 'what transformation?' and all is screechingly recontextualized in some analytic catechism." He listened, and just as we could be hurtling to the brink of disaster, we are not. We are not because he has paused, and I am suddenly unafraid. "I don't have the words yet, but what might it be like to live without fear? Who said 'Cast out fear'? It could be the same as 'Cast out Satan'. Fear is anti-love. Theory and constructs are boundaries and 'non-love'. I want to be unbounded."

"Are you asking that we approach the unknowable, the unspeakable?"

"The 'unknowable' is held in your mind. And it is 'held' in mine. This kind of love is only described as the love of one God for the many. It is non-dyadic. What if this happens between two, like Rumi and Shams? They entered the realm of the unknowable together."

I got the appraisal of my mother's house. I was upset for her, angry that something that she treasured was not treasured, a degradation of her, a humiliation. "I want to protect her across all space and all time." I felt fierce about it. I bought Almond Roca, her favorite candy, while I was waiting for my scripts. It was like tucking her inside of me where no one could hurt her, where she can live out my life safely cherished. I looked up at him. "Is it like this with you and your mother?"

"Yes," he answered without hesitation or elaboration.

"I have tried to regulate my brain just so... so that I would become an attached person without having to attach to anyone, to you. In that way, neurofeedback has been, to use your word, an 'autistic' endeavor, but I can't get free of this. It's almost like my brain has got this, but my mind doesn't." He stirred out there. "I can't experience every feeling I have about you at the same moment, so I experienced them one after another: love, anger, invasion, distrust, trust, separation, wanting. It is a labile attachment." I should have caught on when I wanted to devour the chocolate cake batter. It was not really how much I ate, but how ravenous the hunger was. "I loved her so much, and I will never recover from what she did to me."

"That's true," he said, "you loved her so much, and you will never recover from what she could not do."

"But I will die trying."

"You are missing your mother, and," he said, his voice softening, "you are missing me."

"Very, very much."

As I walked to Arles' office, sadness came in like a front. Who can stand the indelible imprint of horror? That was the only point I wanted to make. "For me, this was two weeks long, not like it was for Merrit or Sabelle or Reggie, and yet it holds my cellular being in its teeth."

"You seem to know the time frame." Surprisingly, it seemed clear to me.

"What, two weeks? Maybe two weeks in the summer." My ears started to ache, and I shut my eyes.

"How hot was it, Sebern?"

That's why we are naked. I couldn't stay present. He confirmed the reality, and when he did, I clicked off. Had he asked, "Is it hot?" we would have stayed in the office. Now, he was on the stairs coming up. I rubbed my eyes.

"What are you seeing?"

"You are not going to hurt me because you are white. There are no rescuers, so you aren't doing that. You are turning and leaving... You're not scared. You are oblivious." He and I have been talking about this, the neurology of PTSD and the freeze response.

"It's not freezing, though," I said, innocent of where this was going. I stared at him. "It was too hot to freeze."

He nodded and sighed. "Yes, Sebern, it was too hot to freeze."

A thought meanders through the day like an Alabama stream, "Does this meditation practice seal over? Is this why so many die young of cancer? Do they sit and not cry?" I looked at Larry, my dharma teacher, sitting in meditation at the front of the zendo. "Who is he?" This is a new question for me to ask. We had our interview. I told him I was well, and he said that was clear. I told him the moment that I realized there was no protection, that I was safe and that in all that followed, I'd lost my fear of death.

"You haven't taken the final yet. But you have lost the fear of the idea of death, and that's no small deal. That allows you your life."

Beca. Her boyfriend came home to tell her that it was over. She was in and out of being overwrought all weekend, but she came in today much more present, much less afraid, more in her life. And it seems to both of us like a quantum shift in her brain. She is taking responsibility for what she did to precipitate this, not idealizing him but expressing real love for him without the usual hallmark of desperation. She is quite surprised. Me too. What is this neurofeedback?

Sabelle takes the eye mask and the earphones off and stretches as if waking up in the sunlight. "I feel so good!"

John ran an Alpha-Theta session for me on my birthday. It was the usual pattern. Two or three times, Theta kisses Alpha chastely. There is no crossover, just deep pockets of bare consciousness.

I feel her fingers along my spine. I am thinking about picking up a pumpkin pie at the farm store on the way home. Her hands move to my neck. A flash streaks through my brain, and my body is elsewhere, dropped, like a corpse. I may have known the moment of impact, and then I blacked out. My body is on the floor of the hospital. I am in a swirl of voices around me. The snap of the gurney, and I slip back into darkness. I held on to Lee with both hands, watching, listening, sobbing.

When I came upstairs, she'd made me tea. "The small muscles between the vertebrae moved for the first time," she said as she offered me a piece of pear cake.

Until Arles asked me where I landed, I'd been suspended in the air, arched in a dive, sitting in the corner on a green plastic chair. I never hit the floor. It seems so sudden when I tell him that I hit him with added force. All those years have weight. I am thrown back into the air, like when a rocket hits the house next door, and I land in my body differently. I can hardly stand straight. I put my T-shirt on backwards, then my sweats.

"Your neck is very different," Sam reports, "more open, more acute, a fresher injury." Inflammation dissipates and returns. All week, I keep it carefully wrapped. When I slipped down into the hot bath, my head fell to the side.

"I think I might have thrown up."

"Yes, it's very possible. Are you feeling that now?"

"I don't know if it is now." I worked to establish the frame of time. "I came to for several hours and then lapsed into the vapor trail of hallucination." I paused. This seemed not connected. "A transcendent sorrow."

"Hmm," he said. "What would that be, a transcendent sorrow?" I didn't know, and I answered slowly.

"It is true that the whole universe is bathed in light. It is also bathed in sorrow." He nodded. "I want to know that sorrow. I don't feel that. My history humiliates me. These stories stack up like crates of eels. I don't want them."

"This memory was a shock."

"It was a shock. It came through me like an electrical charge, like two sweeps of current. And it's the suddenness of neurofeedback."

"What do you mean?"

"How can I remember the feel of the gurney in my back when I am unconscious? I do, Arles."

I flashed on a scene from years ago when I saw Arles get in the passenger side of the new Volvo. I had felt a clutch of anguish. "For me," he said.

"For you." Not really for the unraveling of a relationship. I didn't know. This anguish leapt over that to all the suffering of his innocence. It was for a moment a kind of anguish I have felt only for my mother.

Transcendent sorrow. What could that mean? It could mean that transcendence carries with it all deep human meaning. It could mean that there is light inherent in sadness, light and movement in the inevitability of loss. It could mean that feeling the truth of one's being, embracing it wholly, is the reality of transcendence.

I have stopped fighting. If not welcoming all of this, I am moving toward it.

"I would never do anything to provoke you; that is not in me to do. But I have a lot I have to go through. I need to know in my body that you will not let me go too far, that you will come and make your presence felt."

"I will not leave you alone. I will not let you get away from me. I will be there. Let them all know."

I turned my head away. I cannot look at him. I was four months old. My head had to be far enough away for my eyes to focus, and then I got it.

"Arles, she killed me through my eyes," I can feel exactly where the damage is done behind the eyes. "My brain is injured".

Snow piles up quietly in the neighborhood. It's just past 6 AM. This weekend has been given over to training my stubborn, anorexic Eleanor for 16 hours, trying to hold her brain in a state to help it find a new groove. I sat with her each time she trained in Alpha-Theta, and it seemed likely that my brain flowed with hers, first chattering, then deep plunges, then bobbing up like a cork. One epoch, she went so deep it was hard to reach her, and during this, I felt simultaneously in a deep trance and fully awake.

Forgetting the name of someone so kind to you is like burying someone without a headstone. It comes and darts away. Why do I forget his name, the last name that is also a first?

"Men in white jackets came early in the morning and took people away to Rockland State. They were never told. I was sure I'd be taken away." I clasped my head. "Oh god, Oh god." My mind jumped some lateral gap to the right, and I was in the Holocaust. It could be that this is the only collective experience that speaks to that fear, but it's not that. It seems that I leap over time, and there I am with my old rabbi father hearing the boots in the hall. It was muscular, pulling myself from that ellipsis in time back into his office, back to the story. "I was pounding wildly on the seclusion room door, to get back in. The residents had come onto the floor for morning rounds. I was trying to get away. It was the only place I could go."

"What's happening right now, Sebern? Tell me".

"I can feel myself trying to huddle up against the wall, but it wasn't on Clark 8, it was under a corner of a building, underground, a stone wall, wet. I am huddled there. I have on a sweater and a dress, sturdy shoes and thin white cotton socks."

Sam and I are talking about my foot surgery and the choices of anesthesia. "No matter what they use, you will still be there; you just won't remember." I was there even if I don't remember. This is a profound idea to me, being there and the memory of being there are not the same.

I remember that I did not sleep, or maybe I slept during the day. I didn't play cards. I didn't have conversations. What did they do with me? I refused to get undressed. I didn't brush my hair, and I doubt I brushed my teeth.

I remember his name. Russell. Russell had played in the Negro League. He took me out from under the bed on my first night on Clark 8. He guided me when I emerged suddenly in the seclusion room.

I went snowshoeing with Sammy and his parents into the woods behind the house. I could see the weather system change across his face. He said, as best he could, that he was mad at Philip. But he looked bewildered, sad, overtaken. We were with him in this clearing, but he did not turn to us. He put his arms around a slender tree, rested his face against the smooth bark and kissed the tree.

What has happened to him? What will he form around? He touches me, Reggie touches me, Sabelle, Merrit, Beca, Johnny, they all touch me. A barrier has dissolved. There has always been a part of me that turned away, without awareness, because it was always true; I was stranded in bewilderment.

Sabelle came into my kitchen after her session and asked if I wrote grocery lists. "I love the details of human life," she said, "I love the human condition." As she was leaving, she turned toward me. "Maybe I started neurofeedback too young. Who will I marry?" As her brain deeply organizes, she finds no joy or interest in the playgrounds of her peers. It is not alienation. It is non-delusion.

"This isn't a delusion, Arles, this is time travel. Time travel is just a matter of turning your focus because all time is parallel time." I trailed off. I was inside my mind, I was in the seclusion room, the sun was out now, and Dr. Udel was standing at my bed. He asked me what was happening.

I was looking into the stream of dust motes dancing behind him. "I am disappearing into smoke." I thought I was hallucinating.

"It's not hallucination," he said, "it's delusion." He was matter-of-fact about this distinction. "What do you think? Do you want to go home?"

Inside that mind, it felt like fragments were suddenly and forcefully pulled together, like filings to a giant magnet and there I was back in the real world. The force of this integration was so great that it pushed out into mania.

❧

"Whatever decision you make, you will not lose me. Wherever you go, you will not lose me." I will tether to those words.

My body went numb, and I became space itself. It has become my practice to reenter my body. I tried to locate my fingers. I knew they were there, but I couldn't feel them. It was more like I was energy, up and diffuse or down and dense. In the airy place, I saw into my psychotic mind and the force of sudden cohesion out of chaos when Udel asked if I wanted to go home. I was unable to contain it. It broke through, it had to. I laughed and cried, and I understood Lucy in the Sky with Diamonds. There it was, this former mind, understood from within its own ball of lightning at the moment my sanity was rescued at the brink of forever being lost. Sinking back into my body was an act of enormous will.

When Arles said, "You will not lose me," I wept broken tears, sharp and hot from a deep root knowing of the worst horror of all. How does one get chosen for this, or is this just neurofeedback? It is, however it happens, the opening of the brain and the psyche to what is?

Eleanor left for Cambridge. She said she was "glad for us." She was trying her best to be genuine and "in a relationship." She'd responded to my request to keep me with her from her antisocial position, that lilting degradation. But she was different that night, warmer about her coldness, more mature, and when she left, I felt protective. She seemed so little to be going on such a trip. She described the seductiveness of sociopathy in almost the exact words I had used with Arles after I'd seen her last. Her goodness, she said, is like a shaker bench; her badness, like a gaudy pink sofa that doesn't particularly invite, but once sat on, folds her deeply in its comforts.

Sabelle traverses the equinox, the time of dark and dangerous ritual, almost without notice. Her knee hurt. She is mostly curious, not dragged back into it.

I was floating in brown/sepia tones just below her touch. I didn't think much was happening, and then suddenly I dropped into a deep gray pocket, feeling disorganized, crying, then sobbing, afraid I would pee. I felt as if I had died. I was at the thin transparency between breath and no breath. Shaking, jerking, everything coming apart, everything in my body.

"This is not about losing my mind."

"No," Lee said, "it's about losing your life."

The secrets of the body. Every memory is recorded in the muscle, in the fascia, in the pulse, in the wave.

"You were so uncared for," Lee said, her hands on my sacrum, and, as happens now, I felt a welling up of empathy for my mother.

"It comes in through the eyes. The absence hollowed me out, it burned away tissue right behind my eyes. Something's missing there. It is white where it should be gray, like cryosurgery. If I am not special to you, if you do not remember me, how do I exist?" The Serbs are burning the documents of their victims. These refugees have nothing, only each other to say that they are who they are. The narrative is gone. I have Arles to say, "she is who she is."

"I am afraid that you will disappear when I look up. Maybe not disappear but go vacant and pull away the reality of the last years from under me: that you would actively destroy my perception, that you would murder my mind. With my eyes closed, I can construct you more as you actually are, but when I look up..." I stopped. "I need to know that you know what I have suffered. It is your knowing that allows me to experience a self."

"I do," he whispered, "I do."

My 80-year-old Unitarian neighbors are boiling syrup that they have collected in buckets. The nascence of late March. I have missed its beauty, deferring always to April. But now I appreciate this day, this month, this particular rotation of nearly uncountable turns of the planet.

I have wondered if I lay still enough on the ground, attentive enough, connected enough, would I be able to feel the rotation of the earth in my back?

Johnny's sleep is corrected with Alpha Stim, and my insomnia does not yield.

Arles said, "It's a new sorrow each time, isn't it?"

We are gathered here on the Cape to remember my mother. It came to mind to say "and to be remembered by her," and I feel the cold hollow in my stomach. Our presence here obligates her memory of us—our birthdays were marked in the date book that I found on her desk.

We are at the mercy of the writer's pen. She will be most remembered by what I write, not by who she was. What I include and do not include has vital importance, even if this is never read.

"Do you think you wanted to be dead because she thought you were dead?"

"No, I don't see that exactly. That would require her seeing us."

"Us?"

"Yes, Kevy, Hugh, and me."

"Oh, that 'Us.'"

"She had no perception of us."

"It wasn't like she treated you as things?" He asked this with an air of belief that he'd got this right.

"Well, in that sense, maybe dead, or inanimate. To be seen as dead would imply having been seen as alive, and I don't have that experience. She looked after us and dressed us well, but it was also not as if we were her dolls. We were not her playthings, not her narcissistic objects." He quickly realized that that too conferred "presence" in her psyche. "She just didn't get us."

"How do you imagine she could encapsulate the way she did? She was generous. She supported the orphans' home, but you said you do not remember her ever saying anything kind about the man who started it. She protected him, and it gained her nothing. She did not do it for status. What do you think motivated her?"

I appreciated that he was interested in her, puzzled, intrigued, even empathic. I can't answer his questions. Maybe together we will find her. I told him of my conversation with her and my sense that she does not remember dying, that she is readily able to acknowledge the truth of things without defensiveness, much less the humiliated, withering assaults on my integrity. But she gives it all no meaning. She has gained as little from her death as she did from her life. But she is OK. She just can't help me much in understanding her. No better now than before.

John and Johnny are in South Carolina. He is finally moving home.

I cannot read what I wrote here, but when it begins to be legible, it says... "little girl slamming my head with my hand."

"No, no, you must not do that," and he took my hands. "This is not your fault." But it wasn't about that. It was intense, unmoored affect.

"Moses did this," I said, just to agree with him.

"What did Moses do?"

"...and now there is a threat, now against my mother and against me. He's threatening to kill her. Not just once..." I may have just gone blank.

He interrupted, "And now, he's threatening to kill me." I pushed away, but he held onto me. "That won't happen, Sebern. That won't happen."

I drew a picture mostly with my left hand, looking away from the paper. I asked Arles what he saw.

"Ground zero," he said of the drawing of shards. "Kristallnacht." I cannot get to its root, but it twists in me like a vestigial ingrown umbilicus.

Motherlessness. The soullessness of it; it is out of your reach. It is cellular, remembered and reproduced in every cell division, held in me as elemental. And today, out walking, suddenly and powerfully, I missed my father, for the first time in decades. He was the one who could be proud of me. He could tell me how far I'd come in the world, give me that context, the father's context. I had a glimpse of him.

"My father returned, and when he did, I missed him." I stopped to wonder. "Do you miss your father?"

His eyes clouded over. "Every day," he said.

"Every day?"

"Yes, almost every day."

I realized, like a sudden awakening, that Arles has never been my mother. He was my father from the start, and when he mothered me, he was the loving father of an orphaned baby.

"If I had made you into a mother, the therapy would have failed. There would have been only Mary's slender shoulders to stand on."

I met Charlie for lunch. We went to Lyme to escape the crowds in Hanover. I drove past many fraternity parties, these beautiful Dartmouth buildings filled with the depravity of adolescent men, their ugliness, their penile obsession. Rented tables on the lawn, lined with plastic glasses of beer, the boys in their shorts, music pumped; girls, all of them at some level, afraid. It is such a brutal scene—these are the ones who will rule, and they are the ones who will kill.

He called me "Seebs." It's a childhood nickname, and only one other person does. We caught up and thought back to the Institute.

"You were good," he said, "at being five steps ahead, but it didn't help you. You tried to maneuver me into a pre-existing well-rehearsed script. You were good at it; I think too good."

Driving back to my retreat house, I filled up with gratitude for him. "But Charlie, what else was there? Oedipal drama, is this what drove the madness howling out from the 'quiet room'? The suicide? Was it hysteria that paralyzed Maureen, two doors down? Incest fantasies? Masturbation? Those were the jokes that patients told about themselves. There wasn't anything else to know. That was your training. Maybe I gave you a script so you could stay you."

❧

We work with our bodies to maximize connection and minimize shame. My eating problems come when I feel cut off. I noticed this as I got a kinesthetic sense of myself as spare: it is fighting weight; fleeing weight. It attracts others. It equates with "strong;" I am not humiliated to be naked. Sexuality moves through that body, not the layered one. It is about youth. It is about not needing anyone. I am the one desired. It is exercising control over need. It empowers through envy. Purging allows the rare event, the reversal of consequences. It allows you to be filled up, to have your cake and not eat it. Controlling weight moderates fear. It removes the most potent weapon of shaming, my own body. My size and shape, my very physical being, cannot become the source of my own destruction.

I can't find Arles, and I can't find needing to find him. I imagine today that when I recognized he was the father and had been all along, I quietly turned away from his hard chest as surely as he had turned away from my infant body. There is nothing more to be done. He becomes a witness to events I do not want seen. I don't wish for him to be here. He is fading away in his analytic stillness like a pen drawing in the sun.

He saw the swagger when I came in. He was angry.

"You hate me in this state."

"No, I hate this state in you. You have gotten better at it. It hasn't changed, it has just gotten quieter." This is not true.

"What do you want me to do?"

"I want you to think about it."

"Think about it!" I fought back. "It is as if I have a seizure and you want me to 'think about it'. I recognize it only afterwards, and I am helpless to it." If he is helpless too, if he doesn't recognize it, then we spiral into brinkmanship: who leaves first.

It is incomprehensible that I am here in the midst of my adult children, in the midst of this very life, after the session with Lee. My body felt the beating. I saw a Black hand grip the arm of the man choking me. Lee asked me what I was looking at. I did not die. I felt lifeless, left lying on the floor. The attic floor? The hospital floor? I could hardly move. I was also aware that I was with Lee, that I was entirely safe. I can't drive. I am walking, legs far apart, unsteady. I joined Lee on her deck and saw the books she was reading: a Guide to New England Butterflies and Walking the Tiger: Healing Trauma.

A whole different memory arose when she touched my chest. My feet kicked up, and I wanted, suddenly, to bite her arm. It felt like I'd been given scopolamine. I remembered the young Black man who waited for the Doridan to begin to overtake me, and I could feel the gentleness of his arm leaning lightly on my belly as he unbuttoned my pajama shirt. I yearned for this gentleness. And the sucking on my breasts. He would look at them first. More nursing than sex. As I said this to Lee, I felt a light touch draw down between my legs and the penetration of his finger. I was wet. Sleep was coming on fast. I remember him covering me with the pj's shirt and buttoning it up hurriedly, but still gently, when we heard the sound of a key in the lock of the big outer door. He left my room to tell someone all was well. An innocent exploitation, a tender, driven hunger, all forbidden and oddly chaste. I didn't tell anyone until years later.

"Was he the person who was supposed to look after you at night?" Eva asked. But I was safe. I believed late into my adulthood that I would be safe if I could only sleep.

"Given, I guess, everything else you went through..." Lee said. But, at least at that moment, that wasn't it. I don't think about this as an assault. It is without a category. I doubt I even told Charlie. Maybe I felt responsible. Maybe it was part of why I banged my head against the cinderblock wall. Maybe I thought it was love.

My head feels different. I have a sense that training the left hemisphere instigates inflammatory pain, like it does rage and coldness, and with the Gabapentin, my brain is functioning more normally, so I don't need as much right-side training.

I feel this most with Reggie, who has been in a prolonged abandonment meltdown. Yesterday, she felt all that could not be felt, all that cannot be neurologically, much less psychologically or emotionally, be contained in one body. She feels as if her whole being is going to rip apart, and I cannot move; I feel cold. Arles helped me with this when he asked me how much murder, mayhem, and terror one can see. It could be self-protective, but I think it also could be training. I can't train on the left without risking the very withdrawal that Reggie is reacting to and the fury I feel when she demands more. I summoned a time when Arles said, "Just let it come and pass through you," and it helped me reach across the gulf I wished to put between her torture and mine. I took her hands and guided her. I held her head. She didn't have a convulsion, but it was close. She was trying to hold together the state of being torn apart.

I was as fat and as taunted as Piggy. I would do anything, including die of starvation, not to suffer that shame again. That was why I did not drink a milkshake or eggnog in the hospital when I could not chew and swallow. I was for the first time free of the possibility of ridicule. Eleanor is my height and looks frighteningly thin at 109 pounds. I weighed 79 pounds. John said I looked like someone in Auschwitz. I did not see it. I have no memory of it.

Eleanor is suddenly calmer with T6. She has been in turmoil over why she is so impossible when others with worse histories are doing better. This is her starved brain. I talked with her about "the grandmother effect."

"Some time, generations back, someone was hit by a lightning bolt, and it has been passed through each generation, has set up each generation in its own way, and it has now hit you."

"Yes," she said, "and that's why I have to be the one who stops it." She looked at me and smiled that sweet, genuine, slightly crooked smile, and I knew she knew something for herself, something that took on, at least at the moment, some moral importance. This is true for all of us. Somewhere, it became too much, the circumstances of oppression, cruelty, poverty, or illness, and someone struck out at a vulnerable child at a vulnerable moment, and this was repeated enough that it was taken into the brain as truth. From generation to generation, horror and neglect are handed down like heirlooms.

Johnny moved into the apartment downstairs this weekend. With the use of Gabapentin, he experiences none of the baseline terror, and he is sleeping in his own place on an air mattress. Big move comes Monday. I enjoy being with him and believe this will be an easy tenancy.

I spent time with Sammy and watched him turn toward his mother, a new skill. He ran up to Philip's car to tell him he missed him (!); he is going to school, and the teachers like him. He has been here for seven months. Lara and Philip have done this right, amazingly right. Phil said it was 80% neurofeedback, and I said 50/ 50. "It's neurofeedback that materializes the two of you. You are doing the rest."

Johnny goes off a little with Gabapentin. Training restores him, but it's a fragile ecosystem. I am not too buoyant with this. His madness is now right downstairs. All the mayhem of our child lives, and the question occurs again: what does it take to recover?

"What is the point of psychotherapy if there is no protest?" I think randomly. "I have no protest." And immediately, I know this isn't yet true.

Of course, it was not Gabapentin that was sending Johnny into the terrible loop. He was slipping through a crack in me. I do not see alcohol or depression. All the signs, big signs, are there. It feels more pervasive than denial. It is a lacuna.

He had called from the hospital to tell me he was putting himself into detox. When he got home, he wept in unrelenting psychic pain, and I held him.

I added one minute at FPO2 for myself. Thầy appeared before me in my meditation and moved through me from my head to my feet. After that, the transference to him was over. He was within. The practice was mine. It feels that way with Arles, too. Now he is a man who will help me recover from the atrocities and other injuries. He said I saw his internal state, his separateness as loss and not as potential. Potential! Of course. It went through me like a soft current.

Last night *I saw a black and white photo of mothers and daughters, a summary scene. All the mothers in the back row, babies in the front. Everyone is smiling. My mother was there near the middle, and there was a baby in front of her, but it wasn't me. The narrator read the caption, "Little Sebern kept crawling away, so she is not in the picture." The unseen narrator pointed out, "But your cradle is still there." I couldn't quite see it.*

The gravitational pull felt like a suction force on my forehead. I was hijacked. I try to understand this as it is happening, in a different part of my brain. Is it when I broke my neck? No. There is a searing pain in my clitoris and then a ghastly shock of seeing and then "No," shaking my head "No, no..." I didn't feel this, "No," I didn't see this, "No, this didn't happen, No." My shoulder hurt. It has to do with this time. "How did it end?" I asked this out loud. The scenes are just snatches out of time; they don't begin and don't end. They just are. Cornflakes. That's what came to my mouth, that taste, cornflakes with milk.

"I don't know," I said to him, "what is fair to ask of you. I see the lucidity in you—light beams distorted by the intemperate firing of your brain. I want that to be a clear channel. Your sweet, funny clarity. Open access for you to that. If I went to Make a Wish Foundation, I wouldn't ask to see the Rose Window in Chartres; I would ask for this lucidity. I would want to die knowing that this was how it was for you, this brain, this heart. I do not see you as my child, but I wish it with that kind of intensity. I know the purity in you. I want that open path."

I didn't exactly expect a response, but when there was none, I asked, "How do you feel about what I said, pressured or privileged?"

"From the lucid place, I feel only love. In the places that distort and deform the light waves, I feel pressured."

I wonder if this is the meaning of the transference cure, to see and embrace the reality of your therapist, and in that, to embrace your adult aloneness. Adult aloneness just is; it is not a catastrophe. Arles is incorporated, not internalized. Within me, he has no separate existence – not fused either, but infused, imbibed by thirsty cells and, finally, remembered by generation after generation. Outside of me, he seems a little lost, a little sad.

I was talking about a subclinical seizure, "It is hard to be assaulted by your own brain."

"Yes, that is true. And we all are. We usually think of that as the truth for overarousal, but it is equally the case for underarousal. That too assaults." "Oh," I thought to myself, "you are not underaroused, Arles."

John and I watched *Fruitvale Station*, and then we had to get out of the house, away from such violence. He said we shouldn't bring this into our home. And that's it. I am agitated because I think of the boys I treated in foster care, all of them like those in *Fruitvale Station*, all of them doomed, all of them fatherless. The youngest, who used a jump seat to steal cars at 12, is serving life in prison. When he was 8, his mother sent him from Cape Verde to a father he'd never met in Boston so that he would have a chance. He was in a motel room with a strange man, and the windows were sealed. He lay on the bed trying to figure out how to escape from the room, get through the snow and back to Cape Verde. Solo is even more dangerous, and Kimane is even more lost. I love these boys. As we walked, John said, "Your childhood was no less lethal." He surprised me, but I understand my agitated identification better after John's remark. We talked about my particular ghetto, swamped in drugs, the desperate belief in the material, pushing, hustling, abandoning the kids. Those boys had virtually no choice the moment they were born Black, male and poor. They were murdered many times over by third grade. I get stirred up by the footage of eager little boys in first grade, jumping up, hands high in the air, competing to answer the question who were, by third grade, slumped in their chairs, dispirited and angry. It fills me with a wild hopelessness. They die slowly, indifferently and violently.

I told Arles that I'd done the wrong training, and he commented that I seemed weird. After hesitating, I told him about a brief video I saw last night. It came from a 'baby cam' in an upscale nursery on the Upper East Side. This former nanny is on trial. The baby is standing at the rail of her crib looking at the nanny, and out of nowhere, she hits the baby on the head several times with her fist. The stunned baby just falls down. I asked him to help me grasp the intensity of my response.

"What bothered you the most?"

"First, I thought it was the baby's powerlessness, but this was not the worst. It is how out of the blue, how deranged, it was. It was madness unleashed. It is the insanity of it... There was no reason. She wasn't even crying..." Suddenly, everything shifted. Momentarily, I was the maid. I went cold, expecting the deranged voices calling me whore and bitch, but they didn't come. The cold passed, and everything just stopped. When he asked me, it was almost impossible to remember. I became quiet. The weird feeling was gone. Maybe training; maybe not.

Sabelle described herself as being formed into a pearl. There are no jagged pieces and no hard edges. She grieved the loss of her boyfriend and the impossibility of Merrit. She had seen teachers in them. What happens to the student when she surpasses her teacher? Where is she then?

"It is as if I am coming awake. I see the misery people inhabit. They can't see that I love them unconditionally; that love is there, staring them in the face. Merrit doesn't get it that I would go with her to the flea market every Sunday for the rest of our lives." Sabelle, the empty vessel, the personification of terror, of a life lived only in fragments, is talking about fearlessness and friendship, "I have only you. I am too young."

"I know," I did, "and what is the alternative, six years, 15, 50 years of delirium...?" She interrupted me...

"Of course, that's right. I am just lonely, very lonely."

"Your practice is equanimity. You see the suffering, your heart is open, and now it's how to bear it."

"To learn," she said, "how to help other people." I sit humbly in awe of her and now of what is in store for her.

My early morning conversation in the garden, on the porch, in my bed with Eva on the phone, became the conversation later after the bank, the herbal chai and Pablo Neruda, in Arles's office.

"Maybe you just can't go to that address," I said, quoting Eva.

"What address did she mean?"

"The Alpha-Theta address."

"When I saw you walking in today, you looked like you were walking in Alpha-Theta." I knew what he meant.

"I was walking softly in my grief." I looked at the reality of the bombed-out building, at the reality of no mother that I can't get through. I cannot transcend it. "I will not experience the oceanic mother that you and Eva somehow can feel in Alpha-Theta. But when I look at the bombed-out building, the same gray stone becomes a grotto. It is transformed. I had hoped to transcend the absence of her. I can't. It is the architecture of my brain, of my being."

"Can you embrace this?"

"I think that's the meaning of the grotto. I want to embrace her. I don't want her to be alone anymore, my motherless mother." I paused.

"Eva had asked me if I ever surrendered to you."

"What did you answer?"

"I said I had surrendered after a struggle."

I shared the image I had of him holding a piece of pottery in his hand and shattering it with a jeweler's hammer. "You have appreciated the crude beauty of what I made. You held the shell of me in reverence, and then you destroyed it. I am the cup bell struck for its resonance and for its destruction. There is no duality between destruction and creation, like the iridescent orchid, like the Phoenix. I was not nascent. I did not exist. I was not reborn. I was assembled from pottery shards... I don't know why it's so important that you know the grief. I want this reality of mine to ring, like a church bell beneath your ribs. I am not protesting. I am just seeing, and what I am seeing cannot be seen alone."

THE SUICIDE

Last Friday, Sabelle called to tell me that Dan had hung himself in his empty apartment three blocks away from me. The news was shocking, but I was not shocked. I felt an odd indifference, not cold but removed. Friends were waiting for me downstairs, and it seemed likely that I could go to dinner without saying anything. I was confused by this. Blake called at that moment, and when she asked, I burst out sobbing, no sector of me was unmoved by Dan's death and his hard, short life. I cried many times over the weekend, like water over a warm, immovable stone, saddened, darkened by the image of his hanging. I cannot see his face. I follow his hanging body up to his shoulders. I cannot look.

I did my best, out for dinner. They were alternately foreground and background to Dan. His father, who had never picked Dan up, picked up his body. There are significant and insignificant suicides. When he was hospitalized from the residence, he'd insisted that he would kill himself. It was not a taunt. When I asked him, he told me that after death, there was nothingness.

"What if you're wrong about this, Dan? The vast majority of human beings and every religious tradition would say you are."

He thought briefly and answered almost ruefully, "I'll just kill myself again." I knew then that he would. I couldn't take this away from him. When I saw him last, not long before he did this, I urged him to go back into therapy. "Therapy doesn't help me," he said.

"We were in therapy, Dan."

"You don't understand," he said, "you are different."

I have been struggling with a memorial for Dan in part, I think, as a protest against the anonymity of his death, when Dan's organizing goal in life was his anonymity. He sought the refuge of nothingness within the echoing terror of nothingness. I so hope he found it. I played Ave Maria, my own private Mass, for Dan, for Sabelle. I saw his body lifted by the angels. I capped Sabelle's hands in mine. She leaned her head forward so it was propped on mine. She cried. She read from her journal, "Something stills in me. Something that has been clanging or banging around has gone quiet. A good stillness."

I remembered a dream. *I was visiting a hospital, and I went up to someone on the campus to ask where their unit was for treating attachment disorder. They pointed me vaguely and maybe even irritably in a direction. I followed my instincts and went into a caramel brick stone building. At each floor, going up the back stairs, there was a newly painted metal door like a new prison. As I came to the floor, the door opened, and a staff member came out. I asked him where the unit was. I identified myself as an attachment researcher to alleviate his kindly suspicion and to stop him from turning me away. He took me into the unit, with brightly colored yellow walls, kids of all ages. He introduced me to another man, the unit director, who is very happy to show me around. His wife and two daughters were there. They were Black. The littlest girl was tired and fighting it. They were leaving to put her to bed.* Another fragment. *I was at an Orthopsychiatry conference. A case had been presented. A woman, my age or older, sat with a small, rigid baby standing on her lap. I crouched down next to her, indicating that I might be able to help. She said, "I hope so, this baby has attacked me twice already."*

"There is an entirely different biography from that of need," he said, "the biography of desire."

"The relationship I want is gourmet food. No, healthier than that and less common, harder to find and potentially available at every meal." I live without it, we all live without it and to our various degrees, fail to thrive.

Sabelle wrote me a letter when her car broke down on the Turnpike, "Motels disorient the senses. You are cut off from the world. In motels, the sadness of coming and leaving nearly grows on the walls. How many people have stopped here, escaping something else? In this room, it feels like far too many. How many others have been unable to recognize themselves in the bright lights of the bathroom? I searched my face in the mirror this morning, trying to find an angle that I could see as familiar. Perhaps it was the light, or my weariness, but I looked only at another stranger. It feels like, since Dan's death, I am again starting over in my body. Grief can change your perception of things, and to me, everything is paler, more muted. I don't believe that there is an 'end' to things, but I feel myself wishing that the beginnings weren't so hard." This child has grown into a woman, a person that I respect, who demands an encounter. I am taken off guard because her voice can still have an empty ring. I am somewhere viscerally or habitually misled by it. I read this gem to Arles.

"That is wonderful. She writes like you."

"I read it, maybe that's why."

He shook his head, smiling, "She is very gifted."

Sabelle still approaches me at an angle, glancing away to the right when we could make the deepest contact. It will self-correct as her CNS relaxes into a steady state and into me.

"Would you feel more protected by taking a knife?" I answered "Yes" too quickly to amend it. "What would it protect you from, who?" I felt no bravado, no antisocial flair. I went silent and wept without making a sound. No thought emerged except that time was going, time was up, and I couldn't stop this. Then the thought, "I knew where the knives were. I couldn't get to them. They were two floors down." Arles sat next to me. He doesn't, that often, anymore. I clasped his hand, pushing it down harder on my knee, hoping to feel his presence, hoping to stop crying. But I couldn't. It was time to end, or as he is saying these days, "to pause." He put on my shoes and tied them hard across the top, securing me in them. He put his arm around me, and he asked me to call him on Monday to let him know I landed safely. "And remember you and me." I was able to choke it down, wipe my eyes and leave to meet Blake to drive to Ithaca.

Even when it is not Dan or Johnny, my default mood is sadness. But now it is Johnny. The Thursday night massacre punctured a chamber in my heart, the one that keeps filling up with naïve hope. I am injured and exhausted. Waiting for John to rescue me the night of Johnny's meltdown, I talked with Eva, trying to keep his state separate from all it evoked in me, that he would come breaking through the door, swearing... and then... I can't speak. I don't know what will happen next. My heart is pounding. With Eva, though, I can feel a neuronal sorting out. I cannot face Johnny if I am in some other time in a small body. Once I was able to make Johnny just Johnny, my fear subsided.

John came home, and when Johnny met him with his cold fury, John lost it in an explosion of grief and rage and exhaustion. He told me, later, that it scared him. He had wanted to beat him, to end this endless taunt of alcohol, trauma and psychosis. Eva and I talked about learning that we could not save the other's life, that this is not the same as turning your back.

"It is being addicted to addictive states."

"I am not addicted, Arles, I am enculturated. There has not been a moment in my life that was not back-washed in alcohol. Supersaturated, prenatally until now. I don't want it, except that it is not exactly accurate because, in some places, that is like saying I don't want to live. But every breath is laced. It is the language of my people. The sorrows of gin. I have to extricate. I have to be willing to leave it behind."

Arles asked me to attend to the way I was talking, the odd warmness and slowness and the removed softness. I heard it too. My mother's reserved goodnight kiss smelled of bourbon; my father's was lubricated in it.

I left the silent, shuttered house. Almost everyone I passed walking into town was in trouble. I can't understand my relationship to them. I have no species barrier, and we must, at some level, want the same things, even share the same thoughts. I do not feel superior nor alien, but different. I imagine making a film, a 10-minute, black-and-white documentary with a representative sample, Johnny; the toothless smoker begging for a dollar; the girl with the purple hair, skirt at her crotch; the fat motorcycle rider with a gray ponytail; the girl who won't eat: the girl who cuts; the boy with piercings whose pants fall off his skinny backside, all in a large room doing their particular version of headbanging.

Sue and I weave a closer knit each time we talk. Such different threads. Immense pressures on the company: in demand, in debt, their customers fear that they will lose them. “There must be a mother and a father,” I said. I could hear her momentary silence, their shared reluctance to take it on this way, but of course, this is an archetypal fact. They reassured the affiliates.

I sat with my baby pictures while I used HeartMath, a biofeedback device new to me, to establish a new state of coherence in the rhythms of my heart, like an athlete would have or an old couple comfortably in love. I just looked at her. I was able to do this. For fleeting moments, it was as if everything: time, space, the cardboard, the print disappeared, and there was a three-dimensional baby, alive, breathing. Arles added later, “and with a beating heart.” I had no time to feel anything, just to experience the reality of a baby with nothing separating us, called time or space. “This is an important discovery, Sebern.”

Lee leaned her elbows on my sacrum and worked where the breath is frozen around my ribs.

“Do you feel your spine? Do you have a sense that you are backed up by your backbone?”

I am not sure why it took me so long to answer.

“No. I am searching for it.”

“People who have gotten enough and who haven’t been traumatized live from their spines; everything comes from there. You seem to collect in your ribs.”

“It’s like you were lying in a hammock, Lee and the rope broke, you would never lie in a hammock again the same way. And it is as if the hammock were never there. I don’t have the original experience of that curvature ‘into’.”

“You have the opposite curvature, Sebern. You arch away.”

Lee ended working around the crown and then my nose and eyes. When I came up the stairs after the session, she looked shocked. “Your face!” I was shocked by her shock. Later, she described it. My face was not formed. It was rubbery, plastic, like a baby just born or maybe still in the womb.

I saw the bumper sticker: "Time is what's there so that everything doesn't happen at once." I described these trance states to Arles, that I had a sense when they would be productive and when they would be too diffuse. There is a short route between the muscles of the eyes and the amygdala, not the long route of vision. This is the scanning behavior of frightened and vigilant animals.

I was fighting the states away for most of the session, but then I was jumped by one. Moses' voice at first angry, then plaintive almost, "Why are you telling all of this?" The voice became plaintive after this sequence: these states evaporate time, time presents no barrier; without time, events co-occur, and the old threats are no longer old, they are right now; no, he could not leap through space to kill my mother who is already dead... "I am," I told him, "in this place, both dead and confounded by the fact that I go on living."

I'd come in angry at him.

"What did I do?"

"Nothing. You didn't do anything."

"Maybe that's why you're angry." I followed this chord to an uncontained screaming baby, then quiet, the light leaving, going cold and quiet.

"It is untouchable, far away, empty, like the gap between Moses' finger and the finger of God." I felt cold in the hot office and burrowed under three blankets, trying to see how I might lift this soul of nothingness closer to the perimeter of my skin, nearer to the proximity of touch. I searched everywhere for comfort, and the closest thing there was was bashing my head into a concrete wall. That only helped for a moment. No one, not Lee or Sam, or Arles, no one, nothing, could touch this. When this happened to Reggie, I reassured her that it is transitory, that whatever it is can be nothing other than energy and energy moves. My prayer: "Let it move."

He is silent after I told him of seeing the finger of Moses in the Sistine Chapel. The repeating image made me numb. "There is mind control in these frames." He nodded. "And when things like this happen, I am afraid they've got your mind too." Relief permeates me when he understands.

"You are telling me that Moses fingered you." I felt the outer containment of him even in the shock of this statement. The internal prohibition mounts. He asked me what I was feeling.

"I cannot say it... I could," I said slowly, "I could write it. It's a loophole."

A Baltimore oriole perched on my dead echinacea yesterday, and the cardinals soon will return to their rightful place. I am having trouble with time, fathoming it now that I more truly live within it. It crawls and leaps, and years disappear.

Before I left to paddle through Labyrinth Canyon, I sang a lullaby to Reggie. It touched her, and her suffering, so dark and terrible, was eased. She has enormous courage. And so does my bright-faced girl Sabelle, who goes dark when we talk of her compliance with being sexually exploited. And Beca is haltingly returning, tentatively re-establishing trust, allowing me back.

She'd been doing so well, and there was talk on the Spectrum providers' listserv about marathon Alpha-Theta sessions. Looking back, I think she'd agreed to this mostly to spend the dreaded long weekend with me. We did several sessions, both Saturday and Sunday. She reported only that she heard some chanting or more like moaning and that it just didn't feel good. It wasn't good. She came in for her regular session two days later. This perfectly groomed girl was slightly disheveled, and she had turned away not only from all training but from me. She came to each session, tentatively. Two months later, she told me that her dog was sick. I inquired. Her dog was the only being she could love, and she had not fed him regularly since the Alpha-Theta sessions. He was sick from starvation. She told me that garbage was piling up in her garage. She had canceled pick-ups.

"Beca, where are you?"

"Oh," she said, at first confused by the question, "It's the orphanage, isn't it?"

And now I was leaving her again. It's impossible to be a patient.

❧

Since the river, I experience time like cards stacked sideways in my head, as parallel flows, out to each side of me (more to the right), probably infinite and boundaried by the thinnest veils. In some realm of consciousness, I side-step through them.

"How did I get here?" I asked. "How did I find my way from such a beginning through such deep illness into this grief? How has the neurofeedback, with all else, brought me here? And it all seems just ordinary." There was no better word to describe this ground.

"You are not ordinary," he said quietly. And with eyes welling up again, I told him that I was beginning to see this, at the same time, I found this steady state of being exactly ordinary. Anyone can do exactly what I did. This is what I mean by ordinary. I look around in this state to see my mother and father, thinking they must be in here somewhere, that I am, in this enlightenment, some flame of their spark. But they are not here. They had no glimpse of this. They were the beginning. I see them in a distant landscape, small figures, a long time ago. I am released from them.

I experience each moment as it moves through me, the slow-moving seizure that disrupts me at the deepest core, that may be generated from the deepest core, the "no mother brain."

"Do you think these headaches and these events come from all the head injuries you've had?"

"I'm sure, but I can't really get it. It isn't denial. I think it is that the brain can't quite compute its own injury. There is nothing for it to assess. It can assess the broken arm, but when it is the organ itself that is injured, how does it know? Other than headaches, which seem oddly distant from the brain, it has no markers, no way to feel for its own injury."

"It does seem like a big event. How are you doing with it?"

"It is, and it's tough to ride out. But I've been wondering if a stable brain mitigates against spiritual experience. All mystical traditions, right, engage in practices to dysregulate the brain to some degree? It has to be contained somehow to become something more than dysregulation itself, by the culture in shamanism, tradition in mysticism, meditation practice. I need arms around the vastness that my dysregulation opens to. Particles of the no self of the motherless infant and this Non Self are blending. And who is still recording, who is making such distinctions, or not making them?"

I wondered if the seizure could be part of the dissolving. It rivets me to my body. Perhaps my nervous system is ill-equipped for this level of challenge, or maybe it's all of a piece, both pathology and unfettered awareness. The organized brain is the brain of the religious; the dysregulated brain, the brain of the mystic. It was only madness before Arles, before training.

I see the clock hands and the leaves fall. But we seem trapped in linear time in a way we are not trapped in space. We experience space as three-dimensional, at least three-dimensional. Space is a right hemisphere domain. Time is on the left. We don't conceptualize space and time in the same way at all. I am beginning to experience time as spreading out laterally, infinitely, every moment that ever was or ever will be is now. It takes a slight side step into a different color in the prism, and I am in a different time. The barriers are thin but convincing. I cannot do this at will. But I think of time travel without the sense of the past or going into the past. My rabbi grandfather could not be killed because all time is parallel to itself. Push your arms out in space; push your arms out into time.

This seemingly endless seizure is difficult to manage while trying to keep track of the failure of a treaty ratification or the grocery list. I know this will all change. I want peace, if not that, the absence of horror, if not that, a renewed, strengthened equanimity, for no one relinquishes this suffering without a battle to the death.

"Why do any of us do therapy?" I asked. He stretched his back.

"It is madness. It is truly madness, and it is truly the only way, if there is a way, to encounter the reality of human suffering honestly and deeply. It is perhaps the only way left to be in the community of humanness consciously. All true paths are madness, and it's the only thing to do."

I paused, for the moment deeply satisfied with this.

"How much can you be inside my mind, Arles?"

"That's quite a question for the end of the session," he said, pulling the laces up tight into a lopsided bow. "More than most and probably less than you would wish".

❧

Allan Schore, the attachment theorist, had to cancel, and Siegfried asked me if I would speak in his place. It wasn't hard for me. Nothing grabs me anymore the way it used to.

It is hard for people, for me, to understand that every morning I question who was born to manage this day. Who is born from training the right temporal lobe? It is the return of innocence, the innocence of connection. When I train on the left, I experience an antisocial presence. Is this the true me, suppressed? The unconscious aggression that lies in wait for Arles should he disappoint?

I'd heard of Rae before we met. She was an expert at using neurofeedback for athletes and performers. She and I sat on the dock, our feet in the lake, barely disturbing a large flock of coots, and I saw her, the dailiness of her turmoil, how hard she works to maintain herself. On the other side, Karen leaned against me, whispering, "I wish you lived here so I could see you." Sven tells me of his stay in the incubator and his wish for the bottle. And Lisa says that she, too, could recognize the black hole that people try to climb out of, and I don't remember saying it. People liked the talk, but I think mostly they liked my ease and sense of integration; my lack of presentation.

Arles is impatient with the trances. He doesn't trust them. But without them, I will be left suspended in some space between understanding and not understanding. This space in me has its own energy. I was thinking about this as I pressed my forehead against the warm glass on the 12th floor of the Hilton. At this conference, like the canoe trip, things that I used to experience as discrete events with inherent meaning, bounded meaning, meaning that I could extract and represent to another, dissolve into the flow. I walk there, sit in meditation on the sunstruck terrace, race Siegfried in the pool (and win) or just love Sue; my room is surrounded by trees that attract beautiful birds and it is all swept away along with the debris of alarm over the future and the flotsam of others' discontent—it all just flows, without drama into the river of time and practice. Nothing is separable or remarkable. There is only love, and it is boundless. I press the down button, and the elevator is right there.

At the end of the conference, I had a conversation with David Kaiser, the neurofeedback wunderkind, about getting a ride back to LA.

"Before training," I told him, "I would not have asked, I would've gotten the shuttle."

He said, "I think you would've hitchhiked."

I was floored and asked him how he recognized this in me. He smiled, "I've seen your brain map".

Bob

A fierce wind blew us into the garage. I was walking behind John, just had a thought that he wouldn't lead me into anything dangerous, heard calls of alarm and then the automatic arm crashed across the top of my head, slid down over my forehead and hit my nose at the bridge, knocking me down. John retrieved my broken glasses. I refused an ambulance or the ER. We stopped at McDonald's for a bag of ice, and when I got home, more ice, Arnica, Ibuprofen and rest. John said he felt so badly for me, huddled against the garage wall as defenseless as a young child, bewildered and hurt. Reggie sent me to Bob, her PT, and he has helped.

I met him in his office in an old house in Florence. He welcomes me warmly, says a little bird told him about the accident and takes a blessedly brief history before capping my head lightly with confident hands. I am exhausted from this injury, in some way deeply disabled—I swim and sway in slow waves side to side across my forehead. Post-concussive syndrome. "You have a bruised brain stem. Sleeping better could not be such great news." He said it would take a couple of weeks to really know what had happened and what I would be left with. "You were 1/2 step away from disaster." I felt my old, sad mix of relief and invalidation. "It could have been so much worse" becomes "you weren't hurt."

It has been exhausting to think. I have not read my email. Climbing stairs is formidable. Outbursts of rage come quickly, then burn out. My handwriting is better? My sleep has returned to its old dismal pattern. I have headaches, pressure and ringing in my ears, and my memory is bad.

Arles is away. I imagined not telling him, but I recognized the raw gray structure of the transference, the reality of its steel beams. Can such a building site ever be returned to nature, allowed just to be trees, grasses and wind?

If there are no accidents, then what is this? I have not colluded in it. I wasn't there for it. It just happened. "I was about to step onto the sidewalk when the beam crashed over their heads." This is what I wrote, not over my head. Could be as random and as injured as saying to my doctor that I expected to wake up looking like a kangaroo when I meant to say raccoon. Having a brain injury creates new realities and fear that you were never, or were never quite, sharing the same one as others. I am to see Arles tonight, and I am afraid, afraid that this accident relates most immediately to him and his unwitting betrayals, afraid that I have been injured by my life beyond repair. I am not beyond redemption or transcendence, but the etching of history is deep.

"I don't need to harvest the past; that stony crap is not amber. Since that blow, I have closed a door on the attic. It is time to turn empathic attention to my shoulder. The sphincter that tightens at its center doesn't need to confess to me. It can have its secret in peace. I don't need to know anything more." I was moving fast. "These epochs of disconnection between us are our masterclass. It shows me the landscape without horizon, the gaze unmet turned inward. I have no mother. I accept that. The third epoch has begun, the epoch of transcendence." I took a breath, "It is a solo journey. I want the company of your solo journey." And then I stopped. "I want to go once a week for two hours on Friday if you can do that." I felt both calm and a little restless in this proposal.

"This would be a major shift, perhaps too major, perhaps precocious. We have to think it out."

Arles greeted me with what he characterized as "less than neutrality," and I know that his brain has taken a turn. He was angry. There is coolness behind his eyes, and I tell him what I see.

"Do you see that you ask me to accommodate vastly different states, unpredictably? On Wednesday, you were warm and supportive; today turned away. One day you'll answer my question; another you say it's none of my business."

"Now," he says, "you are organizing what goes on here around my pathological brain states."

"I never use the word 'pathological,' but you do meet me in very different states. It's like Russian roulette. I never know what chamber your brain is in: peace, openness, ease; persecution, abandonment, assault. Do you see this?" He does not answer me. When he is in these bad states, he takes a "love it or leave it" stance. I finally see it for what it is. "I think you believe that you will always be left."

After a brief quiet moment, he said, "You're right, Sebern." He teared up momentarily, and I looked away, feeling only gratitude but wanting to be careful not to shame him by looking too directly at this uncommon exposure. I wanted to embrace his rib cage to contain the lacerated, humiliated heart. I wanted to give him what he had given me.

He'd sat next to me and tied up my boots.

"Thank you," he said, gentle and self-possessed, "for the gift of your being".

Chapter 10

There could be no better way to be in the morning. We walked up the hill in silence, each alone, our way flooded with moonlight, feeling the sharp reminder of the wind as we rose to the crest and no protection. This is the ice-capped landscape of Weston, this mouth full of stars. As the brothers sing, we gather light from their candles to ours, each illuminating a face, the face of God, the Buddha face.

I am turning, less perceptibly than the planet, from warm/dark to warm/light. I'd proposed this simple grid to Arles a long time ago: four sections made by two intersecting lines that could fully represent all personalities: dark, light, warm, and cold. It is a difficult adjustment. I am losing my character. The beech leaves shudder in the wind but hold fast through the winter. I have become disinterested in the dark, and I feel some confusion that it holds no attraction. I am not yet light—more heavy now than dark—a little disoriented, not quite able, almost by habit, to release it, to let it drop away. I doubt this can be willed. It can only be practiced.

Each time I'm here, I encounter the issue of faith. What is the need for faith? It is. It changes. It is. This is where I seek to live, stretched out in the flow, not even needing the comfort of the eddy.

Reggie had an image in meditation. She had sat through a storm wanting to call me, knowing she shouldn't, more she said for me than for her. She doesn't yet see that it is the same. She saw herself entering a stream. She saw the other shore. She looked for me. She could see no one, and then she saw me swimming along right beside her, teaching her the strokes. Like Anne in her canoe up close to mine, to teach me the meditation of the J stroke. Stream enterers, naked in the warm flow, body inseparable from water. The fear that remains is like the fear from caffeine, a neurological habit, an old, well-worn firing.

I talked with Candace, my retreat-mate there every year, about my struggle with the otherness, the kingdom to come. I told her of becoming no one at all, that there were no walls of skin or of self in which to hold God. That I was as tiny as a particle and as vast as all space. I told her about my sudden discovery that I had no protection, and that then I was safe.

"This is a mystical experience, Sebern."

"It was a storm. It was a breaking open. It was a dissolution of self. I still reside there even when I've lost sight of it."

The snow stays suspended in the air, just dancing particles in the breeze. It never seems to fall to earth, but there it is, frosting the orange beech leaves.

❧

At one moment, I am permitted entry, at the next, the door is firmly shut as if it had never been left sweetly ajar. He holds my yearning as an object of interest. His interpretations fall on me like blows. He understands all this when I say it. I am stressed when he withdraws, and I become fierce, cold and unreachable. From there, he can't hear that I don't want this position, this form. I want him.

He repeats the list of things I've said as if they were dissatisfactions with him.

"You are saying I am not good enough to help you."

"No! It's just the opposite, Arles. It is that you are so good that I have a hard time with the barrier that our fears construct, and that this form promotes. Anything can be seen as resistance or envy; anything can be or become dark. I want to cultivate the light. We need a different paradigm."

He held himself back long enough to hear what I was trying to tell him.

"A more mystic me," he said, "perhaps two souls in search of each other."

"Thank you and thank god," I said to myself as I looked at him, my eyes filling with tears. Arles is in constant pain and facing major surgery. As I left, I hugged him.

"I'm sorry for all you're going through right now."

"Thank you, Sebern. And I'm sorry for all you are going through, too."

Two souls in search of each other.

I don't want to be confined by a construct; not absence, not trauma, not repression, not form, not analysis, not transcendence. Not to be confined is not to live within them. This is difficult.

It is January 13, and it is snowing here for the first time this winter. Two kids finally get to wear their snow suits, bundled past gender, but probably boys, they scrape up the snow, leaving the spot clear and lovingly shape their snowballs. I remember Blake, little and bundled, her cold face and fingers when I finally unbundled her, taking off her boots first, then the wet leggings; her body warm and happy to be free. Her face is rosy, her body sprawled on the floor, ringing out reports of Jay and Teresa and Willy, of the snowman or the super slippery slope that is the neighbor's yard. But I don't see the snowsuit or the girl of different ages. Not her face or her eyes. I am like a kitten whose eyes were bandaged during the early window in which one learns to see faces.

I have always somehow seen my patients, but I see them better now. I know their eyes and how their faces fold or crumple or relax into their sadness: Reggie, whose mouth turns down, Beca, whose black eyes just brim and flow with hardly a muscle moving.

"I was a celluloid character watching myself play the parts of me. I know how important it is for people to remember being tucked in or tenderly kissed by their mother. I don't have these memories. Mine are of you covering me with a blanket when I shivered and froze or holding me through hours of flooding grief. These are my memories of maternal tenderness. Your insistent presence in the stark landscape of no mother. My unconscious is the unconscious of you and me. You are the Lucite pole around which the being of me has formed. When we explore my unconscious, we are exploring what formed here. The external became the internal. You became the inner core of me, and the relationship between us is a matter of my unconscious. The relationship between you as my mother and then my father turned on its axis, inverted, and became my internal world. I didn't have one before. I had a hidden world but not an inner one. I became three-dimensional, flesh on the bones, rounded, cellular, through you. I came into being. Transference is spoken of 'as if'. It is kept 'as if'. As if I were a starving child. As if you were my mother. It wasn't 'as if' here. You entered the reciprocal psychosis, and it was beautiful. If the transference had been kept 'as if' I would have remained 'as if.'"

I looked at him over the rim of the white paper cup as I sipped my coffee.

"As I feel my completeness, I begin to feel the enormity of the loss of you as that father. Even though there will be no need, I am grieving that you will never put a blanket over me. At its worst, it has felt like a gripping right beneath my throat, like the sudden realization that my mother is dead. It is that incomprehensible. Maybe more so because there you are sitting right in front of me. You are not dead. And you are no longer the mother or father that I had."

All of this began when he asked how I could feel free to make the decision to go once a week. I put the coffee cup on the floor and lay down on the pillows and wiped away tears, as gently, as tenderly as a father might. I rolled onto my shoulder, toward him, my head still on the pillow.

"It is going into a blank space, not empty somehow, but blank. I don't know where you are, how we are. But your position has changed, and you are over there, apart from me, commenting on me, not as you were, part of me. Maybe I fear that you will pick at, even assault the me that is built around you, because when we approach the terra incognita of my unconscious, we are not talking about my mother."

He nods. He knows our rare discovery, like the skull of the first ancestral woman, that the unconscious is the construction of the two, that the core of my motherlessness was the absence of an inner life. There was a need, and there was high-impact drama, in place of another within me with its richness and complexity. There was a convincing veneer of depth. I constructed a story in place of a self. I understand now the true nature of the deep dive and the Lucite pole, the vow to go beneath the story. I was requesting the destruction of the only me I had, and he did that insistently, tenderly, harshly, mistakenly, beautifully.

"When you left to sit across the room with your tea, I faced the end, and I was facing it alone. I became my mother, distant and competent. I could have her and defend her against the unspeakable loss of never having had her, and now losing you. This isn't a 'defense', it is a complete system. She is the adult template. I slip into her like a red dancing slipper." I paused and sat up. "We have closed the epoch of speaking the unspeakable."

"Yes, it was unspeakable."

I hardly let him say it; I hardly let it out of his mouth. I have no demons now shouting me down, threatening to murder him or me. I want to know he has heard; that he knows even what could not be seen or said. I swerve away as if his confirmation is too much. His validation saves my sanity and challenges it in a single whispered word. I barely hear what he has not agreed to, "the epoch... is closed."

"I thought I would always come to you with, 'daddy look what I made,' that I would always need you more to receive me than to understand me, to say, 'Oh, that's terrific,' not 'What does it mean?'. I can't find you there. This is the blank space. You were that father. Now you are not. You are you. So, I encapsulate this past within it, and plan to move on. I leave you because I don't know how to keep you. I don't have a continuity from then to now."

He closed his eyes and nodded, more, I think, taking it in than agreeing to it.

He tied my boots.

"It gives me my feet, Arles."

"I know Sebern, that's good."

I watched Johnny standing at his new car, smiling broadly as he said goodbye to his dad and went off skiing with his friend. I washed the dishes, looking out of the window of our finally renovated kitchen, in the country, watching the snow falling. I was looking at a miracle, a young man brought back from the dead, stepping into his life ever more fearlessly. He has these moments of happiness that extend into his life and overtake its shadow. But my state was not stable. I feel emptiness, and transitions are bumpy. Maybe that will always be the case that somewhere, however slightly, I meet these micro losses with my amygdala. How else to account for my arousal and irritable edge? Green tea in the morning, one less Gabapentin, weight gain, restricted diet as I try again to kill the yeast, no chocolate milk? I have to rely on a baseline state, the Arles ever-present, the neurofeedback state, the meditation state. And it gets clear for a moment once again that all suffering is delusion, but knowing this is once again eclipsed by the state. It is too simple and not simple enough to trace it all to fear, through its multiple pathways. Fear forges the pathways. The more convinced I am by the "logics" of the state, the more reinforced I am in its practice. It is the well-worn terror of my infancy; it is too much left side training, it is a brain that has been, and not so long ago, drenched in fear.

FP02 today. Awake at 3:30. Since FP02, I am curled up in my bed, not afraid, really, but needing fetal comfort. I have access to deep, nonverbal regions and the sense that something is rising up in me. I have headaches. Last weekend, settling into the deep comfort of Plainfield, I was drawn to art. A poem yesterday. There was intense pressure on my lungs that, I suddenly remember, I used to feel a lot. I have the sense that each side of my body has different agendas. I had difficulty coordinating my eyes to begin writing, very similar to dream states in which I can't see. My mind drifts to worries about money, but no dread follows. I am more centered at the core. Solidity. Reggie reports similar things, including a lift in mood. Eleanor, however, did not show up for her session. Her mother called to report that she had a panic attack in the night, but also that she sees a difference in her. Sabelle reports no fear response to things that would normally trigger it, and that she can feel the place in her brain where the storms begin. She looks radiant, and she is even more articulate emotionally, about herself and others. Johnny reports that FPO2 helps his mood. I asked him to attend to the central issue of fear to see if it touches that. If it does, he can take less Gabapentin.

Sam tells me that my neck is completely different, that the inflammation that has encased it for the whole time of our relationship, and even more tightly before it, is gone. He can touch structures that he could only infer previously. The brainstem is hot, and it is available. He has never seen anything like it. After his work, I feel thrown, nauseous, out of equilibrium. Bob said that I might feel labile, that my stability may have rested in the binding of the basal ganglia. He also said that I was healing from the TBI faster than anyone he'd worked on. I feel a core emotional stability. My body is going through it, headache, yellow shit, short fits of exhaustion, episodes of extreme heat, some restless leg, but I am warmer and more intuitive. Nothing is throwing me.

As my mother got old, particularly in the last year, she became a shape-shifter. She did not become the lynx or the bear; she became who she was meant to be, dumpling-like and human. Nothing sharp left. Even the movement of her elbows was fluid as she went through her forms, and I, trying not to, cried. Her laugh had gotten soft, and she pondered where she used to judge. She wanted me. I was, she told others, her best friend. But she told me nothing about herself, and she did not entrust me with her house. That house, her first mother—of course, she would not leave it. Nor could she die there.

I put my head in my hands. "I came here at the edge of a psychotic break. I was afraid to sit in the waiting room. I used the fire escape to come and go."

"I do remember," he said. "I remember it all."

❧

I awoke early and watched the sky turn from black with one morning star to indigo, and the mountains emerge and turn from gray to gold to pink. It is the last day of the Winter Brain Meeting in Palm Springs, and I noticed the ease in transition, the absence of sadness, as the exhibit hall, once lively with coffee and conversation and brain machines, becomes muted and draped like a forlorn mannequin. I introduced FPO2 privately to some affiliates, and both Siegfried and Sue tried it. Everyone who did felt it, from calm and centering, to the release of a traumatic injury acquired at age 12. She told me she had jumped over a fence and landed on a spike that went through her foot. Nothing she had done had relieved the pain that had now lasted for almost fifty years. The pain was gone. Siegfried reported some FPO2 effects. He told me he'd said "goodbye" on the phone to Sue—he never does. Sue said that for the first time ever, her heart did not pound before asking a question in public. She, too, is quieter and calmer. There were accolades from my colleagues over this discovery. "Quieting fear is my quest," I said to most. I gave a talk. For me, it is most important for Siegfried and Sue to benefit. Sue to venture more deeply into fearlessness and empathy, and Siegfried to perhaps experience living without fear for the first time in his life.

They took me to see the nearly overpowering expanse and strangeness of Joshua Tree. There were three coyotes on the road. We stopped, and they approached us to panhandle. The drought is severe, and food is in short supply. They needed food and water. Siegfried was hurt by it. You could feel it. Sue and I felt more equanimity, she in the science of cycles, me in the taproot of my practice. Siegfried emerged for me. As we wandered in Marengo Park, he told me more of his early life, in Germany, in the war, after the war, never safe. Sue told me of his present difficulties, and as we talked, he emerged more also for her.

It is the sadness and the intolerance of light. I want to penetrate the meaning of this training at FPO2. There is a mystery here. It is not all about being centered and calm. I am both, but there is a sharp edge from 30 seconds on the left (FPO1) that I don't have with training on the right. It leads me to believe that the amygdala is functionally not the same across hemispheres. This may already be known. I tried the left because of a sequential processing problem—it is the province of the left hemisphere. I feel pressure in my chest, a memory of not being able to breathe or escape, but without fear, as if a PTSD experience is attempting to organize but failing to do so, leaving me awash in sadness.

I am astonished by the sacredness of morning. The shadows of trees on the deep woodland snow. This treasured world. The dense, sad stillness deep in me, behind the eyes where all memory is encoded, some enshrined, some hidden, out of recognition, held in the rapid transit firings of time – in the universe which is also my brain. I am edgy and solitary, quick to anger, but I feel no hatred and no degradation. I want only to sit. Not to have a writing group or to walk in the snow. Just to spend time here behind my eyes and with Arles before his surgery. It will be a long stretch without him. He has already begun to leave and needs to lean on our trust that what is most important is that he be real.

The data for FPO2 are very positive. Felix told me that several years ago, a drunk man drove him off the road on his way home from work. The experience disturbed him to such a degree that he never took that way again, even though it was by far the shorter route. He had trained for three minutes at the booth. On the drive home, two days after the conference, a drunk driver came across the divider on the highway heading right at him. He pulled over to the breakdown lane, barely avoiding a head0-on collision. He expected his formidable terror to reignite. He could hardly believe that this had happened once, much less twice. "What are the odds?" he asked. He took a few minutes to collect himself and got back on the road. The next day, he took the short route to work. His PTSD cleared with this training, and yet I am left with his important question, "What are the odds?"

But no data is more compelling than Johnny's. I had blown up at him after I trained at FPO1. When we talked, he said he almost had a panic attack and called my attention to the 'almost'. He'd noticed his breathing and heart rate and was able to regulate, "What is the worst that can happen? I could die. Everyone dies. There's no reason to obsess," and the panic stopped. I apologized to him. He said, "I know that you and I have moments like this and that 24 hours later is 24 hours later. I don't let it get to me."

My old friend, Michelle, was eating dinner at Spoleto's too, and she came over to our table. She sat with us and took us all in, "What a beautiful family!" I have found myself thinking about this. Each one of us has been confined by our own neuronal drama, profoundly constricted by rehearsed patterns deep in our histories and deep in our brains. Families do co-construct a family identity and narrative that reinforces these patterns or at least that allows us to continuously practice them. Homeostasis is built on what is known, and families are our best effort at maintaining the homeostasis of each individual member. Neurofeedback has changed the homeostatic regulation and homeodynamic potential of each of us, and that redefines the dynamic and the deepening stability of the family. I came out of my habit of isolation to join this family. For me, there had been no others, only forms. John clears away the ADD fog and can attend to his family with more clarity, more accuracy. Johnny gathers strength every day and, in being able to care for himself, is able to almost effortlessly care for others. Blake gets quieter, more mature and more genuine. She is less reactive, funnier and able to be here less out of her need and her dedicated role as our savior and more fully from herself. There is more room in her for insight and compassion. And Molly is poking along too. She has only trained a few times, and when she did, she became noticeably more patient, more capable. She has guided me in caring for Johnny. As each of our nervous systems reorganizes away from habit, John and I are finding each other, and this calms the kids. He has become self-respecting and calmly assertive, and I can be, usually am, settled in and content. There is room in me. We have become a family, interdependent, encouraging each other's growth, better at seeing the reality of the other – like laced hands, we can hold each other up.

Reggie is feeling battered by her entry into adulthood. She wondered how many candles I would put on the cake. Six, because I had six that matched. It was arbitrary because she is still of all ages. But desperately she attempts to maintain the status of the child, and I nudge, bully, soothe, cajole, accept, refuse to accept and welcome her to the world of adults, with assurance that she will never be forgotten—the most terrible wound.

There are inklings that Eleanor may be waking after all these years of anorexic somnambulance. I have trained her at FPO2, and perhaps it has made its contribution: instead of bingeing, she came apart. She could not find a way to contain her body; she slammed into walls, wanted to cut, rent and tear, break glass with a hammer, but she went through it all until it was spent, and the feeling at the end, she said, was not to be missed. During this event, she screamed that I had taken it away, that she couldn't go there anymore. Her fear now is that she will become too well and won't get into the inpatient program, a core plot point in this girl's script. She is becoming three-dimensional, psychologically rounder, someone I cannot just struggle to care for but could love.

I am having trouble verbally and sequentially. It is hard to read. The snowstorm squelched my plan to train, but it is clear that FP02 will never be all that is needed.

EEG Spectrum has gone into Chapter 11. Two employees were fired, and Rae tells me Siegfried has been relieved of all official duties. I am worried about Siegfried and Sue. I am, though, completely calm about the money—I will not regret having sent it even if I never see it again. I feel steady, fluid and capable. I owe this and the health of my family to these people. I will do my best for them.

I lay on my belly, everything familiar, describing myself as regular, like other people, not traumatized, no time travel, no dissociation, even and good. I expect nothing from her touch. I expect, without knowing it, that I will feel what I always feel, the resistant knot deep in my shoulder. I had not yet learned that my back plays like a piano with the strings severed. I don't know that nothing has responded until every vertebrae does. I was agitated in a way I had not felt, perhaps because it is a memory, not a threat. When Lee said the time, her voice dropped through dark water, and when I heard it, I was startled. I was interrupted in a reverie, and even the interruption failed to dispel it. Usually, I would (if I had ever gotten that deep) startle out of that state into vigilance, like a cat awakened, suddenly and completely alert. I turned to my side. I didn't know what to do with my legs. I curled them up, and I turned over.

"I couldn't have known."

"Whatever you are doing is working. Your body is completely different."

"This is what they have been saying about you, Lee, that this is what happens. I would never have believed it; I would never have known."

It is Marsha on the phone. This time when she said it, I felt its brutality, its tragedy. "Nothing that happens in my life will make it worth my being born."

Blake and I will go to her presidential address to the Association for Behavioral and Cognitive Therapies. She will talk about suicide.

Johnny called shortly after Marsha. I asked him to speak more softly because I was getting a headache.

"Oh, I'm so sorry." He was not expressing worry over his own actions, which he would then need me to comfort, but concern, spontaneous and genuine for me. "In my work," he said, "I see now that people really suffer, and I know that you have suffered for years."

I must've cut him off, instinctively fearful that he would undo this. These are the first times I've experienced Johnny as empathic in his life. He asked me out to dinner the next day. He's spending more time with Molly and recognizing that it matters. He goes to Jakob's games and last night stayed the night to keep Luke company through the dark of his mother's absence.

He came up to the kitchen. I took his face in my hands,

"Make it, OK?" He nodded. I have lost my desperation because he is doing so much better, but also because I am. We are all gaining on our demons. For John and me, they are gone. We live increasingly simple lives and, without the distraction of turmoil, deeper ones. Eva tried FPO2 and went into a reverie that she had to will herself out of. "It's like being stoned. Images come and go. We took a walk around the fair-grounds. "Maybe it is that I just can't remember what it is that I should be afraid of. I think that's probably it, Sebern."

Eleanor had asked her mother, "If I end up in a two-room apartment over a laundromat in Cambridge and ride my bike to work, and that is my life, will that be OK?" We had both at the same time come to realize that Eleanor has Asperger's. I had focused so entirely on attachment disorder that I'd missed this more clearly neurological reality. Eleanor was not shocked when I told her this, and felt no anguish because, of course, she can't. This is the problem. Her mother cried with grief, and then the relief of knowing. When she repeated what Eleanor had said, I started to cry, stopped, and apologized. "I'm not ready to accept that for her, not ready at all." She smiled at me through her tears and her fear to hope what I hoped. I understand the cross-currents that tumble you in place in a moment of this magnitude. When I saw Eleanor the next day, I had to reorient, I saw her differently, but she was not different. She is disabled, and she needs, nonetheless, the same level of demand as always to come into a 3D world.

"Why don't you just bang your head against the wall?" I asked her.

"Because it doesn't taste good." She constructs her identity through her symptoms. What happens when they disappear?

The kind of snow that plummets. Two days ago, it was 75° and thick. I walked in the evening in shirt sleeves. March is a time of incipience. Hopes and reminders; winter and spring. The purple woods are turning white again. The little song of sap droplets plays in the old buckets. This is a memory even now. The woods are roped, maple plumbed to maple. There are no horses pulling sleds, no harnesses of bells.

Arles's absence rumbles wildly in me. It gains my attention. It is a perturbation that is in the past, and it is surrounded by calm and understanding. It is familiar, both felt and oddly unfelt.

Reggie arrived again, coming apart. She has not been remembering but reliving her childhood, and it has been brutal. She has no protection. I think it is FPO2. At 7.5, it was sheer, boundless, wordless terror; at 8 to 11, it was deprivation and aloneness, starvation and no mother. So I tried 8.5 to 11.5, and she said, "I can feel myself coming out of the dark. It is as if I've been looking through a long hole, and my vision is now widening. I see this room. I see the sunlight." I trained her for four minutes. She felt a laugh trying to rise in her. Her voice lost its tremulousness, and her face changed. She still felt shaky but much better. I, too, feel my body at 8-11 in ways I don't at 8.5-11.5. Eva felt good for two days after her FPO2 training, but then experienced unprovoked episodes of anxiety. The frequency is all-important, unknown before we train and completely individual.

"Dear Arles, I try to understand everything through the fact of your absence, and I can't, except for the tumbling down deep and low and in the dark, and even that is subtle. I am familiar with how the abrupt cut off of your voice cuts through me, more electric than a blade, and I recognized both my vulnerability to loss and the depth of my recovery. My feelings can still be swept along the tornado path of seizure, and there is no possibility for a pause, for a question or a belief. The state of the twister is.' Now, when it touches down, it disperses into my body's memory of being held, into the finally achieved reality of you, into this brain that can no longer pursue that excursion. I am left with a simple missing."

We are buying EEG Spectrum, at least that's how it looks today, Thursday, March 16, a day that will begin at 65 degrees and that will end in snow. There seems to be nothing else to do but to buy this company, but I am not doing it out of obligation, however great, or generosity, although that flows in me as it did in my mother. Perhaps out of morality, which flourishes in gratitude. I feel no greed or aversion to all the inevitable complications and complexities. 10 owners. The business in California. Catastrophic loss if we don't pull this off. "Are you replaced only by acts of this magnitude, Arles?" Even if it were true, this is the right thing to do. I feel adult and keenly responsible for the future of this earth. This is my small contribution. My heroic.

For now, the company is saved.

I know how an infant acquires a self, fleetingly, completely around the presence of her mother. She makes herself in her mother's face. She becomes undone without it. Once I took the cover off a golf ball, I began to unravel it. It was nothing but the constant winding of its own rubber cord, stretching out for a mile just to be at the other end of itself. In the dark, secret nothingness in the center, I unravel myself in the absence of him. My mind could not hold him. There is no understanding powerful enough. My existence in this world is different when Arles is not in it.

Others have described what they feel with Lee when they let go, as memory, a "sense" memory of safe fusion. Infant/mother body. I am learning it, little by little, then distrust the learning, then abdicate the experience, then bring my focus to the reality of her hands on my ribs, try to get it, try not to try. I am more patient. I understand my body's bewilderment, now more its experience than aversion or fear. I am practicing. My skeleton is a ghost of sorrow, a subtle body of sadness that was not now sad. But I started to cry, "That poor kid," and first it was me, but then rapidly not me. Instead, I saw a Black boy about 11, bewildered, in jail. Lee just kept her hands where they were.

Yesterday, I facilitated the owners, the new company, and the group trying to save EEG Spectrum. I didn't intend to; I was drafted. John and I talked last night about how I'd become pivotal and the skill it will take to function in this role thrust on me, and to slowly, over the next year, or constantly in some way, divest it. I have some vague wish not to be doing this, along with complete acceptance of the necessity to do so.

Today, his absence has become too long.

I am wrapped in the red comforter in my garret room, trying to think about the paper on fear, but thinking about Siegfried and Eva and Arles, then thinking about why I can't think about this paper. It is as if I've already said enough about how fear insinuates itself. There is no nature/nurture debate. Nurture sets the fear point, the thud of the terrified heart and the clamping bowel, the cool vault of the depressed mother even before birth, the rage of the mother at the pain this baby caused her, the intolerance of this now helpless body laid across hers, draping her in unrelenting need.

Johnny had another round of drinking. Each time is less of a blow, but it is one. It can feel at least momentarily catastrophic, I said to Molly, "Like watching your house burn down. You are helpless, there is nothing you can do, you know, but that doesn't help." Yet it does. Even though I turned to substances repeatedly for relief, I was not hooked on them. I learned to become curious about my despair and became unrelenting about its causes and its reliefs, and since I never believed it would end, its sources. Like most, Johnny tries to do it.

❧

His office is sunny. I am back on the couch. I felt shy with him.

"I became stabilized in my internalization of you. Now you're back." I was happy to see him and nervous. "Now you could threaten my stability." He is back in his chair. "Your legs are on straight."

He takes this all in quietly.

"And how has this time been for you, Sebern?"

Arles has had major surgery. He has been gone for three months. Has something knitted in me, or torn apart? How is his long absence held?

I am haunted by the image that comes unbidden. It made national news. A five-year-old girl took her mother to see their little poodle floating in the family pool. She had drowned it.

Images well up under Lee's hands. I am sitting on the floor. Moses is sprawled there, spent, asleep, passed out. He has a gold wristwatch. The light is on overhead. Closing my eyes doesn't help. I can't go to sleep. There with Lee, I encourage myself to go to sleep, and my head shakes itself, "No." I saw the watch, but time did not exist. Lee reminded me that I wouldn't have known how to read time anyway.

Marsha had called. She was in a bookstore, convincing herself not to buy any new books, given the thousand stacked up unread next to her bed, and she saw and bought "A Symphony in the Brain." Then she left perhaps a historic message on my machine. "I want to do a pilot study of borderline and neurofeedback because these people get their behavior shaped up, but they continue to live lives of quiet desperation. Maybe neurofeedback can help with their emotions." She wants me to come to train her. We will set up a controlled study, set a budget and submit a grant.

And then there is Eleanor. Eleanor who feels the rush of being with others at the gay pride march, who cried at a film, who sees the absurdity of trying to "regulate through dysregulation," who is recruiting the concern of others. She cut her knee and was surprised that others even saw her when they went to get the Band-Aid. It is a visceral surprise. "It must be about my state, my openness."

"You have used so much energy just keeping your CNS within your body."

"Yes, like an octopus. The body that developed into puberty felt like a cancer." She paused and looked up at me. "I took the word 'nobody' and split it further and further apart to 'No... Body.'"

I am watching someone come awake, create a self and reflect. But, of course, not just watching. I'm in this creation. It is not another autistic exercise of the brain and machine. She experiences a relationship because now she is in one with me.

There are rounded identities where holes used to be in my psyche.

I discourage ants, sometimes by killing them. I hate to do this. I see they feel fear. Each one of them scrambles toward survival, and I pray for each one, an ant-size prayer that they will not drown, that they will find a way out, out of the pipes and back into the ground, like Harry Potter.

I drifted under Lee's hands, getting it that there was another person touching me like this. I eased into dropping away and stayed ever vigilant at the edge of my psyche. Suddenly, I entered the vortex of my own brain's firing, and it is a frightening freefall. I think of going back out into the rain, and I am homeless. Her hands alone save me. She covers my eyes and puts the pillow under my neck. As soon as she touched my head on the left near the crown, I jumped away, and she asked me. At first, I didn't understand, then I said, getting it, "It's not as if I didn't have electric shocks going through my head." This morning, ECT registered as memory, and I understood its place in the damage to my brain. There is no comfort. There was hardly a body to be comforted. More, a series of shocks.

I talked with Arles about how hard these snippets of time are.

"I am standing on a little beach talking with you, and there's a river passing by. I want to divert some of it and let it pool up around us."

"How do you feel as the river passes by?"

It hardly needs to be answered, but I do.

"Mostly it feels alright. It just is. It always is. It also feels lonely." He acknowledged this, expecting it. "I don't feel entitled to your time, Arles. I just need it."

He assures me that he will provide for me as best as he can. Mostly I talk about Milici, about the memory on Lee's table of electric shock, about what it has done to my brain and what it did to my body. The accounts patients give about memory loss, about headache, about not feeling themselves as themselves after ECT are minimized when they are not just ignored.

"Your sacrum is out, but it's as if you had been in a car accident yesterday." Milici did this to me in the last desperate attempt to save me from what I most needed: to be sent away from my home to a secure place.

Johnny was in a padded cell. Signs, "You are being recorded." A cheerful clerk told him he was due for arraignment on Tuesday and that if he were arrested again, he faced months in the Hampshire County House of Corrections. The first cop said he didn't think he had an accident. "But what about the hospital?" I asked. "He asked to go. I can't tell you any more." This was a kind officer, Moriarty. "He seems like a nice guy. Polite when I brought him his meals. The Irish have got him. It's sad." This arrest, this moment, forced access to the horror of his first years, his fear, the harm to his brain and his mind, the enduring tragedy that he has lived out, the sadistic violence of his mother's father. He raped her when she was 10, 11, 12 and 13. She held it together until she gave birth to a boy, and then she went mad and pushed him into the back of a closet and later, watched him slip under the bath water.

He was going for Tabasco sauce after beginning his 2nd pint of vodka. He drove into the rear of a truck. When we went back to see the wreck, I walked next to him, wrapped in generations of inevitability and sadness. He said, "I still love you, Mom." His dark, serious eyes, his own unfathomable sadness, his seriousness and his fear that he could do this again, that it is beyond him to control, all moved me. I touched his head and stroked his hair. "I love you still, too."

"I am better," he said, "I am just not better enough." He describes playing the game, looking good on top of the terror that is somewhat intermittent now, but that builds around even a common stressor. He wonders why life is so much harder for him, and I asked him how he answers this. He has never related this to his mother and still doesn't.

John and I felt this more physically than emotionally. There really is no new way to feel, no outlet in anger, nothing but body sorrow. He is an addict; he is precious to us. Is there something else we can do, something better? Are we making some mistake, dropping into some hole of oblivion common to parents of alcoholics? I would feel embarrassed if I discovered that.

I wasn't embarrassed to be at the police station.

"I've really done it this time, haven't I?" His first words. I coached myself along the way to hold him responsible, not to be empathic. I know the importance of holding him responsible. I know it deeply. It is about forming an identity, being known as an agent, about being. But I am afraid that he is engulfed in shame, and this will drown him, so I walk both paths. As I write this, I know he is gripped with fear in his innermost belly as he is showering and dressing for court. I don't want him to be any more afraid or any more alone or any more humiliated, and I must hold him responsible. None of us quite knows how to do this.

When I first came to Arles, he said I was not suffering, that I was tormented. Slowly, I have transformed the density and immobility of torment into suffering. That was when I started to cry. When I sat in the living room with Blake and John last weekend, another stretch of peace shattered by crisis, I cried without suffering. I was an open channel. All I felt was Johnny's unspeakable torment and his desperate, unwilled exit into alcohol. My sorrow forms no narrative. It doesn't reach back in time for the suffering of Hugh or my father. It does not weave a story about my fate with alcoholics; it does not predict Johnny's bleeding to death. I was, though, approached many times by graphic images of my brother losing blood at every compression of the respirator. I realized something about Johnny. When you strip away the alcohol, if that were not there to cloud the judgment, you have an exceptional man. He is not ordinary. Slowly, it seems that his self-hatred is transmuting to humility, his anger into spine and his fears into kindness. As fear ebbs away, he has glimpses of the other, and he is less alone in the universe. Sometimes there is light in his eyes. He is, beneath the abiding terror, awkwardly gaining his footing. Johnny was comfortable with his rage at what he saw as a Hispanic takeover of Miami. Last week, he started a language class to learn Spanish. He has become curious.

"You are becoming a distant star," I said to Arles. "I am receding from you. I'm in outer space. I am something jet propelled that is moving away from that tiny point of light in the midst of thousands of others and toward me." He is perhaps a guiding star. I distinguish him from all others, but my universe is vast, dark and filled with stars.

As fear drained out of me, I felt the presence of myself, but this inhabitation with its boundaries did not last long. Protesting throughout, I seemed to shed this new "self" like a snake's skin. My body still hugs the earth, but this is "Non self." I have endured this passage that came without warning.

I told him my image of outer space, of his small but clearly known shape as a star, and he spoke to me not of diminishment or of development, but of spaciousness. He is far away on the throne of cushions, now, with one crutch, which hardly seems necessary but that he must use.

"I want you to be proud of me, proud of us."

"It is more than pride, Sebern. It is amazing. Pride is something about the self. This seems beyond that. More of the "ecstatic," beyond anything in either one of us. It is in the meeting. A historical moment." I thought of Rumi and Shams, the dance of their ecstatic love. Are we prophets to one another?

Yesterday, I tried to be coherent with my neurologist about my nearly daily struggle to regulate my brain. Seizure, waking in an altered state, temperature swings, sleep, migraine, dizziness, misidentifying objects, seeing the mixer as my toothbrush, which corrects right away but happens and happens often, not being able to comprehend the accountant, sudden inability to spell or do simple math or recognize the small number of tablets in my hand without counting. Changes in my handwriting. Wheels that roll backwards on cars going forwards. I had come to think that this must be explained by some law of physics that I hadn't learned. She asked how much of the time? I had to think. It may have been an underestimate to say 70%, but that's the figure. So much time devoted to questions—what to eat, what drug now, what is my status? What is this state? I forgot to mention hypoglycemia to her, and that I wake up each morning wondering, who am I today?

I tried Topamax last night. It felt arousing in the night and, like I had trained too low, heavy in my head and body in the day. Joints ache. Very stable, but I was getting there with T3-T4 anyway. So enough of this. I am trusting my body's reactions. Gabapentin feels right. Topamax is not helping with sleep, and it encases me in a drug.

On the Cape with friends, I was aware of myself making the pro-social choice and how different this was from "my nature." The nature that grew like the oak at the edge of the tides and salt winds, twisted and stunted, was admired for its ability to continuously withstand assault. This was not my nature after all, and it was not PTSD but a product of fear. I don't think I have a nature anymore. I'm not even sure I have a history. Transformation of consciousness is different from the transformation of self. Maybe this is part of what attracts me to Thầy. He seems, at least at moments, to be about the transformation of himself, and he is asking his students to be about that too; otherwise, the whole endeavor risks becoming another glittering object.

I am re-committed to my regulation. I am happy in my life.

Last night I had supper at Atlantis, the new rage in Amherst, with Elizabeth Verrill, and afterwards we went to her home office, and she showed me Tomatis. I took the auditory pretest.

"It's really quite amazing that you do as well as you do, given this profile. Frequencies that allow the integration of language, particularly in your right ear, are nearly inaudible to you. Also, in that ear, there is a big discrepancy between bone conduction and your ability to hear through the air. They ideally follow the same curve." Elizabeth is an expert in sound therapies. She brought Tomatis from France to the US.

Sabelle had corrected me, "It is more like the fear is letting go of me." This morning, I couldn't pull free of it, get my head above it, and yet I knew I was at no risk of drowning. I didn't experience the seizure (that I know of) and I had no headache, but at the end I had a hypoglycemic assault, and ate desperately to allay the panic. By night, I was all right. The hard rain arrived like a Savior.

Arles and I fought.

"It's 11:15."

"Yes."

"We start at 11."

He is late to every session, from the beginning. It is worse now. I try to quiet myself as I sit in the waiting room, watching time slip away. He does not yield. I insist that he be the one, trying in effect to reestablish the positions I have forsworn—doctor/savior/father, patient/supplicant/child. I fear that throughout that he will say something that cannot be redeemed, and watch as we get closer to the brink, goading him almost, exploiting this raw vulnerability. And I don't know why. He tries twice to change the track, but I am not easy with it. It feels false. It will be undone between us; it will not be worked through, and I will inflame it. I want him to regain his footing as a man without the boy, which is to say as my therapist, so that I can become the girl in the woman, his patient again. "I pay you for this," I want to say, but I recall even the impulse. I want to be angry too. I want him to bear it and to see what's right in it. I want him not to be hurt, not to have been hurt, not to have never recovered from the long taunt of his childhood. He told me what my tone of superiority did to him. It may be, as he has said, the voice my parents used with an errant servant. He's probably right. I don't hear it except in the echo, hours or days later. In a lull, he calmed me when he acknowledged his unconscious, it was that or an apology for being late that I needed. I asked him to see that every lost minute encodes abandonment and absence, and with it comes my accusation that he causes this unspeakable suffering. This accusation finally topples him, and we are in the fight in the schoolyard dirt, punching, biting and kicking until someone, suddenly tired or frightened of the fray, summons an adult to pull us apart. The door to the waiting room opens. It is noon. We both think someone has come in. We both smile. There is—he checks —no one there. The fight is over, and I can tell him then what it is like to wait. He receives me empathically, and we have risen from the dirt, and, hearing the music of our shared history, we seamlessly begin to dance. At the end, we lingered in time—his apology, my acceptance.

We talked about sleep and EFT.

"How do you learn to sleep when you are left outside your mother's psyche?" he asked me.

"I slept when I was a teenager. I slept in college."

"Before your 'date' at Trinity?"

"Yes." And my hands fly up. "Oh god, I have such a reactive brain. I feel it, like walls of neurons cascading down, and I can't think." It is not that rape, though. We both know this. I have just entered, inexplicably, into the memory where there is no memory, into the atmospherics of memory.

Empathy. My mother's failure was a failure of empathy. I stopped him.

"Do you really feel empathy for me?' He looked slightly put on the spot.

"Yes, I do."

I apologized, knowing I should know this, but the truth was that I was surprised each time.

I had come from the oral surgeon, where he checked on the swelling overtaking my face, flooded in narcotic, strangely alone or more accurately, solitary, moving through all space as if there were no time attached. I looked for fear like a wounded animal, its wound, that raw scrape of skin, for what is gone. I go to all the familiar caves and crevices, and particularly in this altered state, I should find fear. When I don't, it's almost as if my belly tries to stir it up, to find itself again in that familiar territory. The neurons begin to fire and then, like expired fireworks, collapse into quiescence. I walked into town, slowly surprised that I felt no need to hide my grotesque face, as though I didn't inhabit it any more than I inhabited the sidewalk or the walking itself. If this were a pathological state, it would be described as depersonalization or perhaps derealization—being aware of all my surroundings but not of them. It may have been the opiate, too. I don't know why I am speaking as if this were in the past, but it probably will be. It is just another state, but it is not over yet. Arles was in the dark shadow of his hallway when I arrived, in his dark clothes and his new, darker hair. I have come in out of a perfect summer morning, and I am its air, its cloudlessness. He says something about the swelling, and I ask if it's hard to look at me.

"No," he said, "it's not".

I have lost him. He is no longer my transference projection. When I go looking for him, there is no there, there. That room is as dry as a mirage. I want to know where he'll be on vacation.

"When I need you now, it's on this plane, the plane of real geography and shared time."

"This is the last time I will be here in a body, Sebern." I felt a moment of shock, abandonment shock.

"I don't think so. I don't think so because you have not transcended the humiliation of your body. I think you will return because you are still trapped in fear. But this is Buddhist cosmology. You may be speaking from an entirely different one."

"There are other ways to be present, Sebern."

"Arles, are you an angel?"

He didn't answer and then asked, "Have you ever seen an angel, Sebern?"

"I don't know, Arles, have I?"

He smiled and said nothing.

I have moved through the pain and the swelling and the disappointment of my patients in the long, slow night hours as if it were not me. Pain is pain. Time passes in timelessness. I was given an amnesiac drug in an empty office. In and out of that drug, sleeping and waking. Being.

John has cared for me.

I asked him if he believed me, and he did not hesitate.

"Absolutely." Something in me shifted; I could feel it. The moment my mind shattered wasn't when all this was happening in the attic. It was when my parents came home, and it was as if it hadn't.

"It would've been 10 days or maybe 3. It was then that it became a lifetime." He nodded.

I gave Lori, my EFT consultant, the outline of history, and she said, kindly and bluntly, "You have suffered severe trauma." She was surprised because my affect belies this.

It is a strange experience in my good attic room, with my heating pad backing me up, to talk with a woman I have never met about assault in another attic 54 years ago. She commented on my living in an attic with some alarm. We tap and affect drains away, and I almost sleep. I could call it "fox-hole sleep" except I was unaware of any fear in the mix, just the habit of vigilance.

After my first long conversation and a brief session with Lori, my walking was oddly difficult, and I wondered why I had these large glasses on my face.

"It is over," Lori's voice said, with the assurance, perhaps even the arrogance of EFT. There were waves upon waves of attic memory. It had started in a session with Bob. "This is huge", he'd said quietly, "You will feel vulnerable," and then Arles, "Protect yourself from negative energy. You are too wide open." I have rectal pain. It subsided with tapping, but I woke up with it and called Eva. She almost couldn't hear, but then she stopped. "Please tell me, what am I missing?" and then she somehow knew what I was trying to say, what all my life I've been trying to say. It still hurts, like a puncture. The pressure, the feeling that there was something in there, has passed, but the deep bruise and pain are still there. I am wrapped in my red comforter, huddling here against what has happened, and I still feel the depths of peace within me and a new capacity to absorb peace from all the peace around me. I am able to sit with it and let it move. It is over, and it is never over, and it is as it is. I am astonished at my solidity even as I reach out for all the help I can get.

"History and memory are strange places. I think you are in a transition from that place, a place for you, necessarily, of desperation. Hold your place, it will feel new, unfamiliar." Arles was right. I am in an unfamiliar tunnel.

❧

I am working until 11 or 12 at night for this company. Strangely, it is not madness. Keeping perspective is demanding, but it is not madness. It is pure, crucial creativity and a heavy grunt. There is a fervor to it. Every day I assess it, and it is what I want to be doing. It is saving lives.

My troubled, troubled girl from Tri-County is here in her thirty-year-old version. She called me to "try this new thing you're doing." Nieves is afraid she will kill a co-worker, but it seems she's mostly afraid of going to jail if she did. She had reason to be afraid. She came to us through the tortured path of the Department of Youth Services, where one child murderer is judged to be disturbed, the next just judged. She has changed dramatically in three sessions, training her arousal down at C4. She no longer feels at risk, the "asshole" is safe from her, and she is sleeping. I thought to try just a touch at C3 for some cognitive issue, one minute at 15 - 18. She left a message on my machine at 2 in the morning. "This is worse than the worst cocaine trip I've ever been on!" She came in during my lunch hour, and we trained again at C4 around 8 - 11, and she quieted in the chair. There was a killer in this girl, and, like the sociopath in Eleanor, it's in the left hemisphere.

"You were tortured, Sebern." I don't know what to say to Lori and just nod on the phone. Maddie takes Kevy, and he takes me. I get reminders, fleeting images of scenes. My bowel feels like it will explode, and I want to pass out. Bob opened door after door, and I am left exhausted and wanting to be done. Done with being four.

Johnny called to tell us that his viral load is undetectable and that his T cell count is the highest it's been in five years. This is neurofeedback. What else, really?

I noticed again last night that all the cues for fear failed to provoke it—the dark, the cold, being alone. I felt like other people who pull on their coats and go out into the night. It wasn't hard. I had nothing to overcome. I went to buy my juice and soy milk so that I would have them in the morning. I felt no grief at the sunset. The night is just the night, and there I was, slipping into my warm boots and heading out to buy food.

Johnny is afraid again, this time that he will lose Social Security. Fear casts a huge net and pulls in all the little fishes and all the sea monsters without discrimination, and there you are, neck deep in flopping, squirmy, smelly fears.

"This is different this time; this is not a story, this life really happened to me," I said to Arles. "I have no sadness for me, but sadness wells up, and I feel it for all who must endure this. There is no me to receive it, only a large hole in memory."

It is the winter solstice, splendid with stars. I am back at Weston. I am pleased to be here, listening again to the text of their prayers, eating their food, opening to the silence. Each year, I can mark the recession of trauma. I came here beaten and bewildered, Christmas four years ago, shunned and terrified on my way to leaving The Center. But I was comforted here. Tonight, I seek no comfort. I am at peace. I sang Silent Night to the stars. I will see their sisters as I walk up the hill to morning prayer tomorrow. But I have deeper places to go, quieter and more spacious. Each brother greets me warmly. Arles said the monastic life was one of great loneliness. I look to see that because what is apparent here is company – hard work, joy in it and community. But I don't recognize the loneliness for the body of another, that is such a new loneliness in me. Some days and some moments, that is all I want, the skin-to-skin proximity of John's body.

I explored my heart cavity, this gray scooped out socket, and saw the smooth, bloodless interior. I saw my arteries and veins hanging through the fingers. I described this to Arles.

"Who tore your heart out?"

"It was a sacrifice to the appetites of men."

"What men did this to you?"

"All of them, Arles. White collar..." I trailed off.

He asked me again, soft but insistent, "What men, Sebern?"

I dropped my eyes, as if not to see. "These Black savages."

So now I want to encounter the cavity and grow the tender pink bud of heart. No further to go tonight.

Chapter 11

"Is it too much that you are for me the Spirit of God?" I asked cautiously.

"Oh, no, not at all. It is the truth of it."

The bells of Christmas. The warmth of the fire, memories of Weston. Another day of quiet and ease. And then two days after that, I will sit again with Arles and pay attention to my heart and the place between my shoulder blades that Lee cannot move. I feel blessed. I miss Johnny. I don't go close to it. I sit for you, Johnny, and for all those your torment torments. Your father and I are no longer tormented. We are often, not at the same time, angry, sad and apprehensive of the next crisis.

A morning of gold. Deep snow in the woods and memories of our celebration last night. The hour of sitting in which I turned to Metta, a new name on each breath. Then the glass of Korbel and eating the last piece of our cake, muting the TV to keep track of the time, dancing to Bridge Over Troubled Waters and feeling a sense of fusion with his body, the active desire for absorption, for protection, to protect. We dance our vow or more truly, our deep experiential expectation that we are with each other, around each other, increasingly within each other and that this is enough safety. I read him all I wrote about our ceremony. He lay his head on my stomach. I stroked his beautiful head, and soon we were asleep in our beds, next to each other but separate. We will give up the beds passed down and buy a king.

I was watching a bluejay outside my kitchen window when I heard the snowplow coming down the road, and I wondered how the jay heard it —louder, threatening, or more dull? How was the same moment in time, the identical stimulus processed in his brain? I wanted to know the limit to my understanding, the capacity of one brain to know another. I want to know, what could dissolve this barrier?

John just called to tell me that everything is pointing to him as the next president. This is all dramatic and important, but the very instrument that can establish the soul in a person threatens to deprive me of my inner life. His voice is strong, and he is tender. He is with me.

I am experiencing object loss. This is a new feeling and so blindly named as "object." I don't know what to want. "I want my life back" is the call, and "this is my life" is the response. I want John here with me. I want John to run the company. I want John to find someone else to run the company. I want to go with him to California. I don't want to leave my patients. I don't want to leave Arles. I would love working with Sue and writing with Siegfried. It is complicated and compelling. I have put everything on the line for this technology.

I am standing in the beautiful kitchen, looking around to make preparations to abandon our house, and I feel unsettled by the chords of fear playing in my belly. John is on the phone in an executive committee meeting. The cats who have finally made peace with each other may not live together again. John and I may be separated for the better part of next year. We may need to invite a stranger to care for our home, or mice will make nests under the pillows. We are both aware of our near infinite vulnerability. It is a momentous day, both lonely and inevitable. We are caught in a strong tide. Partly we are the moon, partly the driftwood. I will miss John. I will miss him with me, and I will miss knowing he is here, loving his home, caring for it with the same tenderness and frustrations he has with the cats. They will come and live with me. I am packing Bridge Over Troubled Waters and listening to

Respeggi to soothe the troubling tempos in my chest. We will be fine, him and me, but less fine, each of us on our own. I am afraid. I am not afraid. We won't fail, but much is at risk. I will take care of myself; my kids will help me. Arles and I will take one step on the ground and then the next.

We cleared out the refrigerator, sorted bills from receipts; old bills from new ones, washed the last of eight loads of laundry, collected the trash, filled the water jug, cleaned off his bureau and mine and my desk; he finished the second of two meetings—three this weekend. The first was interrupted by an earthquake, a 4.3 that temporarily shook Sue. Almost 6 hours in total: staging, loading laundry, packing my suitcase, his clothes for the next six weeks, a suitcase for his trip to Cuba, the groceries, the cat gym, cat food, kitty litter, trash, water bottle, Zoe and Mieka. We were short one cat carrier, so we taped the little one into a Westatt box. We were expecting snow, sleet, and freezing rain. John followed me in. The cats made it without incident and clearly knew where they were. Mieka was a little clingy, and Zoe stretched out. I only slept until 2:45 and felt wide awake and a little sick from no sleep. It could be just the familiar cycle of insomnia; it could be the disruption of this leaving. I woke up speedy. Three sleeping pills didn't affect me. I am more disrupted than afraid. I don't even feel unquiet, but sleep is not coming back.

He and I talked about my sense of self as fragments in the dark, an endless universe pulled together by the centrifugal force of regulation and why that does not seem to be true in my body. I described it to Arles as a weak force at the periphery and, because of him, a strong force in the center.

"A core!" I exclaimed to him at the moment of discovery. "You gave me a core. There is an empty space between the core and the periphery. I could fill it up with organs. I could bathe them in gold light, but there's also nothing there. Except my heart."

"What is it like for your heart in this emptiness?"

"Scorpion's heart, the star Enterus, blue-red pulsing star like that. When it was the same for my mind as it is now for my body, I was at the edge of madness." He became a strong force, and he has drawn the lines, star to star, in the Milky Way.

Brain injury. It is hard to get outside your brain, but this is what is beginning to happen. I have enough gaps in this dysfunction to recognize how hard I work. Bob referred me for a consultation to a more senior PT. When he put his hands on my head, he asked, "How do you function? If you were a kid with a map like this, you would be in a Special Ed classroom on Ritalin or Dilantin." After the PT session today, it felt like my brain was wobbling on weak knees and my feet felt numb. I can't organize the way I think. I can't get things right, and I am always afraid that something else is true, that I am actually getting worse even as I get better.

"The only redemption is to make it into art."

"That is along the lines of what I have been thinking as you were talking. What about your book?" He is feeling free about it and unafraid.

"I'm not outside of it enough yet. It would mean encountering all of this again."

"I understand. It is important what happened here," Arles said. "It is essential."

I leave for FutureHealth in Miami, and I will see our troubled son there. It's hard looking at the schedule to see exactly when I'll get outside. I just want to be here in the snowy gray north with its sedate winter aloneness. It all seems too loud where I'm headed. My life has changed for good.

How do I talk about Neurofeedback in 10 minutes? I've been invited onto the panel at the Networker Conference "New Visions of Psychotherapy." It is the newest of visions and one which changes for me as my own brain turns another new corner. I hear sound in stereo now. I hear instruments and sounds I've never heard. I can feel riveted to the sensation as if sound is diving into my pleasure center and kicking up, laughing. I listen to the Beatles, and I can hear where each one is on the stage. A new protocol, P5-P6, for the auditory cortex.

He became aware of a subtle difference as we talked. My voice is overtaken by my mother's voice when I speak of business. I organize myself around that pulse of energetic experience, around that power—my successful, popular, impenetrable mother—, and he feels the impossibility of it and says quietly and hopelessly, "Why bother." I see his face now, the darkened beauty of his eyes, the reality of his separate mind, his struggle with the power he experiences in me, all of his associations to class and his own striving, hearing too much about neurofeedback, wanting to be recognized too. He becomes multi-dimensional, and I am beginning to see and begin to learn to trust this person, Arles.

Reggie said, "I desire nothing." I had said the same earlier to Arles. He asked if this was my mother's disconnection or Buddha nature. I was a little dazed by the question. This state, even in its lapses, does not feel regular; ordinary but not regular.

"Do you feel held by the company? Have you handed your infant self into these corporate arms?"

I had wondered that too last February when both he and the company went under the knife. I was not able to save him, but no matter what meaning the coincidence held for me, I would have joined to save the company. All I needed was that call from Siegfried, "Well," he'd said to start the call, "the dream is dead."

"I don't need to be held," I said. "There is nobody in this state, just particles of memory, with near infinite space between them. The space is empty. I have no desire. When all of these particles are drawn together, when they are compressed, I feel that I inhabit a self."

"That's true, isn't it?" he said as if coming in from stage right. "You do not need to be held." He paused briefly. "This could be misconstrued as part of your attachment dilemma or as emotional aloofness. Or it could all be true at once." He will never comprehend how important he has been to me in the elemental, core creation of self that went on in that dark room. And I will never fully understand how alone he was, his poignant statement, "I had no place to take it," through all those years. Arles. Me.

Lee had asked me how old I was when I stopped crying for my mother.

"It is a terrible question," I said, telling him about it.

He smiled gently and said, "Like a terrible flash of light."

"Like a nuclear explosion."

"Yes," he said, "like a nuclear explosion." There I was knowing that Lee had to overcome her hopelessness, and what in me made Arles say, "Why bother?" I am sitting in the Haymarket in the booth behind three people writing a grant for ServiceNet, and I feel a strange compassion for their ignorant repetition of what has never worked. I am so glad to be out of there, that whole terrible delusional world of mental health. My brain has felt like a litter of kittens in a burlap sack.

Reggie talked about seeing her mother on impulse and seeing her for real. She was scared, and she kept waiting for the terrible impact, but there was none.

"It is not about forgiveness, really," she said, "it just is." Her face was clear, and her eyes were steady as she looked directly into the face of her mother's madness. "I didn't cause it. I am free of all the 'what if's'. I could have done nothing that woulda changed it."

The tragedy of mental illness is that the brain's adaptation entombs the mind. It is a world closed in on itself like a planetarium that has been shut for the night: the lights turned off, the janitor's gone home. All there is to see in the shadows are the girders and the gears, the proof of a terrible constraint. It is a structure that can open itself, offer itself to the stars, and be as one with infinity. Instead, we bump it up against our bony, sharp skulls relentlessly, as if the interior bone were the truth of existence. I think of Eleanor most particularly on the night she was walking the dog and, for the first time in her life, stopped and looked up at the stars. I seem to oscillate in and out of these realities, between the closing and the opening of the skull. My left shoulder comes into being, and my head spins.

I want only to sit in the sun. I want only to listen to Arles's heart. I only want to be the Grand Canyon.

"You wanted to get to know those kittens, too."

"Yes, these poor kittens. Otherwise, they are doomed." I paused and looked up at him. "We are all stray kittens, Arles. One will get picked up and live in a house in Brookline; one will roam feral and cold; one will die. Who decides this? They are all cute and all black."

❧

There was fog from the forlorn cranberry bog at Onset Bay and one lane of traffic across the bridge. Before and after, the traffic was fine, light, it seemed to me, for Easter. I kept looking for the feelings I expected to feel. Big memories of the tortured drives down here, the deep sadness leaving, the misery I would inflict on my family when I got home. None arose. My heart is light with the other memories of her last nine months, of the new beauty that enlivened her.

I am here to make peace with the house and talk to her through her dreams, to assure her that it is OK to let it go. There are no nightmares here in this passing on. I told Blake today that Mom is not returning my calls. I can't summon her voice to reassure me. I can remember her words, her ambivalence, her wish that I keep the house, her permission to sell it if that made sense, and my wish not to sell it, to keep her little house, to care for it.

"It is not good," I told Arles, "to die believing that no one holds you in their mind. She died that way."

"My mother too," he said.

"Many people."

"Yes, many people."

"That's what I think is at issue here. She can imagine people remembering the house. She can remember the house. If her rebirth was as a being who dreams, she dreams of this house, and it comforts her. She didn't know I loved her, that I would think of her every day, that I would always see her doing her Tai Chi forms in the den in the sunlight two weeks before she died."

The Tao is here. There is no hot water. The boiler is falling apart, the daffodils are blooming, and I miss her. Yesterday was the fourth anniversary of her death. She is 85 in this life frame. I wonder where she is. She's out of reach. She's not avoiding me. She is re-engaged with living and is just scared to turn over this house to anyone but me. Molly suggested this, and I brought tulips. She said I had to quiet my mother's fears. The tulips are for her and for me. And I have the jellybeans that Blake bought for me at Sweeties before we walked back to Elizabeth Street, before I packed the car and came here.

It is Easter, and I am sitting in her bed with my green tea, looking at the yellow tulips in the blue vase and out to the gray shingled backyards of Summer Street. The upscale oversized cars are spilling onto the street after Easter services at the church. I feel no draw to church, to ritual or to belief. Nor to buffets or baked scrod or family gatherings. I feel only the need for deep quiet, long episodes of silence and birdsong.

Baths in the deep, clawfoot tub were my only comfort here. All kinds of things have gone wrong since we put the house on the market: an ice flood, a condemned heating system, a vernal pool in the kitchen after heavy rains, a dead mouse in the toilet when the realtor showed the house, a gas leak from the stove, a broken vent pipe like that. Sitting in the tepid water, I started to cry. It felt, suddenly, that what might have endured her death is her resentment, that she will not let me sell this house. Whenever my mother was generous with me, which was often, there was a cost to her that I had to pay. She resented giving the gift; she perceived only ingratitude, and she demeaned whoever took it. I smashed my fists into the water, "Why do you hate me?" And I think of when I did not gather her up at the airport, an act that could never be repaired. In the midst of my outburst, I see her beautiful face in the last months, how deeply we were able to love one another, and while drying off, the betrayal of the tub becomes what it probably is, all just a coincidence. But Blake had enough hot water for showers for herself, and three friends, and the hot water heater looks fine. It goes on like this. I don't know where she is. I imagine her reborn somewhere warm. Actually, for some reason, I think she is a beautiful coffee-cream-colored little girl with a ring on her toe, happy and spirited. This morning, Easter

2001, she seems innocent of all the mischief and even perhaps of the clinging. She can let go into her new beginnings, wherever they are, eating mango or swimming alongside the whales. She can look into the deep brown eyes of her grandfather and the smiling eyes of her gentle mother and let go into them. She's unfamiliar with eyes; they will need to help her. But she no longer needs this little house on the chilly Cape. She is not alone anymore; I remember her. She splashes out of the aqua water and runs up on the beach to drop into her mother's lap. They think she is a wonder. They think one day she will go to America. When she dreams, she dreams of this house, not of her mother or of me. It seemed in the bath, in my own little nightmare, a house that I will be forced to care for until I die. And then there is the Tao. I have no idea what is happening. It just is.

John is working for the company in LA. Johnny is hospitalized after several near psychotic episodes, one of which landed him at the Institute. Blake is being broken into social work and is also quite separately very much in love. Molly works too hard for too little, and her boys are fine. I miss John. We are all OK but tired, working too hard and too much. The scope of this neurofeedback endeavor is almost terrible; it is so important. I just want to peacefully say goodbye to this house and reassure my mother that I will hold her forever in my heart. The house does not answer me. At one moment, it feels unyielding, at another neutral and mute, at another, all the lives lived here, absorbed into its cells, vibrate. 1824. Jefferson might have still been alive, and Lincoln was a teenage boy already brewing his madness and his determination. There was no slave trade in this house—for some reason, this is clear to me—but we were a nation trading in slaves. I am coming to understand the lasting wound of slavery in my bones. It has marked us as deeply as the Holocaust has marked Germany, but it is even more deeply denied.

I had eruptions throughout the day, just shouting and cursing, noticing and not noticing and then I was caught in a tirade with John. I was swearing and making accusations, and somewhere, I was a calm witness to it all. I knew I was being irrational. I could watch myself recruit narratives to give these rants both fuel and meaning, knowing they were not true, and I couldn't stop. It was not my unconscious; it was not anything we would hand it off to, it was my brain on a tear. I wasn't frightened by it either, but I was amazed, like anyone in a car on ice as they spin off down into the divide.

Tonight, I am wearing my mom's flannel nightgown with the blue stripes for the last time. It is torn beyond repair at the right shoulder. I hold it to my face, hoping for one last hint of her scent. She is still in this fabric. She'd be creamy and bundled under her quilt, watching TV, dozing, waiting for me when I'd drive down after work. She was pleased to see me, and at the end, I was pleased to see her too. She had stopped setting tiger traps. She wore it to breakfast the morning of her death, so it carries the knowledge that she seemed to have. Tomorrow I will take a swatch from it as a gift to Anne, who is beginning to sew her robes for her ordination. This would deeply please her and deeply pleases me. It will be hard to do.

On Wednesday, Sabelle came in after two hard days overtaken by jealous rage. She had performed a wake. "This part of me is so damaged it will not heal. It has to die." She imagined a little tormented girl in a coffin, finally deceased. Tears rolled off her cheeks. I was moved to be in the presence of an astounding psychic process. We lit a candle to honor her as we would a POW or survivor of the Holocaust. Of course, I think we don't really honor these people except for a brief moment, and then they, too, are forgotten. But I will never forget this part of Sabelle, I have known her too long. We have yet to know if it has really happened all the way down, all the way across, completely. There will be a change, but I am learning that no one is ever really dead.

Arles and I were talking about what it has meant for us that my parents were not sadistic.

"...and things didn't suddenly turn to madness," I said it; I left him. My brain fired wildly, and I could not raise an image. He shifted in his chair. He was coming to rescue me. I saw him as he reached down to pick my body up off the floor. I was slippery with sweat, in white cotton underpants. He stood in the midst of the wreckage and looked around, taking it in. He was not angry. He was not overwhelmed. He held me quietly with only the faintest sadness and then slowly carried me down the stairs. The inquiry stops at the bottom of the stairs; the light changes from gray to white, and the episode is over. My brain is quiet.

On Thursday, I joined a reunion of the Order of Interbeing at the Green Mountain Dharma Center. All of the questions to Thầy were really "please, take care of me, see me, I am suffering, I am abandoned." I had no question or any need for one. I felt open-hearted to the suffering of my sisters and brothers, but I was not there anymore. I don't need Thầy. I went there only to see him, to let him see me, to know that the practice has taken in me and to love him. I wanted to see who he was, to understand, if I could, the man who makes missteps, to see if I could still trust him. He asked us to gather close to him on the lawn, and he talked about walking in the kingdom of God. He moved around the circle, "The kingdom of God is in a flower." As he said this, I was saying, "And in the lines of your face, beneath your eyes." He has always diverted his eyes the second they came across mine. In that circle, this time, he let his eyes rest on my face.

Driving home, I saw a young moose crossing 91, loping over the newly turned field and into the suburbs of Brattleboro. I had been with the Buddha and knew that I still felt strangely, distantly sad.

❧

"I can see all the pieces, but I can't put them together. I can string them like beads along a choker, a narrative, but then I don't stop until there is a new topic. I can't stop and see all of these fragments as a whole."

"What would happen?" he asked without the hard edge of curiosity. I could say first what would not happen.

"I would not go mad; I would not dissociate. I don't think I'd even feel fear. It is the place before dissociation, before it takes form as feeling. It is where the psychological is only neurological. It is that level of disorganization. If I brought all of these elements together in one picture, I would risk status epilepticus. My brain would never recover equilibrium." I realize only as I am writing that I risked seeing the elemental structure of fear without affect; I risked knowing what I experienced at its core, but without the picture, without the affect key to turn it on, I am at no risk at all. The brain stays quiet; the kittens nestle in together and sleep.

When I say I am sad and he asks me about it, I do not feel it for myself. I think surely that must be its source, but when I go there, it isn't me. It is the sorrow of the world, of every human life, and the icon is immediately a Black boy, his bewilderment, his being beaten down, humiliated and hated. It is not me, and it is not female. If I took the time and kept my attention, I could see every soul alive, billions of faces and lives and circumstances. They are, I said, like city lights or like billions of stars. But when I look to include myself, when I go to where my star should be, I get dark matter; there is a hole there. I was born hoping that when I saw my mother's face, I would see myself there, and when I didn't, the implosion began. Until Arles, until training my brain, I did not materialize.

I will see my patients tomorrow and then fly to LA. John will be there to meet me.

I skipped the board meeting. I didn't want to leave the restless harbor of my bed. The meeting with Sue and Siegfried had gone well. Both were warm and reasonable. I said my piece. I reminded them of our interdependence, of the importance of mentioning their gratitude—we often mention ours—and it seemed reasonable to me that they own 30% of the company. I speak only for myself. I am in no actual position of power. I am trusting the process and staying home, trusting the board, leaving this to someone else. I don't want to manage the company. I want to think about how to write the first book. I want to rest and make love to John, watch the mallards preen on the rock, secure in their instinctual monogamy. They must think they have found paradise. I swam this morning and had the small pool to myself. I feel at home here, but I couldn't live here, either in this complex or in the state. I am claustrophobic in these rooms, and outside of them, it is too hard to leave. John drove me the back way through the astounding mountain passes to get downtown, well, to Encino. I am here with these demands that keep me away from myself.

Flying here was easy. The sun was setting in Nebraska. The clouds looked like dinosaur backbones, then rivers, then mountains and beneath them another hidden blue range. Champagne, Emmylou Harris and the clouds, feet up on the bulkhead. I didn't care to be anywhere else. The laundry is in the dryer, the bed is made, I am leading this domestic life in Agoura Hills while history once again is made and perhaps hearts broken at 16500 Ventura. John will be back when he is. That's what he said as he kissed me goodbye this morning.

I asked John what age he was in his deepest core identity. Anywhere, he said, from late twenties to 40. He asked me, and finally it seemed that the age we are is the age at which we know we will die and also feel that life unfolds endlessly before us. That is the age we are internally in the body, and that seems to go with being a young adult. If you don't hold that stasis, perhaps it is then that you begin to age. "No, you always age," John said, "It is then that you begin to fold."

The peonies have lived out most of their short lifespan and bowed to the pelting rain, all their beauty spilled and splattered on the grass. There is no way to shelter them and no way of knowing if they might have wished that. It is the first impulse when their petals look like wounds.

There had been a black coat thrown on the floor. It was a fight I walked into.

"The coat on the floor wasn't Moses." I dropped down in some atmosphere of time.

"No", he said, watching me, "it was Maddy."

I couldn't retract enough, or pull far enough into the pillows, or hide my face or rid myself of the sense that I was an ugly buck-toothed four-year-old with gray hair. It is its own kind of seizure, and then it passes. He left for the bathroom but stopped and touched the top of my head, accepting my gray hair and, in that simple touch, acknowledging all this girl suffered. When he came back, he sat next to me to steady my rapid ascent.

"This arises and passes away. It is as if a small chink of my flesh is cut away and floats down a river until, at the end, I will have no body left at all." He was uncomfortable with the image but then understood it: no self; no suffering.

Gathering myself up to go to visit Eva, I recognized feeling mostly absent, that I lacked essential resources, resources that others had. It is about confidence in the reliability of my brain to perform functions like getting onto the Pike in the right direction, knowing the route, calculating or missing signals of other cars, knowing that the curb is too close, mixing up the signs, suddenly losing all the markers, orientation in space and time, left and right disappearing again, the radio jamming the circuit so I cannot navigate in traffic. I have all of these resources increasingly reliably, but they still fail me unpredictably, and it is this, historically and presently, that can make me a little scared to go out into the world. I still surprise myself when I meet new people. I am no longer awkward, scuttling away from the terrible stimuli of newness, particularly the demanding new person, or the often more demanding encounter with the person I already know. I feel all the impulses subtly to leave before I make the mistakes that will leave me at their mercy. But mostly I am unafraid, open and curious about them. It is as if I bring no history of my own to the encounter, or more precisely, no need to bring my history to bear, to insinuate it into the possibility of intimacy. I haven't been able, quite, to fully inhabit the Now. I couldn't quite stay in the small talk. I would notice it too much, all its punctuation and its detours and my slight impatience with the commerce of daily conversation. And yet my body finally settled into the idleness of looking at the endless sky through the skylight and at her cat's amazing pink nose, and talking of people, of gardens, of nothing at all.

I dreamt of Blake as a forgotten, disturbed foster child. Dreams are fears and wishes. Dreams are always of the self.

Arles asked me to sense into the back of my heart.

"It doesn't look like the rest of my heart, which is rounded and ridged and appropriately muscular. It looks pink like the rest, but it is flat like a skin drawn over an instrument. It is new growth over the whole back of the heart. It is not filling up a hole, and it's not a patch."

"Is it sensitive?"

"It's like a bat's wing, sensitive and strong but new and not yet rounded. I want to go into all of my life wholeheartedly. I have times when I feel no fear, and that's where I want to live." He listened, his legs stretched out toward where I sat. "If I am truly unafraid of death, why am I afraid of memory?" I ask this of myself out loud and answer it, "Maybe because these memories are housed in the chamber that is devoted to fear. They come permeated and wrapped in the membrane of that nucleus. I am not afraid of them, but they are of fear. They must be fear of death," and then I had a different thought. They didn't have to fear death, these quick flashes. Then I felt that odd collapse between my eyes, beneath them, into grey time.

What I felt last night was awful but familiar. The images that came unbidden as the century turned, and primary control mechanisms were predicted to fail. No escape. No thoughts of death because you are faced with no end. One moment of human folly, one careless hate-filled moment, one lapse in cause and effect and the precious jewel, this extraordinary work of creation, orbits as a cinder. The leaves blown off, trees splintered, human flesh and soul, perhaps too, in such heat, evaporate. Hiroshima, but no inch untouched. All that comes now comes unbidden. Neither welcomed nor unwelcomed, but unsought. My unconscious, though, keeps pushing this up and out, and I try to understand my cooperation—why I do this. I do believe that this kind of malignant energy will lodge in my body and make me sick, but this is not the motivation. Strangely, all of the other motivations seem to have disappeared. Perhaps it is for me as inevitable as rocks pushing up to the surface of the New England soil, and even more quickly when the soil is tilled. It is not my process anymore, and it can't be opposed.

My friend Spike, who knows about such things, told me that it is better not to filter your water because when you do, it retains the memory of the pollutants in concentrated form. Like homeopathy dilutes and dilutes at every turn, becoming more powerful until, at its most powerful dilution, it becomes only pure water. We talked about this as analog. I have talked about everything—torture, rape, molestation, bullying, alcohol, maternal neglect, maternal depression, maternal invasion, maternal absence, my extinction, my deadness, her hatred, her generosity, her resentment, her obliviousness, Kevy's and Hugh's deaths, my father's, my responsibility for his death, Johnny, AIDS, my marriage, dissociation, unbearable hunger, brain injury, seizure, near death, wealth, class, privilege, drugs, coma, seclusion, abuse by therapists, Charlie, my practice, Thầy, Buddhism, Christianity, righteousness, dreams and prescience—the full catastrophe. The endless, terrible landscape of no mother—that holocaust. And at times I know what is left: a core darkness, shrinking but powerful enough that when it is active it devours the light that comes up to its edge, and I can't disperse it. It's been active. And there is also the image of the wormhole. Arles has identified this for me, and that this timelessness does end in some experience of time. The blackberry flowers at the very end of the vine are holding against their inevitable conversion into berries. The rest have already experienced their transformations. So, this is where I am, in some late end stage of powerful dilution with moments of knowing the possibility of pure water.

Four psychologists on the board is probably a mistake. Sue wants the power required to maintain and enhance her vision. Siegfried wants to repay his debts, to discharge his humiliation and to reestablish his self-esteem. There is fear that Sue's joining with Siegfried will leave them open to his irrational fears and erratic behavior. He had said he always fired his bosses. And there is gender. Neurofeedback, in its practice, embodies the female principle, the relational. It is delivered in the domain of the male, the engineer. For me, it is about the capacity of the regulated brain to love. And in that room, they are at war over this. They have the future of the world in their hands, and they are fighting because they are afraid. Just like I am, I will breathe and speak in low tones to John to soothe whatever needs soothing.

"I needed to be born to my mother. There was no mistake. The passage into, in, through, and out of her provided a very particular transmission, one I needed. Her genetics, more hers somehow, at least at the moment, than my father's, her cellular memory, infused my foundational being, and it needed to be hers." I felt a little stunned by how clear this was to me. I feel the clear channel, and as soon as there is an impingement or a blockage, I stop as if the river of thought is taking its time to find its new route, pooling in its momentary confusion, then the new channel, or not. But the process has a physicality to it, and it's oddly pleasurable. It is not that this changes all the constructions and knowing that is my mother to me, this discovery does not erase her absence. It doesn't, in some sense, even make her more present to me. There is no more substance to her than I had felt before. This discovery is of the impersonal in her person, the matrix of her isness within mine. It is not the discovery of introject or incorporation. This is not about her within me as much as it is about the inevitable cellular transfusion in conception and even more profoundly, somehow, in the uterine–psychic passage. Her being and all that it held was a precondition, not only the pelvic vessel. All of her shaped me." I stopped and looked at my feet. "I know this already, and I can't take this in," I said, frustrated, almost mumbling to myself.

"What is 'it'?" he wanted to know, "What are you telling me?"

"That I needed to be born to her. That she was the right mother. That I needed her cellular transmission. There must be an analog in physics or in astronomy. It feels as if I am pelted by innumerable particles of her, and my molecules form in this process. It is almost, in thinking this way, that I can feel the squeeze of the birth canal, the tender linings, my almost skin and infusion of her cells. The last pass that my mother's internal body has at its creation. It is not an inert passage. Tight at the top of my arms, pressure on my head, my being, being rubbed up against her most unguarded, most raw. I had hope then, I can sense this. Hope... life force gathered there in the pressure, during the last act of infusion. I have always had hope even at the moments I don't."

"What was your hope, Sebern?"

"To see my face in hers."

Something crashed overhead. I contracted, time collapsed.

"It just has to pass," I said, tears streaming into my hands, the nearly wild, wildly repeated apologies. I am not anywhere. The sound is from the attic. Once the thud registers, I am helpless to the replay; neurological law registers like a somber player-piano. I am not in the attic but of the attic, and it's terrible. Arles sits next to me to remind me of him, to remind me of the reality of place and time; of me.

"It was not just the attic. You had no buffer from sound anywhere."

My mother's lack of density, her impenetrable lack of density.

HYPERBARIC OXYGEN 2

It is the thick early beginning of August. A small group of tired and dirty migrants was harvesting tobacco leaves in the swelter. I saw them on both legs of my drive to the Blue Heron for an elegant brunch. Rae commented on my state of impatience, something she's not seen for a long time. I have started hyperbaric oxygen therapy, and I've been experiencing flashes of memory over the last few days, brief, intense and vivid but also encapsulated. I mostly remember that I have them, they are not all about childhood, but most, and the others about madness.

I swam tonight in the dark river and looked up at Mars and the moon rising and knelt on the sand bottom, offering up my stillness and my gratitude for all the gems, for the presence of my body in the river, for the quality of peace in me that I can almost take for granted, for all the people I love and all the others that I could love. I came back wrapped only in my towel, unafraid. My skin smells of clean river water. I have begun my second week of hyperbaric. I spent the day with Jamie, working on her ad, looking at brain maps and affirming what a good soul she is.

Arles is afraid that this might be a terrible cure.

"There's something different about you, ever since you started the oxygen. It is as though you have a diminished psyche and more personality. Personality lacks the richness of your psychic process."

I know what he is saying and have no words for it and no need to find words for it until he says something, and then I engage again with psyche. But I have to search the palette for colors, hue and tone—all of it feels external to me. I don't know what axis this psyche turns on. If I am no longer pivoting around a history of torment, then what contours will my brain have, what will my psyche be? I am in transition, but perhaps to no psyche: non-self and nothing that observes non-self. Who is to say? It is as if thousands of neurons pop awake; there they are, stunned that they are no longer stunned, with a consciousness of their own, memory of their own. They have been near death while all those around them have been incorporating, expressing and forming my experience. What is the memory of their dormancy? Do they know nothing else but suspension and quietude? Jamie imagines that we are healing the limbic brain, and that could well be. Fear drains out on every exhale, cells stunned into silence by trauma—as I was—come awake in a world that is not alarmed. Whatever memory of trauma they hold seems encapsulated, too weak perhaps to trigger a CNS response. The smell and heat of an iron held up to my face and perhaps to my feet, but it's the smell. And then the thin trace that we would go down to the kitchen to eat sometimes—the strangest sensation is that the light changes from gray to white. The sense is that they ordered food from Gristede's market. I have never remembered that my mother had an account there and ordered her groceries by phone. Why would I?

"Perhaps, it has to do with something other than psyche, with something approaching enlightenment."

He weighed in heavily and carelessly, preoccupied by the call he had to make, disoriented by the inexplicable state changes in me.

"There is no sign of enlightenment," he said. "If cells were waking up, why wouldn't there be joy," as if joy were the only or even the best celebration of life. And he went on like that until he caught up with himself and apologized.

"I am perhaps mourning the loss of something that I think has been unique to you, your enthusiasm." And this could not be denied. Even at the very worst, beneath every breath I have had some element of enthusiasm. I am not apathetic.

Right now, I am in a state of brain. My psyche may be, as Arles fears, foreclosed to me, but I think about this differently. My brain is focused on itself. This is the transitional nature of oxygen waking cells up, cells that all have memory of me and only their microscopic part and of my mother and father and on back, and forward too to my daughter. What have they retained in their dormancy? Have they missed encoding major events? Are they each as innocent as the coma patient opening her eyes, no clue where or who she is? The brain is focused on itself and has no attention left to make up a psyche. Or perhaps this is this form of psyche. I have two images. I am in a white plastic inner tube with neon fish on it, bobbing in a vast ocean. The water is dark and warm and calm. I am aware where I am, aware that the weather could turn, aware that there are potential predators below, and I am unafraid. Arles is able to see me, and I am seeing myself from the same vantage point—way up in the sky, up to the right. I am alone, and although I can be seen, there is no one who knows this experience. When I say this out loud to him, I expect to feel fear, and I don't.

"Do you understand? I am not afraid!" Fear is what follows, "I'm all alone, but it isn't there!"

It comes as a surprise. He nods. He understands this, or at least that this must be. And the other image.

"If you were looking at my psyche, all you would see is a smooth white wall, like the walls of the Aegean, but no marks, nothing at all inscribed on it. When I have experienced being brand new before, it has always been contoured by affect—protest, confusion, fear, or enthusiasm. I knew the shape of the newness because of the effect around it, molding it. Now I have no contours. Just the white unshaded wall."

Arles misses the sweeps of grief and enthusiasm, the accents of torment, my deep subcortical drive to know my own mind. These affective markers signify psyche, and they are gone. Everything seems muted—I am drawn in muted colors—and I am unfamiliar. And then he said,

"I think you are right about everything you are saying. We cannot try to fit this experience into pre-existing paradigms. Who knows what this is?" And I felt my breath become easier and a slight quickening of gratitude. It is no doubt a brain in transition, but it will not leave me the old psyche to return to. It will transform it, and the transformation that began long before hyperbaric is from fear to fearlessness.

My handwriting has deteriorated. It feels very noticeable to me and a little disturbing. I can't remember having reacted to it like this before. It is as if I can't stand any indication of my primary dysregulation. Today, Arles agrees. He thought my brain was so busy attending to itself that it did not have the energy remaining to attend to the psyche.

I careened softly off the walls of the staircase going up from Lee's room, disoriented and dizzy for almost half an hour. "It's a little like the old days, Lee." She was surprised. She had focused on my heart, and it felt as if I were time traveling, metal or glass prisms of experience all together but minutely distinct, as if my heart were a flattened disco ball and each little flat section encoded a different experience. Several places riveted my brain, mostly frontal and prefrontal. The left back side of my brain got cold, the kind of cold you feel in a cave. At one place, I lost all awareness of any separation between mind and body; there was no observer, only experience and then in that state, evidently, I fell asleep. I was aware only of the suspension of any boundary between states. My shoulder discharged in little jerks, which I remembered mostly because Lee asked. At times, my shoulder ached, with pain down my arm. With this, a wash of sensation from left to right in my brain, I would have expected dissociation, but I did not dissociate. This wash feels like a challenge, tiring more than relaxing, demanding—place to place, jerk, screech, time to time, plummet, roll, rise and fall. I asked Lee about her experience. "As soon as it started," she said, "my image was when I was in Finland, in the winter, going into the dark. But specifically, it was a place I visited, an underground church."

I hugged Jamie goodbye.

"We will really miss you. It's not often that we have a Buddha in our midst." I have just finished my last dive in this round. I ended it with a blessing to all the cells of my body and a deepening appreciation of what has happened here. I am not afraid even of the gray, thick air or the man coming up behind me. They held no charge at all.

"I don't have the words to tell you, Arles."

"There may be no words, Sebern. It's OK. Being quiet may be the most important thing. It may be the only thing."

"I wonder if you were in the presence of the Dalai Lama in a small group, if you would feel more his non-attachment to feeling or his love?" Eva asked me over breakfast.

"I don't know if I know the difference, Eva. My heart does not burst with love. I am not in the absence of love, but I don't feel that in my heart."

"What does it feel like to have your attachment history and then to be in this state of non-attachment? To be here without the early experience of being loved. This is the difference between us. I had that. You didn't have that until late in your life."

"I just don't know." I have entered a vacuum of words.

I shut off the computer, turned out the lights and stepped outside. The density of the light, the quality of color at the top of the trees, beckons to me to go beyond my original errand, and I walk. The sky beyond the fields threw up mounds of clouds, the sky of the Renaissance painter, pink and pearly. Color and form in perfection. Two young men and a girl were playing at batting and catching, and I wandered past them into the fairgrounds. The Three County Fair opens tomorrow. The trailers are parked, the community of grifters, class B race horses and fried dough makers is settling in. The purple van with black polka dots is as yet undeclared. The two Black teenage gofers on their two-wheelers, one with dreadlocks and one wearing chaps. I was amazed at myself, walking into this Third World of roustabouts, and no trace of fear or feeling of being out of place. These are America's gypsies. For the most part, they seemed not to see me, busy as they were setting down track for some vertical ride that's undoubtedly maimed or killed at least one child in every 100 county fairs. There was not one inch of beauty. The Ferris wheels were spectacular and not as gaudy as the rest, but nothing could be seen as beautiful. The air was a soft, breathable liquid, languid, like the feel of warm river water over your naked body, a sensual invitation to stay outside as late as possible. I turned a corner at the Farm-A-Rama and there I was in the center of the garish, repetitive, meaningless spectacle, and it was quiet. It was in preparation. The boy stripped to the waist, blonde hair over his eyes, tubercular, potentially menacing, walked by, maybe heading for town, getting out. I did not venture further in. The rides were circled wagons. On the walk home, inside lights were on, and I could see the dens or TV rooms that someone had added, the pride, I thought, of their home. Country curtains, plaid furniture, knick-knacks. The densest core of any culture is its kitsch.

My brain and its processes feel like silk sliding over silk. Another new universe, this oxygenated brain.

With Lee, I had felt the exact spot where it tore and where it felt like he would take my arm off. Bob measures my external rotation. The baseline was 48°, today, 77°. Gains on internal rotation as well. The oxygen is healing my shoulder, and history ebbs out.

9/11

I was on the phone with Bill at Broadside Books, ordering a book of maps for our trip to Mali. He apologized for asking me to spell the name of the publisher for the third time. I laughed a little. "The news on the radio is a little distracting," he said. I asked what was happening. "You haven't heard?!" It was 10:15 on Tuesday morning, September 11th. "Three terrorist attacks— both towers of the World Trade Center, the Pentagon and a crash landing in a field outside of Pittsburgh." I hung up and turned on the TV. Like all of us, Peter Jennings seemed stunned, devastated, grief-stricken, and even bewildered. I took it in, and after a while, I heard myself say, "This is infinitesimal, a spark of consciousness that, like the cell, holds all the information of the cosmos." I was quiet and open-hearted.

Sabelle came for her session, and we walked for two hours, ending up at the Red Cross. Sadly, they will not need our blood. Everyone is dead or escaped. There is constant reference to "body parts." In one moment, we have up to 1 million new cases of PTSD, thousands of orphans, widows, and widowers, bankruptcy and war.

I reminded Jakob to bring any bad dreams or fears to one of us.

"You mean if I had a bad dream that this happened here, to my house?"

"Yes, Jakob. Did you?" He changed the subject.

I drove home through town. There were some scary-looking flag-wavers on the Main St. meridian and then a lone girl with her hand-drawn sign that said "Remember to keep love in your hearts," and she held up her peace symbol. I felt the urgency in her appeal, in her solo counter-demonstration, and she made me cry. I didn't stop. I haven't gone to vigils or to the Sanga meeting. I have felt everything, I have talked to Arles, and to John and to Eva and many friends, so I haven't been isolated. I don't really know why I haven't been drawn, why I haven't felt the need for community. I feel, as Julie, my first neurofeedback patient, put it about herself, "the same as everyone else except I am not angry and this seems, under the circumstances, almost freakish."

"You're feeling an outpouring of Divine Love. You have the sense of an Other that will provide a completion of that love. You have God." I listen to Arles while thinking this is the oxygen and the neurofeedback.

It is as if I have only a receptive heart, not a generative one. I am ready to feel love. This is an infinite potential to be activated. I am on an island, washed up here, tumbled and smooth as sea glass. The ocean that delivers me is seizing with shock and terror and rage and grief and calls for peace and demands for war. Troops are called up, there is a frenzy of flags and love for the country as people help one another, as people stop and notice the thousands of acts of heroism and perform a million acts of kindness. But I wonder when people say "this is an amazing country" if they really expected less. Had we believed about ourselves that we are selfish, uncaring and unkind? And do they believe that other human beings in other countries subjected to such horror would act any other way? Maybe this is why I am not drawn to groups. I don't know what dialogue to enter; I will be held suspect because I am not angry. I don't get this in myself. I can't put a flag out because it doesn't seem like that either. I think I understand the anger and rage. It's pretty simple. I think what people feel is straightforward. I don't quite know where they place it, though. At 19 dead bodies of automaton hijackers who tried, at least in one case, to give themselves away? At bin Laden? That feels like being angry at someone who does not exist. Even Eva talks of killing him, but perhaps that is right. He and others must be contained while we do our best to address all the conditions everywhere that nourish terrorists. How do we do that better than we are doing it now? Only by developing more compassion and engaging in compassionate action, by taking no refuge in virtue, by taking less of the resources of the world, by doing good work, by looking at every child among us who is injured, bereft and vulnerable to hatred and tending to him and to her. The boy across the street is already a terrorist; Sammy would have been.

These planes flew over the Valley. We probably heard them as we prepared to start our day, preoccupied with its anticipated hardships and delights. We would've been eating our toast or stepping into the shower. When one of my patients reminded me that they were so close, I felt sick again at the immediacy, the nearness of this attack. We will all know someone, someone who died, someone who survived or someone who witnessed the carnage. I called Susan, my New York friend, to offer her a respite from the stench and the sick air, but she cannot leave the scene of the battle, that is, the very place she loves most. I have offered sessions to all of my family and will train any other that needs me. Traumatic shock is everywhere.

Now, I remember my irritation at how low these planes flew overhead. I commented on it to myself at the time, sitting drinking green tea at my kitchen table.

I have felt everything but anger and hate. Devastation, grief, gratitude. The mixture of grief and gratitude dissolved into tears. I have felt lonely and without comfort. I am at peace with this and with Johnny and with the company. I am at peace with not knowing who I am, just continuity and even with all the challenges that come with hyperbaric, with the

Rosen heart work, with the carnage 200 miles from here, in the place I used to live, on the flight I used to take and with waking up today to another beautiful dawn, the sun on the tops of the trees turning red and gold. In the darkest times, I feel bewilderment, but even if it isn't dark. I feel bewildered and deeply sad, both old and young, beyond age altogether, unhurt and not different from the ash-covered victims staggering away, just barely escaping.

Unlike Arles, for me, there is no God here. There is no one here, and there is no completion of this love in another. I, the embodiment of yearning at the outset, feel no yearning at all. He felt I was setting myself apart. I had said that he had nothing more to give me. I started to cry.

"I am saying this wrong. I am alienating you when all I want is for you to know what I am feeling, how it is for me. There is no one to set apart. You and I are on different paths."

"Do you have God on yours?"

"I don't. It is not the absence of God either. I am vapor on an island, an ageless person in an inner tube with neon fishes. I am stunned, not shocked but in shock and at peace."

Yesterday, Blake came, and we had lunch, and we talked, and we made pesto and painted her old room. While we were together, living our lives, I was completely here with her and with her smiling dog, Chelsea and with the beauty of the day. When she was not here, I listened to NPR and Scott Simon reading WH Auden, Dylan Thomas and Seamus Heaney. I feel enormous gratitude to NPR for the tone and quality of their coverage. Early on, I had called them to ask them to stop using the Muslim call to prayer as some kind of signifier, "We do not know that this is a religious war. We have to fervently hope not and not contribute to the possibility." There were probably several such calls. They stopped using it.

When I dissolve, such as I am, into the flow of my own tears, into the grief and exhaustion of horror, the renewed torment of my son's mind, Arles dissolves too. He did not cry, but he broke into the space of me, reorganizing molecules. He gathered me into him.

"Oh, Sebern," he said, and I knew he knew.

My responsibility is what it has always been: to recommit myself to helping to prevent terrorist minds, to open my heart, to cultivate fearlessness, to disperse the darkness wherever it attempts to consolidate in me. A little girl in New York, looking out of her window two days after, commented on the smoke clearing away briefly and said, "I think I can see the new opening, Mommy."

The air here is clear and cool, the sun keeps shining and stunned, and we proceed, stagger or walk into it. Everyone needs help. "We are either nurses or patients," Eliot said. I will be the nurse.

Johnny fought off the terror as best he could, but it overtook him, and when it did, he became the other Johnny, the terrorist John, cold and filled with hatred. I forgot somehow that this was his descent into madness. I forgot because I was powerless and overwhelmed with the sheer force of events. I learned later that he had called in a bomb threat to a mosque near him.

The threat of terrorism is always present. It is now manifest. We have joined the rest of the world. Johnny, Molly and Blake are suffering, three of hundreds of millions of victims. When I saw one flag draped in a black ribbon, I felt overcome by grief. The news coverage is coming now with commercials. Sabelle said, "It's becoming a movie."

"Osama bin Laden." It plays like some horrific mantra. It repeats like a gunshot. We are irrevocably changed. I dreamt that *I somehow allowed Jakob/Blake/Kevy to fall into the hands of a sexual predator. I was in the house of this man just waiting for him to return. He is violent, and I am complicit through ignorance, inertia or confusion. I can't quite get what is happening while always knowing what is happening. I think I was organizing an escape just as he arrived in the driveway. We had come there from an ice cream parlor.*

I am amazed again at my non-reactivity. I feel almost quizzical; this can't be my reaction, which is no reaction, just registration. It is profound. I no longer contribute to the emotional burden of the world. I feel the robust nature of the change again after the momentary rearrangement of my brain, the brain breathed into and made whole. Is this neurogenesis, new cells deep in my brain, added to the mix of the dead, the dormant, the errant and the functional? Who am I becoming as I become no one at all? My brain requires itself. It is consumed with its own regeneration.

It was raining hard over the edge of Mount Tom, and it was hard to see in the gathering dusk. Everything felt oddly, slightly unfamiliar. It was as if I were passing through the landscape rather than driving to the airport. A plane overhead was well lit up and seemed to be coming down at a steep angle. I talked calmly to myself, but my voice had a soft echo, and I listened for the explosion. There was none. The rain let up a little, and the garage at Bradley was open and reassuring. Two baggage handlers were playing catch on the empty main concourse at Terminal A. Everything was quiet. There were no planes at the gates; a few people were drinking beer. Two women, overweight and unwell, played a word game. For some reason, they had been in the baggage claim area for three. They were finding names of desserts—almond torte, apple pie, and I felt comforted by them. "Lemon tart!" I just stayed still, trying to return to real time.

John was the embodiment of that. We held each other before heading out into the rain to find the car. He talked about the flight across the country, the long lines at LAX, the pilots greeting the passengers, the camaraderie, his surveillance of the Arab-looking man across the aisle, his acceptance that this kind of vigilance is inevitable, the kind of unfairness that had to be accepted for now. He was determined to continue his life not with arrogance at all or with rage, although he felt some of that. "Out of a kind of generative defiance," he concluded. Walking back to the garage, I felt some normalcy returning, but I still felt a diffuse and distant fear that had to do with darkness and rain, and I learn, only now as I write this, with gas. John drove back. He was exhausted but added "Sleepy exhausted," and I breathed in again, reassured, even knowing somehow, we were still not breathing the same air.

Gas attacks are predicted. A pervasive low-level fear spreads through me, like gas. A deep nausea. I feel like an old, gnarled Jew who will die. No resistance is possible. Something in me had collapsed. Arles asked if it would help if I had a gas mask. I could not comprehend at first what he was saying. I cried like an old person, "I cannot get enough gas masks for everyone I love. We are all going to die." More a squeal and a whimper than a cry. More in grief and exhaustion than in protest, I said, "I have fought so hard to overcome so much trauma and for this? For extermination?"

Being with him eased my fear, but it would return abruptly—a dark, rainy, ash-covered dread. It isn't about now, and it seems stupidly indulgent to be talking of the past. This fear is of the Holocaust, past the point of being hunted down, on the way into the camp, to the chamber. The smoke. The awful smoke.

I am writing to try to bring myself into the present, as threatening as it is. But in this war, I am here with everyone around me and on my side. I might even be a lieutenant. We are rallying against this unleashed evil, and we are strong. I am not in the attic, singled out for attack. My brain twists—I feel it, and this is somehow about the other memory. This is where we huddle together naked, where we can feel no shelter or warmth in each other's bodies, no safety in numbers, no defiance or strength. Slowly, as I thought about the gas masks, I realized that if such an assault came, it would be survivable, and as I write now, I can pull myself out of this paralyzing fear enough to go to the computer and order them.

And still, equanimity prevails alongside the "other time dread."

"But I know someone in the building. It's different when you know someone who died." Jamie was explaining her entitlement to outrage that she really didn't need to explain. I acknowledged that she must be feeling hate and said I would hope that even if I had lost someone very close to me, I would not feel rage.

"Why not?" she questioned, her voice raised, "It's natural!"

I breathed. I could feel some discomfort in my own position—it is unfamiliar.

"How do you think the Dalai Lama would respond, or the Buddha? I am just trying to approach that, Jamie." She was quiet for a long time. "My mind is clear, Jamie."

"Yes, I hear that. I love you, Sebern."

I am living in parallel states of Now and Then.

Last night, in the frozen bones of my skull, I started to mourn the end of normalcy. I cried it out and now can hardly imagine what that was about. What is normalcy? There is no before September 11 except in calendar time and illusion. Arles said there is no outside and inside now. That blew up. It is absolutely impossible to comprehend all the forms that this will take, even in one human mind. We were savaged, brutalized. We were awash in blood that was quickly and horrifically cauterized. It will take a year to clear the rubble. We made plans to go to the site. As we emerge from the first round of shock, many of us will take this pilgrimage.

Yesterday, after supper in the golden end of the day, I walked toward town. I saw a young woman getting into her car. A cat had gotten in through the open window and was walking along the top of the back seat, and she didn't seem to know it was there. I was beginning to speak when the car raced forward, the woman screaming in terror. I yelled, "Stop! Stop! Stop!" and she heard me somehow and slammed her foot on the brakes. I went to her, told her that it was a cat, to put her handbrake on and to put the car in park. She was a foot away from a parked car. She was shaking and crying, her face contorted with terror and confusion. I helped her out of the car, rubbed her back and repeated, "It was a scared cat. All of our nerves are like that." She began to calm a little, a tear still rolling down her face, and she said, "He was just scared, wasn't he?" "Yes, he was just scared." She apologized for the garlic on her breath and laughed shakily. The American nervous system, two weeks after the assault, which we are calling the bombing.

I asked Sam again about our session. The only thing I could remember at first was that he said it was "atypical."

"I have never seen this pattern of response before. It has to do with the lizard brain level. It doesn't have anything directly to do with the hyperbaric or even recognizable PTSD stuff, although there is some element of trauma. I just don't get what I am feeling because this is new to me." I told him my reaction when Arles talked about gas attacks, the terrified Jew who said, "We will all die." I remembered my strange voice and my stooped posture and the slight registry, "Who is this?"

"That's it!" He exclaimed, "What I am feeling is a response to a neurotoxin!" He kept his hands where they were at the back of my head. "This gives me the shivers."

"Who am I? What is this that I am experiencing?" It feels like the weight of fog in my marrow. I turn for help. I was not someone who sought help. I collapsed to the force of the heel. I would not have known how to turn toward the underground. I would not have imagined the possibility of escape or sanctuary or kindness. I could neither seek nor offer comfort. I died in the gas chamber, huddled together with other women, not feeling the touch of even one body.

Just as I think that nothing will ever be the same, sameness seems to be slipping back through the seams of trauma. Life seems possible even as you, at some level not so deep, brace for the next assault. This town is peaceful, perhaps more so than before September 11. September 10th, business went on at the World Trade Center, but their destruction was assured. There is no protection. Incipient violence is always. So is incipient peace. September 10th was a time of ignorance, not of innocence. We are no longer ignorant. Or innocent of our own vulnerability. 60 bodies yesterday. Firefighters. A sign in Union Square reads, 'As I was going out, you were going in.' And tears come. We must hold the souls of these men with great tenderness forever.

"My brain vibrates, and when it vibrates at the same frequency as the membrane, I slip through time."

"An eerie knowing," Arles says.

Stress outs on my skin, I have hives. This company will not work. I held the phone a little away from my ear and took in all the implications of John's report. I once again had to accept its death. That is what became clear. And reincarnation. There was life after death. John and I would live our lives, simply and deeply in our home, coming into the knowing of one another. I doubt that there will ever be a life without neurofeedback for me. I told Eva that I would give up my car before I would give up this system. All of this comes at the same time, and I must learn to surrender. Surrender to the airplanes and all the dead, surrender to the deep wounded psyche of all Americans, surrender to the inevitability of this company's failure, surrender to the loss of these friends.

I trained the night of that dread, remembering only as long as I needed to that this was a brain state. At first it was better, then worse, then better. I felt the surround of the bath, the embrace of deep, warm water as my brain shifted. I mistakenly trained with an Alpha inhibit, which made it harder than usual for me to sleep, then drifted into twilight, dozing with compelling and sometimes disturbing images. Very little urine. I pee 3 to 4 times a day and then not much. I have much less appetite, as if appetite were in 8-11 Hz, and no hypoglycemia or response to sugar with the usual bloom of yeast.

Blake and I flew to Philadelphia to be with Marsha for her presidential address to ABCT. We met her after a long, comforting lunch at Maggiano's. Blake and I were at ease in each other's company, just happy. I was carefree. I am never carefree. When he heard we were from the Springfield area, the manager, a former native, bought our desserts.

Marsha's suite was large, almost gangly, but I felt no ambivalence about being exactly where I was. I realized when I saw her and hugged her that I missed her deeply, that I was just as glad to be with her as she was glad that I was there. She looked beautiful in her black suit with red stripes across the bottom of her jacket, just right. 2000 people came to hear her talk on suicide and the need for research—a good talk, but, as she had predicted, without passion. She did say that locking people up who wanted to commit suicide was discrimination against mental patients and, worse, not effective in preventing their deaths. She did say she believed in the right of people to kill themselves. Neither of us, of course, would be alive if that right had existed. Her voice quavered when she referred to 9/11. She received a standing ovation, and I saw her, her history, her suffering, the suffering she can inflict, the moment that should have been one of triumph, but in some way felt mostly sad. Most moving to me, Marsha seemed humble, receptive to all this appreciation, but not filled by it. She has made so much of a life she didn't mean to live. We had dinner with her sister, then joined her again for her party. All of us wanted most to go to bed. I left and caught the last hour of A Time to Kill. Blake slept, and I drifted through the night to another dawn. The Pleiades, I was told, were spectacular somewhere but not on 12th and Market.

I went from the airport to see Lee. The left side of my sacrum was a little sore, and then my feet went numb. I turned over, and she took my feet in her hands. I started to tremble. She held the tops, and I thought I could go mad, pulling my feet away, arching into muted howls. I was there hanging over the banister. I could feel the top of my head, and it was at the bottom. I wasn't on the table prone, but swinging above the two-story stairwell. Lee asked me if he held me by both feet. I seem clear on this. But there is a difference this time. When it was over, it was over.

I was with Arles when I recognized that part of being hung by my feet was the baby as a trophy, the cold delivery where you are turned upside down and spanked to cry. This marked the end of her motherhood. She had done what was expected of her. There was a war.

"What war?" he asked me.

"THE war," he left this ambiguous. After 9/11, planes crashed into our heads. We are in a state of war. Nothing else is spoken of. John and I will go to the site early tomorrow after celebrating our thankfulness today.

❧

We reached Ground Zero by seven, before the commuters, before the tourists, as the crews arrived, the rescue teams, the demolition crews, the medical groups, the National Guard, OSHA, the forensic teams, cops and firemen, Verizon workers, and hose crews for another day of confrontation with the evil in men's hearts and the immense sorrow and stark horror it creates. A weary firefighter, still in his black slicker, approached us, standing at the gates, trying to take it in, "It is horror. That is all it is." He has and will forever have a memory of this that is continuous—it may begin before the second tower was hit, it may include collecting parts of bodies and putting them in plastic bags, or coming to the circle of heat that radiates from the thousand foot crater, the screams as people ran or couldn't run, the bodies that looked like dolls to me on the small screen, the funerals and worse the memorials without bodies, the stench, the dailiness of most of this and how it reflects in every face inside the site and those that now gather at the perimeter. There was no one there yet taking pictures. The green canvas over the fencing now would make this difficult, and the yellow police tape keeps you at a distance from that. Those like us who came to see are kept away from seeing, even those like us who have come to pay our respects not at the shrines but at the gates. The necessary exclusion contains the horror. It begins to make the site sacred.

We look at the twisted metal, the hanging ash of an American flag, the five or six stories still standing, the concrete wrecker's ball (rectangular) plunging repeatedly, and a large chunk of wall and debris giving way. Perhaps this section has been searched, and the crane operator can know he is not crushing or burying anyone. There could be satisfaction in the demolition if you knew this, but what must they feel not knowing? Some buildings still stand. In one behind us, there was a bar, open, with a large banner across the windows: "Infidels welcomed." I felt welcomed. Other buildings stand charred and awaiting demolition. This is what war looks like – twisted beams, twisted lives, twisted faces, and minds that will never know innocence again. I strangely wanted to see more, still trying to get it, to feel, without muting it, the full impact of what I was seeing; I do not want to leave them behind in their grim work. The air still turns bad, hot and poisonous. As we drive home, there are signs in big red lettering, "Heroes Highway," and in black and green just "Thank You." And for one moment, I feel it all, the universal terror of those morning hours, the risks of knowing and then just as quickly of not knowing, forsaking knowing for reaction. The enormity of all the grief and rage and terror, the concentration of it right there behind us.

I am in this place, the USA, and I am glad to have been born here, but I feel no "I" now, and this kind of identification is all "I." The "I" of me has disappeared. It arises only in moments of sudden distress, and it forms completely when I feel dread or grief or fear. But it is only then. Wave becomes particle. High arousal, negative affect, reactivity defines or is "The Self." It is from here that the narrative of self begins.

Our day in New York was warm and clear. It's been raining since, and feeling like November.

I am told about work to help survivors of the earthquake in Turkey. They were using EMDR with a mostly elderly population to help them in the aftermath. What came up for most of them was genocide committed against their parents' or grandparents' generation. Most were not alive then, but that's what kept arising, not the earthquake. Arles tells me that 98% of DNA is unspecified, that scientists don't know its purpose, and it is unassigned. They call it "junk DNA." This is where cellular transmission has happened and where it is held. Access is granted through trauma, seizure, and meditation. There it is.

The exposure was too great. Arles's voice held me and led me through, into and out.

"Men at the windows; how many?" I held up three fingers fast.

"Three?" and I nodded a young, heavy head.

"They aren't just looking, they are crashing in." My whole body knew this. Everything was happening on the left side of my brain. I was dragged down by that fist of trance, like hair being pulled, little jerks down. I didn't fight it exactly, but I didn't succumb to it. It wasn't fruitful where it took me; it was toward a deadening. I saw the three men playing cards, and I remembered it smelled bad.

"What do you smell?"

"Cigars. Sweet. Sickening." I could've said the smell of Black skin. I smelled that too, but that smell is as sweet as Nivea cream. I could have said the smell that erupts with rage and sex.

"What about sex?"

"It wasn't sex. I don't know about sex. They had my body. They took off my clothes."

"How did that feel?" he asked, carefully.

"It wasn't different; that didn't scare me..." I considered this. "Four-year-olds have people dress and undress them."

He nodded, "That's so, isn't it?"

"But they didn't dress me. I put on my own underpants." I was looking.

"What are you seeing?" I looked harder.

"I was dressed when he hung me from the banister and before that when he grabbed my arm, and something tore. 'This is what will happen to you.'" I could feel the air passing under my head. I looked across to the corner. "They were playing poker. I was on the floor. I was the prize."

Gently, softly, he asked more of me.

"What did they win?" Beneath my answer, I blacked out.

"I don't know. I couldn't get out," I looked at the floor. I had crawled beneath the floorboards. I felt the concussion of boots right on top of my body, the weight bringing the floor to touch my shoulder. I couldn't lie flat. I was curled, like later under the covers at the foot of my bed, when I heard his footsteps overhead. There was a lot of noise.

"Is this from the movies, Arles?"

My old father is sheltering his head from their assault. I described it all as best I could. Today, the world is at war, but it is not this war that I am in. In the war I am in, there is incessant bombing, here where I live, a rain of small incendiary devices.

"I don't think so," he said. We both sat quietly, perhaps neither of us "all here." "This is not an ordinary mind." He sat down next to me. I felt the change in the cushion. He pulled the boot laces tight and strapped me into my feet. "Why do you think you were chosen for these memories? To open this channel?"

I left thinking about this question. The "Why" I don't know. But I think everyone has their constellations of deep memory, and these are some of mine. They want to be known, not to be obscured; they want me to tell Arles about them. They want not to be forgotten. That is the single wish that endures; memory is the vehicle of transmission. But most people with more stable brains are not crossing these time barriers. These repeating chords of trauma hold me back; they are obstacles. I am compassionate toward them, and they stand between me and transcendence, all of them, the old Jew, Moses, my mother, the "others," the seclusion rooms, the burly Jew who yanked me out of the crawlspace, all of them grasp for memory. They demand to materialize there, to hold me in time—theirs, or mine then, or mine now, it hardly matters.

I woke early in an unfamiliar state. It was as if my brain were knitting itself together. I could feel it; pull one, gather the stitch inward. And I lay still for hours and observed it, slipping into it, out of it again. At one point today, it felt as if I would erupt. I try to imagine some possibility of neurological comfort. The shades are drawn to the sills. There is no psychological part to this, no panic, no catastrophe. I sat this morning, but had to do it in bed, the red comforter tented under my chin. I am cold, clammy, and anxious, but there is no story. The train came through, and I felt rocked in its rhythms, all the cars the same length, the predictable pause in the vibration at each juncture of track. I love this and noticed that I feel it most in my hips and sacrum—synovial fluid bathing these joints as the train lumbers on to Detroit. Exercising made the situation worse. I could not figure out what to do. There was no one to call. It was comforting to run hot water over my hands and rub them hard together. Tonight, before I trained (and wrong!) I was pounding my stomach, ribs and chest with my fist. Every break during the day, I came to bed, to the heating pad and the pillows around my head. I could do nothing but observe. I had somehow arrived in the regulatory system of a seven-year-old autistic girl. My brain was banging inside my head. There was nothing to do except get through it. All the mistakes I made today I made on myself. I trained for 9 1/2 minutes on the left, 6 1/2 of it at 10.5. When I saw my mistake, my heart dropped and then the dull flare of rage, which took the form of deciding not to see Arles and Sam tomorrow. In that flare, this antisocial, imperious withdrawal made sense to me. After seven more right-side sessions and one at T3-T4, it is hard to breathe, and articulation is messy, but I don't feel like a serial killer. And I don't feel autistic either.

Reggie is doing her second week of hyperbaric oxygen. She called, weeping and fleeing the whole experiment. When she came for her session, she was almost multiple again. It was as if I could see the array of alters and family members behind her, all of them bloody, like Halloween ghosts. She was swarmed by ghosts. She felt suicidal and filled with a nearly unspeakable despair. She was wretched, and she could see no other reality. She wanted to quit. She wanted to protect all of those behind her from me, and she was fierce about it. Her rage was palpable but not scary because, somehow, she was containing it. She was protecting me from them. Everything shifted for her when I assigned all of this to the HBOT, to the effects of the oxygen on the amygdala. It is the healing crisis. Her body relaxed. The next day, she described herself as "a small boat, like a dinghy in a calm ocean." She feels detached. Things seemed flattened today, and she realized that she couldn't find any joy in Christmas. She had no desire. "Not depression," she said, "just no interest." In our now two-person exploration, I recognize another familiar HBOT landmark.

I am flying to LA. My back still aches, but the severe pain is over.

"When you break, you break bad," Sam had said, "But you heal well. There are three ways a sacrum goes out, and yours went out all three ways at once. Whatever you were working through is in this injury, and the source of it is very, very big."

"I have never seen anything like it," Bob told me, his hands there. For one week until Christmas day, I lay in bed in indescribable pain, unable to move, walk or sit. We did not go to Weston. John cared for me, but he needed the retreat. His grief and exhaustion around Johnny and the company had made their claim.

It began, I think, with Lee, with my decision to begin the work at my pelvis. I felt the impact of the boot and my fetal contraction. How can I really ever know this, ever really inhabit the young, bewildered body that experienced this? But I feel it, and perhaps it numbs me almost as much as the original long-standing dissociation. These are rapid glimpses, body memory as jagged and incomplete as all other memory, more compelling yet less believable because it is not a product of what one believes, not of the mind. The body does not encode experience as belief. It just holds it innocently and insistently like it was first experienced.

Bob ended the cranial sacral adjustment. "Nothing is moving here. You are completely shut down." Was that the nature of my equanimity being shut down? "This is post-traumatic." I think this, too. It is about demons left behind in my most sacred core, and my hubris in casually asking Lee to address this. I wore my soft pale corduroy pajamas and a long sleeve cotton top. When she rocked my hips, I first felt rage and an urge not to ever speak to grab her hands and throw them off me, screaming, "Don't do that, no!" That passed quickly, and then it was as if a soft bullet thudded into the center of my brain and all was quiet. Quiet, I felt the rocking, I was not alarmed; at times, I drifted into serenity. It felt as if she touched only the very surface, as quiet as the regulated breath. I did not sense the thing lurking that could shatter the structures in all directions at once.

Chapter 12

Arles leaves on New Year's Eve, and my exploration will stop here. I need a rest. After Bob, I may have gone through a red light, mistaking it for green and by the end of the day, I was holding my nervous system together with Gabapentin and the deepest acceptance, even wonder, over the resolve of my body. I was cold, it was hard to focus, I was trembling and at times close to throwing up. Maybe it was the shaking off of trauma, the prey animal realizing that it has survived, discharging and getting up. The natural thing seemed to be to try to stop this, but I didn't. I nearly caused a collision on my way to see Sam. I was too young to drive.

"Angels never seem to come in pairs. They are each one complete."

He was taken by this thought and talked of the heroic journeys one takes only to find themselves at home. Not back at home but there, never having left. On the train, through the snows, the eclipsing clouds, we are there looking for the one within us. Psychoanalysis and certain Western religions have decided where the energies of despair begin, and I have agreed. It is not a pagan myth, not evil spirits, but something from within us. We are only possessed if we believe we are possessed, and the task is to purge the belief, not the demon. But it is all energy and attempts to describe what feels true. Is this an energy from within the terrible unconscious, unrelenting conflict in which, like the dream, every actor is really you; or from without the sexual demon, the evil spirit of the other's all-powerful rage and appetite?

"Demons," he said, "are our projective identifications." I feel my brain wilt momentarily. It is the native tongue that I no longer want to speak.

"I think," I say tentatively, "that it is all energy and these are descriptions about how things are felt. Moses is a force outside me. My sacrum blew apart because of that force now in me."

He stretched out his long legs, leaned over them and said, "Sybil's mother was not crazy."

"Do you think she was evil?" He nodded. I don't think so. Or Moses.

"I don't want evil planted in me. And I can't see him. I feel the energy, but I don't see him, particularly not his face. I see his chest. I smell the cigarette and the cigar smoke. I don't see myself either. I can't inhabit the body that keeps insisting on its own history." We both went still.

"Don't forget me, Arles. Don't leave me here in the attic. Don't forget me."

He looped his cashmere scarf around my neck.

"I won't forget you. I will think of you every day."

Moses was crazy. What he did was evil. What Sybil's mother did was evil. Sybil died young. I want to die old, with a beautiful mind.

There is a great tragedy unfolding here, and we are powerless to stop it. Sue is near collapse, her thinking is conspiratorial, and she feels friendless. She won't speak with me except to say that she can't, not right now. Her vision is narrowed, the prey watching the movement of its predator. Her narrative is post traumatic and reductionist. She has been brutalized, not just by the most recent events, but by the entire 15 years. And although they have been the key players in this history, she does not see that either she or Siegfried played a part, not to mention what that part was. They are not privy to their own unconscious; they are as we all were at The Center, mystified victims of circumstances. They are once again on the brink of losing it all, and no one there seems able to draw back from the brink. After all the hours of nearly fruitless meetings, John and I went home. We were aimless, desultory. Neither of us felt ennui or despair, although it is not clear exactly why not. We had done our best, and now the vacation is over, the meetings are over, the dinner at the Greek restaurant is over, and I am too tired to go to the movies. We scrambled through channels, and we settled on watching an interview with Giuliani that was done in September, in which he seemed strangely untouched. He had the air of a boy giving a "show and tell," but it was about the collapse of the World Trade Center, his brush with death, all the death, the aftermath of the assault. He told it eagerly and cooperated easily with the interruption of the commercials, "Celebrate, celebrate, Celebrate."

Sue called me, and she reassured me of her trust in me. We don't talk about our differences in perception. Everyone who says to me, "You are not here," meaning in the room, in the center of this conflict, is right, and I silently respond, "Thank god."

"You don't need to do anything differently. But..." and then I started to cry, not over anything but the sheer beauty of possibility, "you know I live in an unpredictable brainscape." He laughed gently. "There is great richness there and so much that I want to share. I want to go very deep, John," and I almost whispered this, "I want your company. I want to learn together what it is to open our hearts. I want to be with you until there is no 'me' left. Or 'you'. I want to lie here hip to hip with you and fall backwards into the universe." He turned into me, around me, lay his head on my chest, he may have cried briefly, and we began to fall.

The 101, the 405, Calabasas Highway, the extraordinary rouge-red flare of dawn. California feels too much like home. I left the deep, warm embrace of John's body. I felt a kind of little girl bravery, traveling out alone, back to the stark winter of our other home in Massachusetts.

Johnny was dumped back into the Bougainvillea, discharged with no plan. It is as if the entire profession of psychiatry, when confronted with severe mental illness, drops into either magical thinking or hopelessness.

Or maybe that's us, John and me. The fear of AIDS dementia creeps in. Neither of us said this, but after the altercation and hang-up two hours earlier, Johnny called to ask, "How are you both doing?" He has been in restraints, on Haldol, speech slurred with Klonopin, and we are in no different place.

I lay on my back and talked with Lee.

"What I am in touch with is terrible. It is something my body has to deal with; it has no choice. Bodies are literal and concrete and prone to somatization. My body is finally knowing what happened during that fraudulent process of dissociation. It is as if they did not cut you open during anesthesia. Your body holds no such belief; it holds experience. So, it reveals what it knows, almost, it seems, cell by cell. As a collective, they know the same experiences and as individuals, the story of their ancestors. It is as if my body has finally found someone, me, who wants to know and every part has a story to tell, even the black tarry stool on Tuesday. The questions Sam had asked were about blows to my belly. I had no answer to this, no image formed until today. I would have seen my doctor if it continued, my belief is not *that* strong. All of these events are momentary. Although my body needed all this and I had no choice or felt no choice but to embrace it, it wasn't mine. I am not dissociating from my body, but this is not 'my' past. There is no 'me-ness' in it. It was; it is, and knowing it this way protects me."

Eva asked if I thought it would ever end. I answered, "Yes!" without hesitating. Emphatically. "I expect," I said, "the clearest and most powerful decade of my life." (I keep starting to say century.)

John's snoring woke me. I threw my dreams back in the water. We are out in the country, both happy to be here, but he is particularly delighted to be home. I love his delight. I fell asleep to Carlos Nakai, in John's arms. I only left when his body felt hot as a stove, and my back ached, deep in the night. These are the miracles of neurofeedback.

I felt bewildered during Arles's absence. There was no fear to mask it. I would look at the space he was supposed to fill, and it was empty. He was not somewhere else; he wasn't anything but the space itself.

Two mornings after Arles returned, I woke up and looked into a cloudless night sky, and there were no stars. He was gone. Arles is a missing constellation. I think of him many times a day, but the magnetic necessity of our being together has disappeared. I love him when I am with him. I don't yearn for him. He is an Other in my life. I would expect to feel loss, a fall from grace, disappointment, something here, something that matches the starless sky. Perhaps I do, somewhere. Perhaps the fear is so momentous, and my defense is so strong... But I just do not find any truth in this. It is fear that requires defenses, and I don't fear. I wish he would join me here, help me to discover these intersections between regulation and psyche. I do still tend to default to the belief that he is just not hearing me, that if I jump up and down, say it more convincingly, that he will join me. This is the remnant of transference until I learn again, recognize his other-ness, his right to his own path, the necessity of it, the loneliness of mine.

I awake these recent mornings in a large empty room that echoes. Even as I write this, I know there is no one to tell. Arles seems to think there is nothing left to explore in the realms where I most need his company, the terrain discovered through the body. He is interested in developing meaning, and there is none here for him.

"Don't leave my feet, Lee," I cry out, suddenly alarmed.

She reassures me and moves to take hold of both ankles, and my body/mind erupts into a double terror. Arching—is it the stairwell? No, the smell of ether? No, something about these movements themselves. It is layers of experience, and in the memory, I am twisted, screaming, biting my hand, almost choking on a clot of mucus, crying. She moved to my head to comfort me. "Quiet, here now in this room, on this table, safe in the present," I whispered inside my ear. But my legs tuck in almost under me, helpless. The brief episode seems to be entirely encapsulated, but a friend says I sound strange, and another asks if I am alright. The muscles of my lower abdomen are pulled and sore.

Arles and I have agreed that my body has its own journey to make, but somehow this round it has recruited my mind. And it has no words. Arles wants words. So, this is what we must talk about, he and I. Why has he dropped out of the sky?

None of this felt true once I was with him again, telling him about all of this. As I was getting ready to leave, I said, "And none of this adds meaning."

"The events themselves don't, no, but how they affect the course of a life, how they register, does."

How do they register? Knowing them is not as I have long hoped, salvation itself.

Today I am sixty. The morning is beautiful, and I was only slightly churlish when I came home, and there was no breakfast and no spontaneous Happy Birthday. John was consumed by the computer. I reacted as if I were injured by it. There is almost no other choice in the habit repertoire. Habit has formed, and it must be used. Inside, I look blankly at myself and allow the habit to take its righteous course, flapping like a moth at the light.

Yesterday, Bob had one hand on my chest and the other on my chin, and my body thumped up off the table, as if, I thought, it was under paddles. Maybe they used them when I arrived at St. Luke's in a coma? Something happened. It could've been ECT, but I don't think so. It's focused on my heart, and somehow, my skin is being pulled. I mentioned this to Bob. "That's interesting," he said. "Today, the rhythms between your atrial and ventricular systems were strange. I haven't quite seen it like that before. The rhythms re-regulated smoothly."

I was talking with Arles today about the letter from Sue and Siegfried, and he asked if their son had Asperger's, too. I reacted against this characterization, and we explored the strength of my reaction. They are not so 'other' as that diagnosis makes them.

"They are not so different. It is I who is different. I have forgotten how to participate in the common commerce of reactivity. I have no one to talk to from this place of singular regulation. I don't have a vocabulary. It is not even that I think you wouldn't understand, it is that I don't have the words and you don't have the experience." Arles asked why I hadn't pursued Sue, that this was not typical of me.

"I don't know anymore what our common ground is, what my standing is in her realm, who she is. I am no longer feeling the compulsion to save that family." I kept feeling I should say that I feel betrayed by Sue. I could righteously say this. Or hurt. But I don't. I feel that I am on an island, a beautiful island, but an island nonetheless. I have no protest, but I would like company here. I would mostly like Eva's and his. But I also accept that everyone takes their own path. I just need to soak up the rays and radiate them as best I can. I am ok with that.

I wanted the safety of him. The door is locked. I knocked. I knock again, but I know it's faint. I think he must've gone out. I sit on the stairs and wait as confusion, desperation, and anger begin; and he comes to find me.

"It's not locked. I wouldn't lock it." He has me try it, and it opens. I struggle to tell him what is true this time about these feelings. I do not experience this as catastrophic but as a known stimulus for catastrophe. I tell him of the sense that now that I have returned from the demands of the conference and of the company, I am in for another round. He understands. I tell him it occurs to me to protest, but that it falls on my own deaf ears.

"If I could have just gotten her to look in my direction, to look at me. The most heartbreaking of the pictures is the one on the changing table. There is still hope, and it's going to get even worse."

I am quiet, and after a while, he asked me to tell him where I was.

"I am within the core of dissociation. It is silent, a state of constriction into matter so dense that there can be no movement, no sound. All the noise of mental illness is above this; even the noise and movement of breathing is above this. I am closer to knowing this is real, but there is still a buffer between me and that realness. I don't doubt anymore, it is nothing quite as simple or concrete as doubt. I don't know if I could bear the absolute ground zero realness." Even as I say this, I don't see the terrible consequences, it is no longer psychosis or being shattered. But there is that moment of consciousness right before one is dissolved by the detonation of the nuclear bomb. That absolute knowing of the absolute realness, not of the events but of that state of mind, is like inviting that moment into consciousness forever. Arles sits in an almost reverent silence as I say this. "I am at a new level," I said, and he nodded. "I don't want this lodged in my body, not as it feels today, a metal rod jammed between my pelvic bones. That cannot happen."

We were in the presence of something.

"Knowing requires naming, and this is beyond naming." He paused and then asked, "How is your heart?"

"It is peaceful and pale." Pale was the right but surprising word. "As pale as the moon when the sun is still out. Light. A white light around it. Very little feeling in it, but I am able to fill it. When it fills up, it is tidal and foaming and teeming with glittery little fishes, and then it drains, it is pale, collapsed." My brain feels as if it is trying to re-organize and in a whisper, it comes to me. "It is like the interior of my mother's chest, slimy brown and pale, and her heart is a thin disc, as thin as a communion wafer. I put it on my tongue, and it disappears."

"Does it leave you wanting more, or is that even possible?" he asked.

"There's no 'more' there. It isn't even enough to be tantalizing. It is gone as soon as it is tasted." I covered my nose and my mouth softly with my cuffed hand. "And then the wine. I always liked swallowing the wine. And the prayer was said over my head. And all of this just in tones, in Latin, so I couldn't be reminded that this was about 'remember me.'"

As I left, Arles spoke to me in Ukrainian.

"Is that 'Go in peace, my child?'"

"Almost. It is 'you have a beautiful heart.'"

At some moment before I'd stopped, and from some place slightly apart from me, I looked at my brain and my heart. I felt admiration for them that they had endured. Appreciation and a light, moonlit joy.

Yesterday I turned the car stereo up so that sound filled my brain at just the right level, and I drove in the exact moment, the fluid muscle, the Now of absolute regulation.

BRONXVILLE

I've begun to talk about going back, imagining walking up the stairs. Eva cautioned me. It could be completely renovated; it could be unrecognizable. She worried that this would feel invalidating and confusing. It could. But I hope it has been renovated and that the walls are painted sky blue and lavender. I would go there to assure my body that it's over. Moses is gone. There are no blood stains.

"I think it was pretty drab when they lived there."

"There will be something there," Arles said, "that is beyond architecture," and suddenly I feel the tugging in my brain, the pooling into trance, the strange fullness in my head and blackness in my mind, staring at nothing—what's there? It is very quiet. I am not frightened. The light changes. It is darker, and all systems are on alert. My jaw hurts. I don't know how to name this experience. All cues are gone. Maybe I am in the attic, but less in it. A switch is thrown. It happened twice or three times during the session. There is no action, no real scene, no people, just an evacuation and response.

"In this space," I finally said to him, "It is hard to speak. I would clutch your arm. I don't know what state I would inhabit."

My dreams are about houses with many rooms. Arles is in some of them, and he is, in them, always in the process of moving or planning to move. Movement from the complex to the simple, from the history to the Now. Sam said that when he works on my body after a new training protocol, it is a profoundly different body. He still recognizes it as me. "It is not like multiple personality disorder," he assures me.

When I turned into Elizabeth Street the other day, I realized the huge nature of the mind that is the Antichrist. It is not Satan's despair and bent toward evil. It is the absence of 'mother', the absence of God. It is the state of non-love, not the state of hate.

Arles and I talked more about Bronxville. When we first spoke, I was in a state that could negotiate the stairs. I knew that I could not reliably predict my response. It was state-bound, and it responded to the rules of that state. I had a flash of the episode when I went into the bathroom at his office and couldn't leave the hard reassurance of the walls.

"What if that happens, Arles? What if I react like that in the stranger's house? I will embarrass you."

"You won't embarrass me. I will hold you." He is big enough. If the scene is hard, it just is. I will send apologies and flowers.

"I am not bringing anything into the house."

"No," he said, "it is already there."

There is something about three days. My body suddenly turns cold. But this would be impossible. There would be evidence, and nothing was ever said or done. Maybe they lied about symptoms. I had bruises from a fall, and I lost my first baby tooth like that. But it doesn't quite fit right. Arles said that in mystical traditions, three days stand in for eternity. Perhaps this is the meaning of three days, endless.

"It is Good Friday in two days," I said. "On Easter, the banner will go up on St. John's church—Christ Is Risen. I have always loved that banner, the bold and delighted proclamation of no death."

Bob could see me early. He worked mostly on my stomach. "Everything comes here," he said. "It is as if you were curled in the fetal position." I knew this was true. "There has been serious trauma here, some kind of kick or a blow with a blunt instrument." He didn't want to tell me, but I insisted. I couldn't feel anything there. He moved his hand gently from my stomach to my heart. "I think you went into shock," I'd been in shock since my first waking at 2:30, chilled beyond getting warm. "And this is probably why you don't remember. You were hemorrhaging, and you went into shock." Bob told me later that he had only twice "blended" with a patient, once when he was working on a woman who had been struck by lightning and this time with me. "It was huge," he said, "and your affect didn't match at all the magnitude of what happened."

I lay on Arles' couch, exhausted and still shivering. I was better than before, Bob. He'd encouraged me to rest. He'd wondered how I survived. He'd wondered how they could not have noticed. Other details seem to come clearer. It was three days. Maddie was away. She lay me in my bed gently. She put soft clothes on me. She gave me water, and I sipped it through the side of my mouth. I have no details about getting downstairs. She gave me orange aspirin, and she sat with me in a chair next to the bed.

❧

I am on the plane to Dallas and then to LA. I need to be gathered up in John's arms and sheltered. I need to rest in the sun and take B vitamins, arnica, and possibly something for bone healing and hemorrhage. There really is no passage of time in this experience. The extreme inflammation and swelling all around my stomach were gone, but still, these remedies seem important. And bed rest and water. I trained my usual protocol to help me along and saw when I reviewed the screen that I had forgotten to use a 2-6 inhibit for the first round at F7-F8 during my last training. Was this the source of this new information?

I talked with Arles about the power of this experience, the effect on Bob. He works with trauma survivors, he has surely encountered worse.

"Moses' force was ancestral. Part of the reason I have so much trouble getting that this was me, apart from dissociation, apart from shock, was that it wasn't me. It was some monster, some White monster in Moses' mind. I was the surrogate for my mother. I imagined myself lying almost dead, Maddie there. And suddenly something goes flat in my brain and takes on a pale blue color, and I whisper, 'It's only a story. Nothing happened here. You know nothing.'"

"That's Maddie's mind," Arles said. Oh god, Maddie knew what had happened.

I am withdrawn in California, unable to justify or align my experience, and it's so much harder to do here than at home. I was glad to see him. As we drove to Agora, he came to understand that he was picking up a child who had been savagely beaten. It's impossible that I'd flown to LA; he should have flown home. He asked us to stay together in the grocery store. I am not steady on my feet; my legs are weak, and this morning it's hard to get myself showered. Nothing that I can do meets the situation, except writing this.

Driving down Ventura, we were talking about my feelings after the first episode with Bob, that I didn't want to tell anyone. He said, "Like you did the first time," and I reacted.

"No, I didn't do anything or decide anything! There's no narrative; no speaker, and no one to hear. There is a form that I get from the details of the beating around the outsides of my body, the back of my head, the cold whiteness of my feet retracting. There is form in the limpness being laid down on the bed and limbs free-falling. I hear as much as I see Maddie and smell the fragrance of her skin, sitting, paging through a magazine with bright colors. No words belong here." He sat with me as if his mind too were cleared of thoughts. "It is different from repression, there was no decision not to know. There was no saying that this thing happened, and I would not know it. It could not be known; it could only be experienced."

They are using the leaf blowers outside to clear the condo walks, less efficient and harder to use than brooms and rakes, loud and polluting. Why's this?

Everyone I see—and I look now—is not there. They make no sense to me. Siegfried is not there, and it bores me. Sue is not there, and she is training herself into a kind of cold, reactive madness that excludes everything but neurofeedback. She does not recognize how she is driving herself further and further from human warmth and kindness.

Yesterday, when I could not communicate with John—he seemed absent to me—I started to yell, "I don't care about Neurofeedback!" repeatedly. And I was surprised how true that was to me. "Sue is imprisoned by her training; we will not be imprisoned by Sue!" It opened a door for John.

We are going to Seattle to introduce neurofeedback to Marsha and her team at UW. It has the endorsement, she tells me, of Martin Bohus in Germany. I asked Siegfried to tell me about the factors that mitigate against the double-blind, and he assaults me and insults Marsha without recognizing that he is doing it. I don't want this. He does not change, and Sue changes for the worse. It does not interest me.

I kissed John goodbye. We have become familiar with separations. He dropped me at SeaTac for my earlier flight, and on the way, we assessed our visit. We understand the complexity and work of a research study; Marsha will help us, did help us design it; she will introduce us to Martin Bohus; she will get us human subjects; we know about small business grants and consultants to help us get them. We need preliminary data. I feel fatigued. Marsha fed us pork roast and explained her lack of response to 0-3 @T3-T4 or 5-8 @T4 by saying that she was already in an ideal state. She had just a day earlier returned from a meditation retreat in Arizona, and it felt "like meditation" to her. She didn't understand the model, and we did not do our best in describing it. They want data to study it; we want them to study it to get data.

Marsha's students seem distantly at ease with her, there on the weekends, walking barefoot among the chaos of computer cables, stacks of boxes and piles of videotapes. Her office is long, cluttered and without any charm or distinction. Her interview room is cherry red. Everyone she treats, she videotapes—them and herself. They're all giving exit interviews about their treatment experience. Someone thought to ask them if being videotaped affected how they behaved in session. They report feeling safer because everything is on tape. Marsha is deeply ensconced both in her treatment research and in the cold, beautiful surround of Seattle. She won't leave there. She cherishes the idea of her siblings as a bulwark against her loneliness, but they do not invite her for Christmas. She has no place where they have to take her in. All too often or maybe not often enough, she breaks my heart.

Until what happened with Sam, I'd only been able to put one foot in front of the other. It was near the end.

"Everything is moving," he said, "but like cold molasses." Bob had told me that the sympathetic and parasympathetic systems were not cycling but coming up against each other and leaving me in some strange energetic stasis. Sam feels this too. He was working on my left foot, where he always works, and I told him, almost offhandedly, that I was feeling increased heat across my back around the kidneys. He put his hands there and said the adrenals are releasing, and at the same moment, I started to sob, and I couldn't breathe.

"Now is when I want to pass out." He took the back of my head in his hands.

"Breathe and try to breathe through your heart." It is amazing how you can stop breathing and breathe at the same time. I did that, and slowly it did pass through. I heard the next patient arrive downstairs. Like the dive master in Belize who checked my too rapid ascent, he said, "No, not yet." He almost lifted me up, and I was surprised that I was not meeting the same air resistance that I'd become used to. I could sit up and stand. I could be present on the spring morning.

Arles was sick. He was trying to be there but couldn't. I gave him the couch.

"You can't reassure me about this, Arles. There are times I am worried that I make you sick. You have been having these strange flus, and you are attuned to me." He did not refute or agree. He asked weakly if I was worrying about this now. "Yes, I am, but there is nothing to be done."

He must learn what I am learning, what he in part has taught me, let it pass through.

"Do you see how this would have to lead to sickness?" I asked John. "Do you think that a body's memory has a frequency and might that be Theta?" He could see.

"Did this happen to me?" That is the first question.

"Yes, Sebern, this happened to you. You are not making this up."

"You have been here each time, haven't you?" He knew what I was asking. The evidence is not even circumstantial. I went mad without knowing why—everything looked just right, and from the moment I was carried down the stairs and laid in my bed, I drifted away and into the thick, polluted crawl of forgetting. I know that, and I still cannot know. It is as if the body memory rises as far as my nose and then just when it could take root as a reality in my mind, it disperses. There is nothing.

On the phone that night, Alan, my NeuroOptimal colleague, asked, "Does all of this make you question the idea of repression?" Training my brain has begun to pry me away from this idea. There is nothing to repress. Or maybe it is known only in the frequencies it happened, like for Billie. All is in the service of the relationship, not the ego. And, of course, survival.

"I feel movement in my brain."

"It is the ligature between the brain and the skull. The brain is too soupy," Bob said, holding the cranium of soup.

"Imagine," I said, "a large school of fish, silver ones as they swim and then in the absolute grace of simultaneity change direction as one body. What would that feel like? That is what it feels like in my brain." Something more than metaphor. It feels different to me than the powerful movements of cranial sacral work—I can feel this too in my brain—but this neurofeedback sensation is the swirling of sleek silver fishes. The energy of the sea and the squalor of languid muddy streams, this is where I am.

But who did this happen to? There are levels to that, too. Dissociation. No mother. No other to say it. I was psychotic. And now, I am asking it from no "I" at all. There is no language for it, no pronouns at all, and even "spaciousness" is too boundaried, too personal. I cannot root any of this in mental imagery. There is no Me to claim it.

I told him how grateful I was that I was registered in his mind.

"You are not registered in my mind..." I felt the beginning of the long ago red queen fear... "You are registered in my being."

The room was instantly transformed.

"You have just made this into a sacred grotto, Arles." It was leafy, fragrant, dappled and holy. I remembered a caution I'd heard early into my exposure to the dharma. "Do not sit for hours looking at a wall if you are not willing to see the face of God." "You brought God here."

All that feels right to do is to kneel but not to him, not to anybody or anything at all, just the body's reverence, the body's sudden experience of God.

It is like a virus that you expect to leave you in three days, and is still around in three weeks. You have a relationship with it. You begin to resent the virus. It is useless but inevitable that you resent it. The virus wins. It stays as long as it needs. Body memory arose again after what felt to me like a closure. Arles said there are no words for that kind of brutality, and suddenly, softly, almost, it was completed. Like the tortured Rubix cube, all the colors in their rows and the one missing square, a blue one, slipped into place and locked in. I don't know what the position is, but he found the right place. And even then, I don't actually leave his office free of it. I couldn't quite get through to the sky. It begins again to erupt like a slow-moving volcano. I take Gabapentin and 1/4 Percodan. The cocktail. "Don't worry," I say, "it will be over in 45 minutes." Arles asked me what "over" was. It is subdued. It roils, but it does not break through.

"What would you be doing if you weren't dealing with this 'virus?'"

"I would be creative."

"Oh, I think you are enormously creative. Your exploration and articulation of psychic states is very rare—your willingness to pay attention. This feels very creative to me. You are willing to stand in the eye of the storm, unflinching."

He made me reconsider. I had been adding production value.

"But I am not in the eye of the storm, I am the eye of the storm and the storm. There is no flinching involved." He knew immediately. "This is the creativity that we co-create. I use your energy as a grappling hook; it holds me down, it pulls ideas forth." He nodded. "It comes easier, every day, even as I want to gag and maybe even scream."

Last night, my left foot suddenly went numb. Bob had been working on my toe, and he began breathing deeply.

"What, Bob?"

"Well, there is no simple dysfunction in you. This leads up to here, the inside of my thigh, and pulls outward. The implication of that... I don't even want to go there."

How does my body prioritize memory? It has the feeling of archaeology, but is more truly one of yielding up, rather than digging down. I am waiting for the next stone or rock or boulder to surface, to make itself known as if it hadn't been there all the time.

"You will not self-destruct, Sue, not without a fight. The two of you are too important. I don't know exactly how to do this, but I intend to try."

"It feels as if you are brushing a feather across an exposed surface of my brain." Bob was hesitant to press harder, but he did. I felt his hot breath on my face and opened my eyes to see that he was sitting straight, his face far from mine. I can feel it even now, the heat, the exhaled breath as it falls on my nose and around my mouth. I was, oddly, I think, unafraid of this little hallucination. It was very brief. Very real. Later, as he worked on my face, my throat got sore.

"We are at the tip of something," he said.

"Don't forget," I said almost plaintively. "One of us has to remember."

Today I said hello, and Arles smiled. I described the unfolding of body memory, the way this goes with Bob. I lie on the table and begin to drift in and out of states pretty readily. My attention is idling on some future event or a conversation, a patient, and then suddenly, under his hands, it is drawn into the room. Physical pain is rarely the issue. Most of the time, it is just a change in the focus of attention. There is no strong valence to the shift, I am "in wait" for something. Usually, I drift back out, but sometimes the waiting becomes more intensely focused on my breathing, which I notice has changed. Something is beginning to arise, something is beginning to take form. When there is a form, I try assignments of meaning and if something resonates— which is usually no more than "when" or "where," rarely "what"—that is close enough to memory but not memory, I stay there. Sometimes it is more of an inference. I draw something out; something seems to suggest itself to me. Either of these paths can lead to the rare experience of memory, and this always includes some visual, usually a partial representation of a form. This is what happened when I remembered the banister, but it happened very fast and while I was training, and being kicked, which I remembered like this when I was with Lee. If it gets as far as memory like this, then discharge or abreaction has to happen.

"I dreamt *of a bird that dove into the ocean and became a fish, then instantly a sea mammal, but when I looked closely, it had neither feathers nor fur. The transmutation was seamless, but the tone and colors suggest it is utilitarian, it is work. There is some joy in being able to do this, but this is about survival. The sea is dark, and the skies are cloudy."*

"It reminds me," he said, "of the baby diving into the depressed mother."

I felt revulsion. I cannot imagine this without feeling sick. I try to stay with it. Eventually, it's a gray baby—no other, no landscape, no context. It involves a resolve to need no mother. I probably did not get what most people meant by "mother," what the link is that they feel, even if they were bound in some destructive way. Some of my patients have sadistic mothers with the intent to harm them. My mother was not this. She did not attack us. We did not form in her; we were not the objects of her projections because she didn't have objects. In that way, she left us alone, too. I was afraid of her until near the end. She would organize to shame me. She needed to control me. All of us. But she was not engaged in psychic murder or the slaughter of the soul. We did not have them.

I remember a fragment of last night's dream. *I was in a café or a nightclub, and a woman walked in who immediately had everybody's attention. It was my mother in her 40s clothes: gray suit, gray hat, but beautiful—not radiant but with a spotlight on her and her entourage. "Who is that?" Someone asked. I answered in a tone that assumes that her beauty bestows esteem on me, 'That's my mother.'* I felt a moment of tenderness in telling the dream, or recognition of how difficult and, in a certain way, how trivial a life she had led with all that special beauty.

"It is really me who has lifted my family out of trivial existence."

He laughed gently, "That's true, isn't it?"

That dream of the bird is really the whole story. The story of depression, dissociation, refusal to die, insistence on transformation, and still the absence of joy. He asked where I got the capacity for transformation, and I knew in a way that he didn't that I developed it with him. Life force is one thing—miracle enough, the weed in the crack and in me—but it is not the same as the desire for transformation. There was a seed, but the transformation grew with him, with his insistence. I would have lived a competent life, but I would not have changed without him and without training my brain.

"You are in my cells, and that makes my life possible. But still, every time I leave, I leave you behind. I step out into the world alone."

He tied my shoes to help with a peaceful transition.

Blake asked if she could come up for a hug. I said yes without hesitation, but I also recognize my accommodating heart, not really an open one. She opened herself to me, and I warmed to her in a way that felt new, in a certain way horrifyingly new. I have always loved this child. I have been open with her, shared the narrative of my central contribution to her sorrow, and somehow, we stopped there. We, mostly I, fashioned her into a beautiful golden girl who was confused when she didn't feel loved. I prized her. I thought she was beautiful and special, and all of this gave rise to the myth that none of this history, none of what I have learned about myself, really touched her. She alone of the children escaped the dark currents. How could that be possible to ever believe, much less to persistently believe?

"Mom, this is me," her tears spilled onto the page of I Know Why A Caged Bird Sings. I didn't hear what she read. I saw her, with a sudden jerk of recognition, the being of this young woman before me.

"Yes, it is you." I could recognize her for the first time, perhaps, and here she was before me, grieving. Blake is suffering. I felt it so deeply I thought I would scream in agony. I have been matter-of-fact about it. I have been impatient with it. Last night, with the courage of her request, I embraced it for the first time.

She was talking to me about the hopes that her boyfriend, Ryan, continued to dash. "This dream is a prison. I am trying to get something filled up by things outside me that can't be filled that way, and I don't know why I do it. I have to learn from this."

"How will you do that?" I asked. "Is your therapist helping you?"

"I don't think I'll tell her." Her therapist may have come to see her as we have, as the one "untouched", the one unhurt, even when she is torn apart.

"The depth of this sadness," I said, beginning to cry, "has to be about me. It has to be before Ryan."

She blinks; she tries to take this in. She desperately wanted to make it all right. That was her job. She recognized her rage at Johnny for taking all that we had to give and then threatening to leave her forever. She tries to recognize me, and I see her again for the first time and welcome her into this agonized growth. She smiled sadly as if it shouldn't be this way. Last night I took her into my arms and held her like I could have all night, like I wish I could have all her life.

"You helped to heal me, Blake, now I will help to heal you."

On retreat, Blake, Sue and others passed through. I set Sue aside, but Blake was there. I wondered if I had envied her: her beauty, her country home, her feminist upbringing, her sober father, her mother? I wonder what I did to make her feel just not quite secure, and then confused about it. "Not smart enough, not deep enough," she'd said.

Last night, during the meditation period, my left hemisphere was more active, more full, than my right. In fact, the right side felt pale, almost empty. The left was a vibrant soft gray, fully alive. The left is text and chatter. The right is the feeling of being alive. It was like a gauze outline or an anatomical three-dimensional model, a representation of a brain or a hemisphere, not an actual one. I would dismiss it, then see it again, and finally, it occurred to me to work with it. I failed at first to shift energy. That seemed to be the task, to balance these hemispheres. Suddenly it happened. I could feel the shift. I was very pleased that I could do this. And then my shoulders froze up, hard and painful, registering the terrible wordless knowing of that silent hemisphere. After half an hour, I felt all this tension give way.

"The ambulance crashed," the first line of a chapter came to me when one drove past the meditation center, and I listened to it down many blocks. "This is what must never happen, but always could: the crash of the ambulance."

My new patient tries valiantly to manage her wild despair, and now I understand why I would train her out of terror but not out of sadness. Terror, panic, rage, and anger are all emotions that get their power from kindling. They only have meaning at the first moment of being felt; all the rest is just repetition, amplitude, agitation in the brain-kindling. Depression is self-stoking as well. They are feelings that become brain dysregulation or that begin there. Sadness and grief do not kindle; they flow. They are rivers that run out either to the sea or that sink into thirsty ground. Sadness regulates. Sadness is true, or it isn't sadness.

Sue is in desperate trouble, and I want her to hear this and to be able to recognize who her friends are, who will help her. She won't. She retreats deeper each day into the dark cave of delusion with Siegfried. Some believe that she has always been like this. I don't. I remember her warm delight when I would call her. I remember her T-shirt that read, "Chocolate. It's not just for breakfast anymore." I don't, oddly, feel used by Sue even though I was so apparently used. I do not even feel discarded. She refuses my entries because she has rewritten our history to justify her bitterness and anger. She reads my treatise on "the power of the state" and tells me it's brilliant. She wouldn't think it was brilliant if she understood it was written for her.

I re-introduced P3-P4 at a lower frequency, and it feels as if I am pooling in the back of my brain. There are no thoughts; there are just pools that ripple with the perturbations of the universe and disappear. There is no intensity there, at least not at 4.5, but there is a kind of aimlessness or even quiet restlessness. Frontal training brings me out, forward into the dialogue, into the fray. I do that quietly, too. But back here, I can't organize any forward motion. There is no self back here either, just organization and pooling. This is when I miss Sue. It is now when I would call her, and mostly, she would exclaim mildly and then tell me something akin to her own experience, like feeling her brain moving or the fact that to navigate in traffic, she too has to turn off the radio. But there was someone who had at least one way to hear what I was saying or what I was discovering, someone who would want to put it to use, who would be knowledgeably intrigued. I miss this collaboration. These "changes" (like "the troubles" in Ireland) turned me toward others. When Les Fehmi says that he thinks Alpha Synchrony would be good for Sue, I feel something relax in me because he says this with fatherly concern and without deference or disrespect. Someone else sees the trouble she's in. They may have seen it all along.

Self feels located separate from agency, and in my brain, it is in the temporal lobes. Self is not in executive functioning, nor is God. Candace Pert is wrong about this, the mistake of a scientist. The ego may get distributed and be manifest mostly in the functions we execute, but the ego is not the Self. The ego is a construction based on arousal. As fear diminishes, so does ego. Self then distinguishes itself from ego and becomes, at the same time, harder for me to recognize because there are no hurt feelings, ambition or rage to define it. No false self to reflect self. No comparison to others. No strategies. No observer of the self, no self-consciousness. The observer is fear constructed, and when fear is deconstructed, there is no observer, and when there is no observer, then even the self, the self at least as a construct, begins to disappear. Non Self. That has become the default position. Of course, in a way, it is everyone's default position. Affect, reactivity obscure it.

P3-P4 sets me back in my head. It feels new, neither intelligent nor dumb. It's a setting or a baseline. There is something that leaves me restless. It seems to want feeding without hunger. I could assign this to the time with Lee, the end of the session, when I couldn't sit up or turn over. I was too weak. Are there blows that bleed somewhere, that fill up some reservoir beneath consciousness that will rupture in the ultimate refusal to be forgotten? Or is this all just energy, energy locked in the cells being released into a large and forgiving universe? This universe can absorb it and neutralize it, letting it become again just energy? That is somehow what neurofeedback is doing in my psyche. It does not seem to extend the same beneficence to my body. The physical body holds its memories physically, recognizes them physically and requires their release, if this is possible, physically.

There is no mystery to map onto P3-P4, just the warm, cool, inviting pooling of the brain. There is no God. No self. No intensity, only an incomplete calm.

All along, I hoped for a witness. But more than that, a witness who would supply and bear the effect and the aftermath of the events. Supply it for me. Now I wonder who they would see.

❧

I'd expected the train ride would bore me, but I found it beautiful with the rivers, wetlands, black geese, the little upscale New England towns, and the Sound, sparkling with its little white boats. Penn Station was IMAX, a marvel of shape and movement coming and going and color that I was slipping through without resistance in time, without apprehension, perhaps without being. In the cab, easy. Up Eighth, a near collision, but grabbed by the seat belt. Each block is teaming. Not even one block is governable. It is benign; it is teaming with terrorist intention—organized and individual—, and it is held together by the wish, if not for peace, for being left alone.

Sue is looking at me across the room and making me invisible. I recognized this shrill chord, and I left, shedding it as I crossed Central Park South to enter the park. I was entranced by a surround-sound experience of all parks in all time: the promenade, the children in the playground, five baseball games in one field, ardent play in 86 degrees and high humidity. The shade comforted old people and nursing mothers and the exhausted homeless who don't dare sleep at night. I lost my sense of direction and maybe time. I watched the Black boys break dancing and gave them money for their fine acrobatics and hip-hop choreography, or perhaps just for their endurance in the heat. I lost my way. With help from a stranger, I finally came out across from the corner of 79th and Fifth. I looked up. It was Milici's office. Strange, the unconscious. I have always been confused about the geography of the park. I had no way to navigate it from inside my head. I couldn't form a map. I stayed on the street to find my way back to the hotel.

I left the hotel around 10 to walk over. It was hot and thick, and I felt disoriented. I could not stop the wobbly vibration in my head. The humidity? What have I eaten? The solution seems only to be found in food. I fixed on cold chai and walked to the little Starbucks on Columbus. My head buzzes with energy that I cannot quiet or organize into a process. I can only address it somehow like a wound. The chai doesn't help, reading the Times didn't organize me, it was hard to concentrate. I couldn't enter the fray of enthusiasm and demand that is the training Sue is putting on. I am too restless. I put the paper on the windowsill. The scene across from me formulated itself first as a montage and then slowly as memory. I'd just swallowed a second Gabapentin when I saw the inscription on the building St. Luke's Roosevelt Hospital. That was, at the time, just Roosevelt Hospital. I was there. These were most likely the residence quarters. We had a date. His name was Vince, and he invited me up to his quarters, flattened me to the bed, put his hand over my mouth and nose, pushed my dress up, grabbed the crotch of my underpants, pulled them down to my ankles, rolled his weight onto me and raped me.

I could walk over there and find the deli in among the looming buildings crowded in on each other, where we went to eat, after he washed his hands like a surgeon and apologized. I didn't eat. I repeated the location of my car to myself over and over silently as he talked, I think,

about becoming an OBGYN. It had happened in the heat and in the long torpid shadows of this neighborhood. When I realized where I was, my head cleared. The wobbly static disappeared. It is as if I had become acquainted with the neurology of traumatic memory, the infrastructure of disturbance. It doesn't kindle the emotional fear centers now, but it does disrupt the smooth operation of the brain.

We have the day together before John leaves for Australia. Continents. What will it be like when you get back? What time will have passed? It could be more like an age, the passing of the dinosaurs, the melting of the ice caps, the eclipse of the sun. Terror may have struck. All that is left of us is a shadow. Or it might be a minute or the rapid flick of an eye, and no time passes, the timelessness of a soap opera, time crammed with events and nothing happening, no forward movement. I will miss him, and I will yearn for Arles.

"In this new brain, I am no longer negotiating the tragedy of comings and goings, but I am missing you. Your leaving used to be a black hole that would swallow my whole being." I made a tight circle with my thumb and index finger, "Now it is very small. It is as if you drilled to the center of the earth with a fine bit—it is as molten as that and as deep. If I were a tiny Alice, I could tumble down, but it would not end. There is no threat. It is cellular knowing more than memory, as though a seal breaks beneath my heart, behind my stomach, and there it is, the dark chute to the molten core. These feelings become the arching back, biting the hand reached out to grab my collar, a protest or demonstration of rage at abandonment, my attempt to secure the presence of a ghost. At the bottom of the bottomless chute is madness."

He said he heard this in my voicemail message. He pointed it out, creating a safe, cool distance:

"Your unconscious is a specimen, not a tender nakedness, or vulnerability that seeks housing in my hands."

When I drove to Whole Foods, I knew I'd see Sammy. He was in the aisle in front of the checkout lanes. I called his name. He turned around, looked for a moment and said, "Seboin?" then ran into my arms. I held him, his legs around my waist. There was no resistance in either body. He was absolutely there. His fingers drummed on my ribs in his excitement and completeness. He has stories to tell me of going horseback riding and being 7. He still can look stricken with fear; he is still too thin. But he is connected and warm. He and Phil unloaded my cart. He still had the neurofeedback paste in his hair. He complained about the games. I invited him to come and train with me, maybe even stay with us.

"That was dangerous!" I had driven down a one-way street and knew it only when I nearly missed a crash. "You are not organized in your body. It has been a long time since you have been held." When I feel so deep and wild, I have some distant body hope for containment. A proprioceptive yearning. It is the only thing that will help. There is no holding in that office. It is open to the air, to people at the windows, to the swerving of skateboards down below. I plod through it. It is appropriate. I can do this. I can organize him in me with words, but it is not this. I am not playing out an old script. I can't feel his presence. He slips away. He opens the windows and goes for coffee. He brings a coffee for me, decaf.

"It should be chocolate milk," he said, sitting down next to me on the couch. He registers the time I am in, and he settles there to listen. I am slipping away into a fugue, and when he asks me what I am experiencing, I press the question, I turn it all angles and try to discern its essential element. What am I trying to say? No act now is mere discharge or acting out.

"It is about the collision, Arles. It is to tell you that things are still colliding in my head." As I left, he took my head in his large hands, and we stood there for a while in the embrace of this singular journey.

A monk who was oddly referred to as a performer stood stage right in meditation for 90 minutes in a gold funnel of light under a shute spilling golden rice on his head like rain. 500 pounds of rice flow softly, bouncing off him and the stage. It creates a river. The worker rakes it away, stage left. The first month of their rehearsal, we were told, was meditation: sitting meditation with bowls of fire and prostrations in the rice. Rice rains down in sheets and explodes up from the dancers in arcs, and all the time the monk stands and the rake rakes. The audience is wild with appreciation. They are fans now of Cloud Gate Dance Company of Taiwan. They clap and yell when the monk arrives as if he has entertained them, as if it has not been what it's been. That monk was the Buddha. Peggy agreed. The quality of his meditation, the fact of his meditation was extraordinary. I was worried for his brain, but his stability and serenity were unbroken. Clapping for this? So strange, but what else does an audience do?

Beneath every impulse is an evoked potential. Beneath every traumatic memory arising from the body is the wild firing of neuronal pools in the belly, in the heart, most painfully in the head.

"It's like an elephant sat on me," she said. "When I try to get up, I am weak. I feel flattened." Reggie is convulsed with memory, defiled by memory, rope around her neck, oral rape, the slaughter of a kitten. No human being can endure this cruelty. We have two paths, dissociation or convulsion. It started up in her again the next day. It was right, it was authentic, she needed to tell me and will again today, and I feel like a trapped animal. "I can't do this," I have to tell her; "I can't hear this" and I look into her face at the abject terror of this brutalized child, her powerlessness and her innocent and complete trust. I know I have only one choice, and my voice drops, and I say to myself, "Bring it on, you bastards, give it your best shot, I can take anything!" I held her as her body re-lived it, jerking, choking, head thrown back. I was there in the density of it. There was no other place to be. I cannot discharge what builds in me as it builds in her. It is my responsibility to shelter her. I went into phase lock with her, trapped as one magnet to another. Only a thin membrane of role divides us. I was her only containment: my body and my psyche, her only protection. These missiles were falling on both of us equally, muscle torn from bone, throats seared, eyes stinging, but my body was thrown over hers to protect her from the firestorm that her life, her memory, was bringing down on us.

My body contracted. This weekend I have withdrawn to the spinal cord. I grieved the retraction of all that life, the oceanic transcendence drawn back into bone. There is no possibility for intelligence, vision or spaciousness. I am my central nervous system, primitive, where life is about only one thing: survival. It is somehow a spinal cord that swims, a primitive eel-like creature. It swims in the darker pools of the ocean, but I can see it where the sun still filters through.

"What about your heart?" Arles noticed I was rubbing it.

"It feels agitated, but I did Heartmath to calm it, and I had very high synchrony scores."

"Maybe it isn't *your* heart."

I didn't hear the rest of what he said. When I visualize my heart, it is red, pumping evenly and filled with health. Then I felt another heart beneath it, a sick dark heart. I kept feeling and looking into this cavity. There was a small heart attached to the end of mine. It was grey with black splotches. This was hard to see, but it became clear that this heart was made of penis tissue—it was sick and weak, vestigial, and it still beat weakly when mine pumped vigorously. It was attached, like a tumor with a heartbeat. Moses' heart.

"How did Moses' heart get there?"

I sighed. I don't look for the exits anymore, it just is. "It happened this way. How is this possible? It was awful what happened to me."

But I said to him, "It got there through my mouth." Several times during body work, I'd felt the thick pressure at the back of my throat. It gets bigger. It makes it harder to breathe. I want to pass out. This gets confused with Leonard.

"Is this what Leonard made you do?"

I was surprised that he said "made me," and I felt something relax. "Lick it. Suck it. Like a lollipop." I tried to refuse. He pulled it out and pressed my head. I am gone then. I don't remember. I am not sure I remember any of it, but this is a repetitive insistence of my body.

I try to understand my relationship to these fragments of memory. I cannot collect them, they flow out of me. It used to be that Arles collected them, that he contained the fragments with his body, with his prescient understanding, but now they flow through him too. They are all too ephemeral, and they become too light. It is difficult for the 'me' that lives in the place where none of this happened. I can't transcend this. An image begins to form in the back of my brain. I have never been able to see myself as a child except in photographs. I ask him how he does this.

"What are you seeing now?"

"I think it must be like a movie, but I never see that." A small figure arises in my brain, deep in the back. I don't see any clothes on her, but she is not clearly naked either. I pause, waiting, I think, for him to come. "It's me, Arles," but when I go to say "it is the beginning of registry," my distress begins to rise. "You will need to hold my wrists if I say this." He will, but I know if he does, I will try to punch him.

"You won't be able to punch me," he said, and this is a relief.

"Can you see how I looked then?" He had images of red swellings. I asked again later.

"Can you see how I must have looked?" and it was clear he could, and so could I, because she was right there in the back of my brain, and she just stood there, like evidence.

"I was four." I counted it out on my fingers against his back, "One, two, three, four. Only this many years. I was four. I was four."

I remembered cardiac resuscitation, those hands on a heart that was fading into death in the ER. I knew that he had done this without anger, something more like urgent sorrow. He had looked at my face. I was not just 'another one' to him. He did not want me to die. I know this to be true, and I felt deep gratitude to him almost as much for leaving me with this impression of his hands as for saving my life. I sent it out to him with such pure force that he must have felt it, must've wondered, "Where did that come from?" He was sitting in a chair, a comfortable chair and off duty, whatever that duty is now. I will never know his name. Such an important person in my life, and I never thought of him before this moment. I had never thought to thank him.

I am here with Alan to try Alpha-Theta on Neuro Care, or as it will always be called, Val's system. It is, as promised, an entirely different event. We began with Beta/SMR, and both times, I felt a lot of activity on the left side, clearing into the sinuses, and it felt as if the right hemisphere was supporting this. No over-arousal. Some slight ticking of my head to the left. The action was unstoppable in Alpha-Theta. It reminded me of the epoch with Arles when I couldn't stop the takeover of fugue states. I woke up yesterday feeling that my brain was less jagged, things that usually took bumper car turns moved smoothly in gear. I had a stiff neck and still do as I write this in the downtrodden Ramada in Beachwood, Ohio, among the southern families here for their vacations at Six Flags, the Rock 'n' Roll Hall of Fame and perhaps even the Ramada itself. Sitting with different groups of these Black families, I noticed two things: my comfort at being with them—these are warm people—and my sense that since I am White, I have come to the wrong hotel. I wandered into the Inn at Chagrin Falls—another possibility—it felt awful to me. It was White, privileged Westchester County, and I couldn't get out fast enough.

Alan is thinking very important thoughts: sacred geometry, neurofeedback as the paramount control system, and Wolfram's New Kind of Science. He imagines the possibility of constructing a mathematical model, three dimensions that must in some way suggest a fourth dimension or beyond. He is trying to think his way to the most accurate model, plugging in Siegfried's ideas and Val's system to provide the best possible reflection of the brain to the brain. I am less smooth after the second training. On the phone, Rae notices stuttering and irritable responses. I am over-aroused and don't see how to address this with Val's system.

I drove from the airport to my appointment with Lee.

"What I most feel," she said, "is the absence of vacancy." She spoke of her friends with a two-month-old baby not fully present yet still making vital synaptic connections. "This is how I feel about you." I agreed, the potential of presence is there in my body. There are no obstacles, just the need for new synaptic connections, for arms and hands, for the opportunity to suck my toe.

She can't do much for my stiff neck that keeps jerking to the left until it stops at the edge of a cliff.

The starting point for my 'episodes' is almost irrelevant. Sometimes it is a thought or a perception, sometimes it is a slight rise in blood pressure or a hit of caffeine and then the process kindles. It is all about kindling. Information triggers neurons which, if possible, recruit other neurons and they take their familiar pathway, for Jamie to blood pressure, for me to convulsion, for Eleanor to binge, for Sabelle to fall over the edge into dissociation.

HBOT 3

My first week back in hyperbaric. I am diving with a woman whose son had 100 seizures a day and, after 50 neurofeedback sessions, has none. Here is the cutting edge of medicine in the former nine-car garage of a former millionaire at the end of a mile-long driveway in Great Barrington, Massachusetts.

By the end of the first session, I felt as if my hips were locked in place and my sacrum was out— the pressure, weight and the pain were intense. Again, my mind refuses this and orphans my body. For the first few days, I thought that if I could only shit, I could move this out, but I was locked there, too. I couldn't move. It wasn't so much because a bowel movement would hurt; it was that the fullness and pressure were part of the information. And the tearing and twisting of small bones. I could not turn over. I was too hurt.

Lee felt helpless and confused. "I don't know why this is happening. We have done this already." She will understand when she gets there; this is different; this is sodomy. But I am not sure. Maybe the EFT experience doesn't count outside its meridians, or perhaps somehow its energy settled back into my muscle rather than being dispersed. The EFT experience, I think now, could be what women are actually experiencing who report the visit of the incubus. On the phone in the night, I told Lori, "I need to do EFT on EFT!" The body's memory is tenacious and determined. Lee lifted my head with a pillow so I could blow my nose. I needed to be in a hospital in a white-sheeted crib with the railing down and the nurse there. I could feel myself begin to regain strength. I was in the great eternal drift, meeting all kinds of people and seeing images float up and by. There was a young Japanese girl with bones like glass lying on the table, recovering.

My sacrum still reverberates. The bottoms of my feet are numb. Jamie will recommend more oxygen, but I have to return to my patients and my other life of competencies.

The second week, my skin is filled out, my brain is more stable, and my sacrum is still out. My head pivots from or through 01, in sudden, dramatic but smooth shifts, 2° to the left.

"We are codebreakers, John. Neurofeedback is a code-breaking system: brain becomes mind; brain to mind to universal consciousness. To understand how the brain works. The meaning of symptoms. Where they originate and how. Trauma and kindling. Kindling is the model."

Arles asked me about the Japanese girl, and I noticed the subtle vapor of dismissal that surrounded my response. I didn't trust his question. I am measuring—is he with me? Is he taking me somewhere? But I answered.

"Her frame is small. I think, you know... You see these petite young women with babies, and it seems impossible that they could have given birth without breaking. She is naked on the bed or a table, and she is being attended to by someone who is in Lee's position. She is neither alive nor dead."

"What happened to her brain?"

"I don't know." I paused to find out what had happened. "When the bones of glass in her pelvis broke, it broke the bones in her head." I paused again. "She's intact."

"Is there a hemorrhage?"

"No, she is clean or as clean as a body being prepared for burial, but she is not dead. She is not in a room, or if she is, it's a large room, and the walls are far away, and they cannot be felt."

"What kind of light?" I had to look more deeply.

"It is a white-gray, thin light, wan, but it doesn't wash out the color of her skin. If the light comes from anywhere, it is from an operating room light that is so far up I can't see it. The attendant is folding sheets. The focus of trauma is her pelvis, the sacrum of glass. It shattered. She is 14 or 15 and Japanese."

"How do you know she is Japanese?"

"That's a given."

"Are you looking at her or through her or from her?" This question is hard to answer. I look more closely.

"None seems quite right except that I can't see her face because I am beneath it. I don't have a position related to her. When I turned over on Lee's table, she, alone, was there."

"Where am I?" he asks. This question allows me to begin to relax into his other questions. I realized that I had not expected his presence when I arrived. In all this trauma work, I expect only to be alone. Not desperately or tragically alone—not anymore—but all together alone, without company. No one to catch me in the freefall. It feels as if there are shards of glass in my own bowel. This does not surprise him or me either. I did not suck exhaust from a car in a closed garage or shoot myself. I ate glass. It was about shattering.

"This girl is as fragile as glass. Her pelvic bones are like those blown glass deer you find in gift shops, like those glass legs."

"Why is she Japanese?" I didn't know. I made guesses.

"The episode in the attic happened in 1946."

"The '*episode??!*'"

"I don't know what to call it." I felt a little embarrassed on my own behalf. "I grew up with 'Japs' in newsreel footage of the war they started. I think we hated Japs. I only imagine this; I don't remember it. I do remember being confused because my cap gun had 'Made in Japan' pressed into the handle, and the caps came from Japan." He nodded.

"The girl is not reviled or hated, but perhaps this is the confusion, the reason." When he begins to close in from the perimeter, I begin to feel what happened then in those rooms on the third floor. My brain begins to burn, and the thought—no, it isn't even close to thought—the near sensation of knowing incinerates me. It is spontaneous combustion.

"What is your relationship to this girl?" Every question takes me a few seconds longer to answer.

"She is my spontaneous creation, the creation of turning over from my stomach to my back." Brutality, he'd called it. Such brutality. His naming that, his empathic laying on of words, I had thought would be enough. As I thought, the boulder dream would be enough.

The more questions he asked and the more I ventured into the details of the image, the less Arles had to say. I begin to feel alone, being just beyond the stretch of his arm. But not entirely. He is not afraid to ask these questions. This glass girl has meaning to him, which helps me to protect her meaning to me.

"Why don't I turn over just as me or even as the child?" He waits for me to answer. "I can't. If I stayed that little girl, I could not turn over. She represents how small I was and maybe how hated." For some reason, I can't feel this at all. "She is beautiful, pubescent, innocent and suspended between living and dying. Maybe it is an image arising recently in the deep unconscious where all of this is held—not made then. Not a creation of that time or of my four-year-old self. It doesn't seem likely to be the creation of a child's mind."

He was quiet before he spoke, "It was nuclear."

It was a revelation, not insight. I did not say "No."

"This isn't happening the way I thought it would."

"It is discovery."

"It is not what I expected. It isn't memories arising, cohering into a narrative or something that could give rise to a narrative, spoken and then released. It could never have been like that. It could never be like that, but that is not just the Hollywood version; it is the trauma experts' version."

Beloved. The word arrives inside the oxygen hood. Beloved. And with it, a memory that he was cradling me, furtive and overwhelmed. As I try to describe this to Arles, I have images of King Kong and Fay Ray.

"It is like that." He asked me what I felt. I was reporting, not feeling. "It's the oxygen, Arles." He grants me this, but he doesn't understand. The memory is thin as vapor, embracing it is like walking off the wing to hold a cloud. I think this happened. It comes in a flash across the front of my consciousness, but it disappears. It has no substance. There is no limbic culture to nourish this.

Arles seemed almost to amble into this. It left me riveted, psychically staring straight ahead, maybe physically too stunned. "With all the brutality, degradation and horror, you seem to have more attachment to Moses than I have ever heard toward your mother."

There was no moment of reflection. It came as sudden as a bomb. "Oh, god, oh, god, I am seeing Ground Zero." It exploded in my brainstem. It shot through my brain in waves of white light through my eyes. That is what I am looking at. He sat over there, but close enough that I could feel his attention. "Have you ever boiled an egg and opened it and found a chicken fetus?" My stomach turns, and my head throbs just below the skull in the tender transition between body and brain. "This is like that. I can't describe my experience any other way." All the familiar words for state or affect have dissolved. "I have no feeling, just registration and barely that." Or, I thought, "completely that," but without any possibility to comprehend it. "This is a lot to take in."

He realized immediately, I think, that I had landed somewhere other than he had anticipated, that he had not really measured or anticipated at all. He tied my shoes and rubbed my back as I bent to the task of leaving. Without knowing it, I expected that the real world of people on the street would be warped beyond recognition, that I would have slipped out of time. It looked both familiar and new but benign.

This moment slips into the background. It is not something I can step around or work through. It is Isness. It is my private ground zero. The device exploded in my brainstem. Did this begin with my training in Cleveland? It feels like a blow there, a blow that shattered consciousness. It is the image on the small black-and-white TV that Maddie watched in the afternoon, the image of the bomb, it never seemed Hiroshima or Nagasaki but Nevada, and it is looking directly into the nuclear explosion that blinds you. Never look directly into it. The image is just like that. It burns back into my eyes. I cannot look away; it won't blind me exactly, but it hurts my eyes. I can't look at it long enough to take it in. It will have to be absorbed, somehow.

"Arles", I asked with some urgency, "hold the statue, the one carrying the rigid baby/Buddha." He stood up, gracefully, without any urgency of his own, took the small Indonesian carving from the bookcase and sat down cradling it across his large hands. It has come to represent being carried. In one moment, it is Moses turning me over gently after the other two have left, picking me up like the Pieta, sitting down with me in his lap, his tears landing on my face and my naked chest. "I can feel his rocking. He is not rocking me." Arles seems to get even more still. "It's as though I await instruction. Will you lay me down and stretch out my legs and lay my head down with your hands under the back of my head and my neck until it touches the pillow?"

Holding is now confusing. It has King Kong in it. When these memories arise, Moses' chest becomes black leather. I do not want to be crumpled into the massive black arms. He doesn't hold me like Fay Wray, but he is that scared, that confused, that hunted. The statue is being carried downstairs, out; it is over. Taken into my bed. Moses is upstairs. I want this to be in Arles's hands. There was a flash of urgency and then the stark rigidity, the image: Nothingness. Isness.

Over tofu at Paul and Elizabeth's, Eva asked me about hate. Arles had asked too. "I do not hate anyone." I wondered with him if this has to do with objectlessness, the original one and the one now gaining in me. He seemed to lean in this direction but was not at all convinced, believing, I guess, in hatred—a pure, Biblical hatred. But in objectlessness, hate disappears. Eva thought this was the dharma teaching and that it must be true of love as well. "I don't think so," I said, after swallowing the last bite and wiping the corners of my mouth. "There is something irreducible about love." She immediately agreed. She called it appreciation, though, I think, to take the arousal out of love. Arousal that keeps us troubled, even about love.

It is the anniversary of 9/11. Before I could sleep, I turned the TV on again. The New York Symphony Orchestra is performing Verdi's Requiem, the New York City skyline behind them, thousands of empty seats in front of them. "They were," I said to Arles, "playing to the dead."

Memory is a confound. The only memory that can be trusted is that which is not memory. King Kong. When did he enter this field? Is this fiction proof of a larger fiction or a salient clue to the reality of all that my body brings forward, memories as reliable as the stones in my New England garden? They were not there last year or even last month. Oxygen shoves them up from the healing limbic brain. It may be that we encode everything, that everything is memory, and it slips in and interweaves its firings in tidal pools of neuronal communication. King Kong. Everyone felt for King Kong. I cried when he was finally killed hundreds of times over to rescue the squirming white worm of a thing that was no one at all but blonde and not to my mind worth saving.

"More attached to Moses than my mother." I started to say, "Well of course," but I didn't have time to agree before shock set in.

My body holds back. I am not opposed, but my psyche-soma gates memory, wisely or unwisely; reflectively or reactively, I don't know. But in the morning, when I saw Bob, I had to push against the energy I was left with. I needed to lie right there where I was. In that state, I could not get up. I was sprawled across the floor, unconscious or dissociated. My mind is not so much a part of this. No narrative, no explanation, just the heaviness of the blow to the back of my head, the injury to my neck, the impossibility of getting up on my own. In these times when I learn again how badly I have been hurt, I wonder why I have to. Memory keeps digging a grave, then refuses to be buried. All learning is repetition, and each repetition gains on the last one and alters it, but still, it is not real.

Reggie has settled into an equanimity that is genuine but that I have learned not to trust. It's not fragile exactly, more like an internally timed explosive. Her peace has been of short duration. This time, it was someone else's strange paroxysmal event. When she bent down to attend to him at the sheltered workshop, her violent client punched her in the face. She got through that, but when he came back the next day, her fear had her. She fell apart. It came clear to me.

"Reggie, punch him back!" I coached her. It was watching a switch turn on. Her eyes brightened. This command changed a whole set of perceptions. She saw how startled he would be, that it would probably be good for him, that it had never occurred to her that she would not precipitate a worse attack; that she could stop him. This morning, we will see how much this holds in her. That and FPO2. We trained there at 2-5 Hz for two minutes, no changes reported; 1 to 4 for one minute, no change reported. The next day, she was in a state of equanimity. She had been getting there before the incident, but she was now more settled into it. The distress was gone. Her short-term memory was also impaired, but it seems to be coming back, and there is no re-emergence of traumatic fear. She felt her memory would return, but not the fear. Over the weekend, she'd watched Schindler's List. It was the second time, but for her, very different. She felt "of that time."

"How old are you?" I asked.

"I am no longer little." There is a pause. I think to myself, she is 17. "I am an adolescent." She describes a wooden room. There are other girls there. She was raped by the soldiers. They are laughing. Her whole body jumps in terror as she experiences this. "They slit my throat." Almost as if she hadn't said this, she went on, "Today it is like a toggle switch. I can be focused and stay in my work, be with people, but then I return to the Holocaust." She looked to the side, collecting her narrative. "There were mix-ups in scheduling today," she said. "I feel like the whole world collaborated against me today." I was struck and asked her about the word "collaborated." She said it had struck her, too. It wasn't what she intended to say. She knew it meant working together, but when I asked, she did not know any other meaning. I'd begun to wonder if she was telling me about rape and murder by the partisans, not by the Nazis. I shared this dark meaning of "collaborator." She began to feel that this was not her, not a past life memory, that this was a spirit in the room with us, wanting, she thought, to inhabit her. I asked if the spirit could be a collaborator. Again, a quick body reaction, Reggie couldn't say exactly what it was.

"She has run away from me."

"After what I said?"

She nodded.

"You know, most collaborators were forced to collaborate." At the same moment, Reggie heard her say, "I had to do it. I didn't want to." That poor girl, I thought, and I then thought, "I am being a therapist for this ghost as well."

"You could look at this as an intrusion, and that would be true. You could look at this as a privileged encounter, in which you were chosen. You could look on her as someone to be feared and perhaps as someone who needs forgiveness. She has come to you. Ask her what she needs."

"She just looks scared," She concentrated, "Terrified and confused."

I spoke directly to the 17-year-old collaborator. "You have come here for a reason. You have a decision to make."

Reggie translated the buzzing silence in the room. "She is afraid that her parents hate her."

"I know this is what you're afraid of, but you have to face them or forever be a ghost. It has been many years. They understand now what you have understood, that you didn't want to collaborate, that you had to."

She seemed to look away.

"See if you can feel them. I sense that they are waiting to hold you in their arms."

Two days later, and Reggie is still harboring the spirit and all the Holocaust suffering. She felt an exhausted protest. She had asked what the spirit needed. All she could come up with was that she needed a bath, warm clothes and tucking in.

"No, Reggie, that is what you need. She is dead. She is beyond all that."

She closed her eyes. "She came to ask... all I can see or feel... it is as if she needs protection."

"She is beyond that, too. She might think that's what she needs, but that's not it." I was talking as much to the ghost. Reggie looks deeply again, trying to make communication with the unrooted and terrified spirit. She wanted 'protection' to be the answer.

"I am thinking about what you said last time about forgiveness. She is Judas. She denied someone."

"It was Peter who denied Christ, not Judas."

"I know, but what she thinks is that she's Judas. She thinks she lives in eternal damnation. She'd denied being Jewish after her parents were killed. She was marked as a collaborator."

"Sometimes, people are killed or die before they have time to understand why they did something or why they did something against their own conscience. Some people think that this is the explanation of ghosts. They wander between life and death without resolution. This one finds herself caught in her own belief. But she has come here for a reason. She has come here because of you."

"You could be doing this so much better than me."

"But she came to you, Reggie, and like you, she has to make a critical decision. Will she live in a state of eternal damnation or use this opportunity to be understood and understand, to free herself? It is her choice. If she chooses eternal damnation, then this is just a visit; she is taking up your session, and it is time for her to leave and continue to wander. There is nothing for her here. That's fine. That is her choice."

"I just want this over and for you to hold me."

"I will hold you, Reggie, but I cannot hold the spirit."

When I told Arles about this, I realized that I was blocking the transfer of the spirit to me, Reggie's wish, probably unconscious and perhaps that of the spirit as well. Reggie closed her eyes and described entering a state of forgiveness. The spirit rose over her head, above the couch, above the clouds and there, Reggie saw, she was received by her parents, openly, eagerly, without malice and by hundreds of other Jewish souls as well. "Homecoming," Arles said. He had been guiding me. His voice played a soft chord in my resonance with this entire situation. I commented on my own sense of ease, my lack of fear, the second nature of this, the simultaneous therapy, the confidence, the responsibility for believing Reggie, watching that I did not lead her and did not leave her in the dark.

"You have learned not to idealize these events."

"Some people summon angels; I seem to summon the hungry ghosts of the Holocaust."

"Reclamation," he said, "divine healing."

❧

At dinner in LA, my colleague Dave was laying out his latest ideas about neurofeedback and waiting for me to respond.

"You're worrying me, Sebern. I didn't think this was such a bad idea." I couldn't track what he was saying. Just as I was leaving to catch the plane for LA, I got a phone call from Colleen, my friend who is a private detective on the Cape. She had found Vince. I thanked her, stunned. I had not anticipated my response. I snapped back into the present time, and I apologized.

"A long flight," I said, "not a bad idea." I plan what I will say to the others should I have to talk with them. Somehow, none of this affects my talk. The news that both men who had raped me, Vince and Leonard, are alive runs on a magnetic track in my mind. I can participate in the day-to-day social functioning and my talks. I can't, though, quite find my footing at the CIC, and everyone, rightly and wrongly, assumed that the intrigue with the Othmers explains it. They are oddly secondary. Not easy, very sad, but not it. I don't want to be there, but where else? Siegfried insists that there was no bankruptcy. "That's where you are wrong," he shouts when I say the simple fact and turns and walks away, only to greet me later with a warm smile. He'd trained in Alpha Synchrony with Les and Susan. Sue avoids eye contact, and I don't know how to greet her until finally I just say, "Are you not going to say hello to me?"

"I have tried twice, and you haven't responded."

"I would never do that to you, Sue. Never."

"That's good," she said.

We embraced like the old friends we used to be before she trained herself out of her mind and into a needless crusade.

❧

After we'd sat together for awhile, I said to Reggie,

"I have a quiet mind."

"Yes, I can feel that," and she laughed. "I don't have such a quiet mind, but I can get a sense of what it is like, being with you. I look forward to it." I have returned with a new resolve, and we'll see if, once again, John and I can try to save the company. The world cannot lose neurofeedback.

I walked into town, noticing all the signs that it was the end of November. Thanksgiving yesterday, snow flurries, 29°, snow already on the ground. I am wearing my ski jacket, mittens, warm hat and scarf. I need evidence. I need to see the temperature display at the intersection of King and Main because I am not entirely in this loop of time. I am beside it, gathering the data I need to move with it. This time is outside of me. In me, it could be any season, any day of any month, anywhere. And then, too, there are these strange dreams. I feel myself transported more than dreaming. I seem to inhabit some other geography—time is unclear—and to be in the middle of the ongoing lives of other people. I am both a part of these lives and apart from them. They both encounter me and don't. Arles has no trouble with all of this. I don't think he considers it in the hard realm of fact, perhaps because he doesn't live much in that realm anyway.

Chapter 13

At the Advent services at the Priory, I try to penetrate the experience of belief. I am in emptiness. God is the meaning and the order, the gravity of this unknown, the rules of mystery. I suddenly feel—and with this feeling there is a vague organization of hope—that I have landed in a corridor between universes. At the other side, very close, is another universe with God there and gravity. I will open a door, and there will be a whole new sky filled with stars. Post emptiness. Could I make a god of that? Is that God beyond God, God? Perhaps it is because ideas don't exist here either, just sensation or sensate knowing, without senses at all, or anything for them to sense. I Am Not.

God creates God creates God. Universe creates universe, creates universe. Anything static is a delusion. Maybe not a corridor between anything at all, but falling into this never-ending, never-stopping, never-defining creation.

"I know the terrain of trauma."

"Oh yes, that is true."

Containment was all that was possible. This was the pathway to the subcortical events, through the body. Arles began forming at the outer limits. After the fugue states came memory. I inhabited terror in the memory of terror. And then fear ebbs away: Arles, neurofeedback, body work and hyperbaric. And now the brainstem. It is as if I have eyes there. I cover their hands with scarves. Everything is encoded there. It is no longer mute, but this memory unfolds only in sensation and eruption. No words. No pictures. No alchemy of meaning. Information is lodged there in my body and gibberish, cut off, sparks again and then stops cold.

I try to ride along the rail of nerve, to follow the sensation in faithful detail as closely as I can. It eventually has its own voice: POOR MOTHER APE. So I begin there. The only advantage of wordless memory is that there is no narrative of doubt. Bob and Sam are focused on my brainstem – that primitive part that has assigned to it the basic functions of breathing, sleeping, waking and fucking. That morning with Arles, I sat at the far end of the couch. He said I had the fleeting look of a wild animal. I was caught in some harmonic of earlier states, almost paralyzed in them. All I can think of doing is banging my head. He sat next to me. I am in the throes. There is nothing in me that wants this; nothing in me that protests. Will has no part.

I train FPO2, and the dread disappears. Sam reports that my adrenals have quieted down, they have been inflamed for weeks.

I would try to speak and shake my head no. I searched for ways to represent this to him without telling.

Arles asks me to follow the only words I have: Poor Mother Ape. Moses is rocking. I am limp. He is crying. My neck and head are back over his arm.

"Moses was passionate about you." My head swims.

"No. No." I pushed away. I saw him, massive and my small worm body. "It isn't me. His history, slavery, race, class, sex, alcohol, insanity. There is nothing about me. I am the vacant baby in the photo." I stopped.

"Don't stop, Sebern. Follow this out." I listened to my breathing.

"He was motherless... he knew me... passionate, psychotic. He wanted to destroy me, degrade me and rescue me." As soon as I see it like this, my vision changes. I leaned back against the couch. "I am not caught in the tide, but I can feel the pull under my heels. There was a wash over everything, even the snowfall felt like a catastrophe, and that wash just went away. Seeing it this way makes things different."

"He's not so 'other,'" he said.

"It's not so incomprehensible. It's clear in my right eye, not so much in my left. My left eye doesn't think this is quite over." Earlier, a car alarm went off, honking for a minute or so, and it would stop and then start again. I'd felt desperate and young and unsheltered. "This is what this is, you think it is over, and you can relax, then it starts again. In the silence, you want so much to believe it won't happen again, but you can't allow yourself to believe it because it starts again. There is no respite even in the respite."

"Is this the assault of your own mind?"

"I hadn't been thinking that, but, yes, I think so and the assault itself." I had been thinking of the respite in the arms of Poor Mother Ape.

"What does your left eye see?"

"I don't know." The brainstem was mute by its nature. Trying to see what the left eye saw, I felt the paralyzed voice. I would try to speak, and my head shakes, "No." There was only one way. I ignored everything in me.

"Do you see? No, Arles, don't see. My head is pulled back by the hair, my neck is arched, and my back too. He used my mouth. It would choke me. They held me, someone forced my mouth open."

His response was dispassionate, almost disconnected.

"You don't believe me. You find me disgusting!" He was taken aback.

"Oh, no," he said quietly, "I think this is entirely possible." Where had he gone? "I think this is entirely possible".

The human Moses, the monster Moses. Poor mother ape.

❧

Udine. The seventh annual conference of the Biofeedback Federation of Europe. After 30 hours awake, two planes, a bus, a train, a cab and 12 hours without food, we staggered into a crowded, smoky and friendly café. John loves his thick hot chocolate, and we both manage the only thing on offer here, ham sandwiches. It is clear to me that I am having a different experience of this café than anyone else, different from the collective reality, a reality that I have also experienced in other settings, in other settings, in fact, like this. The individual brain joins with all the others in a neural network of the moment. My brain is somewhat off, not quite in the synchronous rhythm of the whole. I hear every voice separately, even as they join and blend into the happy ruckus. The scene looks different, feels different to me. This is the kind of sensation that would have caused fearfulness not long ago. Now I recognize it, feel it, mention it to John and look to see this experience in other faces. All the sensations are present, the talk, loud and never ceasing, the smoke, the movement of the waiter and the scrub of chairs across the floor, the high white lighting, the dusk darkening the windows, but the sensations don't quite cohere into a common place. I am exhausted, and my brain has lost its hard-won cohesiveness. We walked back to the Astoria. It is 8 PM, and we sleep in until eight the next morning.

The first two days I spent in a workshop with Yuri Kropotov. We were in some way quite taken by each other. He seemed to be teaching the seminar to me. We met in a room of the library at the Physical Medicine and Rehabilitation Institute, deep in the aroma of old books. I understood it as he spoke and have retained the general implications, but I was left mostly with the way I loved Yuri. Jay Gunkelman compared himself, "I'm like Yuri, a nerd who knows nothing of interacting with other people." Since Jay was disqualifying himself as he characterized himself, I felt no need to protest. I wondered how much that is true, though, who is it that studies brains over human behavior? But he was warm and spontaneous, reachable and funny; enthusiastic and humble.

It is so different from what it used to be. I am no longer left to figure out the social rules and try to abide by them through imitation. I've become one who helps make them. I had a hallway conversation with Joe Kamiya after his talk, given to remind us about consciousness and human experience as the raison d'être of the field—a fact lost to many here. I was the last to speak, and about a half hour before the talk, I felt quietly seized by fear. After it was over and I'd told them that FPO2 could quiet fear, there was applause. I spoke with John Gruzelier about comparisons with Alpha-Theta. "I think Alpha-Theta returns one to an early state, most probably to one of blissful union between infant and mother, but if that was missing, if that hadn't happened for this baby, then Alpha-Theta might not be helpful. It is not a de novo experience." He was interested in the idea of "a known state." Joe told me that he thought it was an excellent presentation; "Important." Tanju Surmeli, a psychiatrist from Istanbul, came up to me. "People asked me if I could help them with fear. Now I can say 'Yes.'" "Now you can say Yes," I repeated, and he double checked the position of the electrode.

A panel of men was forming in the front, and their lack of self-consciousness about this feels like the 60s. I went up to say goodbye to Yuri.

"I felt a little like a dog thrown in the ocean." He looked concerned and a little surprised.

"Oh, no, we need to hear everything, everything goes into the flux." I kissed his soft cheek and left with John to grab a pizza, and then to reverse the pattern: taxi, train, bus, two planes, shuttle, car to the airport Hyatt where Marsha and I stay. The FPO2 seed was planted in the rocky soil of Udine.

❧

I am not making a story. I am talking to my body.

I would not remember any of what I am to write, even by tomorrow night—this is one of the reasons to write it. I don't want to remember, I don't want to remember, but most clearly, I don't want to forget. It tries to slip away like a dream. It felt to me that I could hurry its passage.

Arles told me that I had to let go of the wish to tell him of Udine for now.

"It is hopeless to cry."

"Why is it hopeless to cry?"

"There is no appeal. It evaporates. I am beyond crying."

We sat, each on our own side of my evacuation.

"My brain feels split down the middle. I can't remember the name of the book... 'Locked in', finding whatever way possible to communicate, to tell the story. He woke up. I keep remembering 'The Bell Jar', so I can't remember the book's name. He comes out of his coma as they are sewing his eyelids closed. He can't tell them he feels this. He can't scream. Neither can I. This is not as thin as a metaphor. It feels as if it's in my left eye."

"What did you see?"

It had never occurred to me that I saw anything. I am helpless to these episodes, except for their presence. I stay present now almost entirely, and he does episodically and then exquisitely.

"There is wave after wave crashing down on me, and I just want you to come along, grab me by the collar and drag me out of the surf."

"I know you wish I could do this. Instead, you must remember that this tide will ebb."

The engine turned over, and a beautiful trumpet solo played on the car radio. It took me a moment to recognize it, "Sometimes I feel like a motherless child".

I am settled with attic events. There may be more I must know, and if this is so, I will learn it without the energy of pursuit. Arles reminds me that I have declared it "over" before. I remember most vividly the way I felt after the boulder dream, and that I knew then nothing else was required. The boulder rumbled down through my dreams and tore open consciousness. The shift is still there. I am sitting back on my hips. I am more drawn to settling than to discovery.

Sam asked me what happened. His hands hovered over my lower back. "Your adrenals are numb. This is different for you."

"What does it mean?"

"Shock." I don't want to hear this. It was a discovery; it came out of the blue. I have the Networker conference, then the New Jersey presentation. I can't have shock, not now.

"There is a lot here, Sebern." I barely hear Sam. This is the "settling in" time. Enough is known, and here is the difference between the timing of the mind and the body. Arles seemed to challenge my growing conviction that for me, it is this body work or it is catastrophic illness. I think this is wholly true. It seems such a salient hypothesis to me. It is difficult to account for this constant discharging of body memory if it were not akin to detoxification—bad information, extruding from muscle and fascia. Nothing much after these events in the attic seems to have been coded as trauma, not the rapes, or the car accidents, or being held up in the elevator. I never seem to end up at the edge of the road in the Black Forest or in the elevator with a knife at my throat. Those circuits were blown when I was four. This phenomenon is reported every day but not recognized. Replay does not re-traumatize. It is only a pathway back to the original events. There is only one opportunity for traumatic learning so deep in the body. There just couldn't be another.

It is 6 in the early spring morning. I walked up the road to the hermit's house. Everyone is still sleeping, but the chickadees and the woodpeckers are not. The streams have opened up a little, and the snow is crusty from melting in the day and freezing in the night.

Bob talks to me about his struggle against blending. "You are dumping, and it's very big." He asked me to warn Lee and Sam. I had told him he should wear latex gloves. "With others with trauma, it is as if they reach a place, the motherload, as it were, of trauma, and there is emotional release, and it is processed. With you, it is more like a shattered window. I don't know what... this is something, some higher order processing..."

"It has meaning that the only other person who evoked Bob's fear of blending was a woman who was nearly electrocuted," Arles said.

After the night closed in around us, the rain froze into jewels. Everywhere around me, the trees are embedded with diamonds, more encrusted with precious gems than the entirety of the Russian court.

❧

"This energy is far worse than anything in you." That's what he said later. At the time, 18 hours after it happened, he sat for less than 30 seconds in my office. "This energy is terrible! It is the worst I have ever felt." He left the office, and we sat in the waiting room. "Do you have Gregorian chants? Put on Gregorian chants. Male voices are best. Sai baba incense." We opened the windows. Later, I got a mirror and put it at the door and a fan to blow the energy out the window. I lit a candle. I thought it had passed through me, but Arles doubted it. By the afternoon, I could not think clearly. I am vibrating with the concussive shock. My soles were hot.

I want to clear the vibrational field, but I do not feel penetrated by what happened here Tuesday night; I am concussed by it.

I have never witnessed nor read about anything more terrible. The force of depravity and degradation. The force of evil. It blew out of her, out of her chest, out of her face, exploding into the little consultation room. The door slammed open in her brain. I have to remember to say that she had trained at FP02, and first it was the rape, remembered and worked out, but that was nothing.

Tuesday night, when I came into the waiting room, I knew something was very wrong. Reggie's cup was still on the table. When I saw her, she was recognizable, but I didn't know who was sitting there. I asked her, but the question confused her, and the confusion I feared would frighten her even more. In a voice I didn't recognize, she told me that she didn't want to come, but she did so because that was the contract. We had never used that language. I wanted to say, "You don't have to be crazy," but I couldn't. It wasn't true. She had no choice. I had called her uncle a murderer. She had fractured.

"Who tells an eight-year-old girl her uncle is a murderer?! How could you do that!" She screamed. She realized even as she made the accusation that there was now an unbridgeable gap of us and them, of those willing to kill—she was in that group, I in the other. I had known nothing of the letters he sent her, the letters that helped her survive the ice-cold house, the frozen parrot, the dog run over, the mother never home. She probably took those letters behind the only chair to read them "in privacy." She said on the phone that she hadn't known. She realized later that she did know all along, every grizzly detail, that she'd heard her mother scream when it came over the news on TV. Relatives gathered there. She'd been told. She heard me call *her* a murderer. I could watch her try to grasp why I would hurt her so.

"You said you understood about the shock of the word 'murderer'!"

"Yes, but what you feel and what I understand you feel are not true." She started to cry.

"I never killed anyone!"

"No, that's true, you never killed anyone. I know."

And then the "subs" are there, and although she identifies these subs as her, they were unholy and disembodied. Then, she told me later, the room turned orange, and she laughed. It was sociopathic but even less human. It was her uncle's energy fused to her child's murderous rage, encapsulated, projected and exploding into here and now, into my chest. I breathed. There was nothing else to do but sit there. There was no escape. I had, without experience or intention, performed an exorcism. When it had worn itself out a bit, I asked her what she needed. Her face crumpled, and she began to cry, and both adult and child had returned. "I need you." I held her. It wasn't hard. Easier in fact than ever. She was quieting. The tremor was more in me.

She gave her talk that night, amazing given what had just happened an hour before, and I attended. Back home, I couldn't focus; I wandered. I smudged the room but in a kind of Protestant way; I watched TV; I took all medication early. I somehow didn't think to take a bath. The next day, she returned. She had slept well (!) but was drained, too exhausted to walk longer than a mile. She smelled the incense as she came up the stairs, and when she got in the room, she was met with the chanting, and she felt at home. As she pulled her jacket on, she said, "I am beginning to fill with grace." She credited me—it could've been me —and the next day smudged her house for three hours, praying, opening windows, cleansing herself, her clothes and her home of this dark, dark energy. I want to cleanse with the chants, but the CD player is busted, so the vibrations will ebb out, not flow away in these voices as I would have wished.

But Tuesday, I had faced down evil—no, I faced evil, I sat through it more than with it. I wasn't terrified, I was chilled. I was pinned, and I kept my focus on her and on the clock. This would end. Yesterday, knowing it was not the same force that I had met in the attic, I learned that it was also not different. The energy in my consultation room was evil. Moses' energy was crazy and demented. She asked about her uncle,

"How could I have loved him?"

"You loved his letters, Reggie."

But I can't say that about Moses. Trying to put these things together creates a crack in my brain. It vaguely hurts, and it makes me feel wild enough to bite the arm of the sofa. Oh, that was about a seizure, too. I don't have this evil in me. But my shoulder cramps. I am confused by comfort, rocking, tears falling on my body, and near death. There was, I just realized now, no blood. Her horror was filled with blood. Mine was dry, hot and humid with his tears.

"Keep your feet on the earth," Arles instructed, "feel the energy of the earth."

Bob had my left foot.

"This is challenging," I said.

"I have never seen this before. Didn't think memory was held in a foot, but this foot is purging."

"But the banister, you know about that."

"I thought that was the ankle." The terrible recognition, sudden and nearly breathless, and I started to cry. He had held me over the banister by my foot.

Then he focused on my chest.

"This is going to sound bizarre, but you have cigar smoke in your lungs, a lot of it, yellowish, blue smoke." I knew that was right. I imagine the room dense with smoke while they played cards. "It is almost as if it had been blown into your lungs."

Sam says that the whole right side of my body is "up," that something is coming up, and my sacrum is swollen.

Lee has the sense of purging too, of catharsis, as if memory worked that way. She's moved the sheet over my feet, and they jump away from her touch. "I wondered where that was," she said softly. I asked her just to hold them. I was dangling. I wanted her to take her hands off my feet, to leave me alone, to stop and if she took her hands off my feet...? I was caught, suspended. She couldn't take her hands off; I would fall three stories. She moved up under my legs, holding them close to her body, then she put her arm under my back. I tried to form the image of being laid down on the floor—I didn't have that part of this memory—but I could feel it. "It is the Pieta, Lee," and she knew this.

I thought Lee would bring her hands up my shins. Instead, she created a form for this Christ energy. She was part of this. I was draped across her body.

"Christ became the lens that focused all trauma that was and all trauma that is yet inevitably to come, into that moment."

"It was not me there, Arles. This did not happen to me. Energy formed. It had to do with experiencing this trauma, bearing it and transcending it all at once. It was the Pieta in the painting, legs held by the Holy Spirit, the infinite mother, the mother of God. It's hard to tell whether he is alive or dead; he was both. Even Jesus could not be protected."

"Should he have been protected?"

He stuns me with this question.

"No." I had to think to be sure this was right, that he wouldn't disagree, "But I should have been."

"Yes," he said with no hesitation, "You should have been."

As I tried to describe my state, he reminded me that this day was the anniversary of Chernobyl. He spoke of it: 500 Atom bombs never exploded, shrouded in concrete, threatening the worst nuclear event ever, remembered better in the cells of unborn Ukrainian babies than in the minds of bureaucrats anywhere. It could have been that.

"My nuclear event is more like an Anasazi vase, the only remnant left of an ancient civilization. An urn, a beautiful ceremonial burial urn, is all that is remaining. It is cracked, shattered. All those veins are nerves that hold memory, and I am not free of it. The spaciousness within it, the 'not me' space, presses against the insides of my body, the inside of the urn, the smooth burgundy clay of it, lifeless but for memory, a representation of a whole civilization that has mysteriously disappeared. It is kept behind shatterproof glass, locked up by the museum staff. It is preserved in its shattered wholeness. There is no desire to restore it, only to preserve it. It's all we have left." I read this to Arles, cradling the journal. "And what would happen, Arles, if we just tapped it with a small hammer, a jeweler's hammer or a restorer's hammer? It would collapse along the nerve lines into tiny shards, the last rubble. The vessel that is still me would lie at my feet. My body would be only a body."

I imagine asking him to tap at the rounded shoulders below the full open neck. What would happen then? Just the smallest tap of the hammer. It cannot be me who taps the urn. It is so beautiful, ancient, burgundy with white patterns.

Traumatic memories do not pile up. They live in me like circles within circles.

"In a way, Arles, I have only 'then' and 'now', nothing in between of the nuanced life of pain, sorrow and joy, all the relationships that make up a life. They are barely recalled and only in broad strokes." "Motherlessness and the early assault bleach memory, like bones on the desert floor."

"What is it like to read this to me?" he asked.

It is the fetal curve of my mind in his. It is coming to and lying against the cool, glazed burgundy wall of his consciousness. He is a vessel.

"I am exposed to the elements, and you shelter me." Mater Dolorosa. Not grief and not sadness but sorrow. He asked about this.

"Grief and sadness nourish us. Sorrow doesn't. It is not fluid or static. It is transpersonal; beyond. Sorrow is the soft gray membrane across all of eternity. It exists outside the psyche, perhaps outside of time. But it is 'of humanness.' The apes and the elephants begin to feel it. It becomes our collective contribution to the cosmos that soaks back into us like fog."

As we talked more about what I hadn't written, I asked,

"Is this the exhaustion of transforming death into life? Is this analogous to what the Tibetans describe as the Bárdos, the stations of transformation, what is required of everyone? And why is the image of the Anasazi, of these people who disappeared when they looked like they were about to sit down for dinner?" I know it's an urn. It is reassuring to see this so clearly, and he understands this too. Of course, it is an urn, not a vase. Of course. It is suicide, perhaps even genocide if I were to use the hammer. In his hands, it is liberation.

As this consciousness fades, there is one last image that stays with me about my relationship to Arles. It is my back up against the smooth surface of the interior, the burgundy interior of his consciousness. It feels cool, sheltered, comforting, my warm bare back against this cool internal form. This is a vase or a pot, not an urn.

It is rainy and cool, and everything is greening up outside. Soon, my bedroom, so long exposed to the street, will become my tree house.

Bob has, it seems, held back.

"We can decide to do this, to remove the linchpin; I know you will be alright, but it will be walking across a minefield. It could undo you for a while." He thinks that I am held together by intelligence. What else is there to do once presented with this? Neurofeedback plays a big part here, and I can't know what that is. But I trust it. It will collect my brain.

Last night, we expected to celebrate Molly's birthday at the Hofbrau House with the odd crowd she collects. Her 40th. Instead, John and I spent it in the ER with Johnny. He didn't know where he was, at the airport, in Miami, he didn't know the year. He couldn't walk. He tried to get up, to pull out the catheter, to smoke the rubber oxygen sensor or pull it off every minute, which made the monitor go mad. John finally just put it on his own finger. He fought the IV; he was severely dehydrated. I would quiet him and secure his cooperation for one invasive process after another. We were with him next to him on a gurney in the linen supply room. The table next to him held the 24 bottles of medications—the source of this crisis, this round. One nurse looked at the array of orange bottles and exclaimed, "This is medical malpractice!" Johnny broke every agreement he made within a minute. He was weak, so I could hold him down, but I had to do that every 90 seconds. John kept the doctor from giving Johnny a spinal tap. Our family physician noticed us from the hallway and came to help. He admitted Johnny to critical care. I asked him if he wanted us to stay and go with him up to the room. He reflected. "I would actually." Another 45 minutes trying to keep him from exposing himself and the machine from beeping. It was like Memento. It was not known; it was just experienced, and it had ramifications. The neurons in my brain were dancing in a mosh pit. But I felt open to him, to this experience. I just loved him. There was no separation; it was just as it should be, and it took a toll.

He is in critical care, still slurring and saying things like he just wants to go out and go about his business. He apologizes, but without awareness of the impact of what he does. Talking about that never engages him. It is as if you push through to blank, numbed terror. He has a hazy self, but he has no center. He has a beautiful soul, but he is obliterated by fear and even more now fear of fear. He needs care beyond our means to provide and beyond his capacity to receive.

On his way to the shower, John came and sat with me on the bed. "This is beyond your reach. It is beyond mine."

"Were you afraid that no one would understand you?" Arles asked me.

"It isn't that, but I do feel that I can't make myself understood. Something profound has happened. I have had an experience that I thank Johnny for. After the ER, I entered into the memory of my own psychotic states. I knew the terrible feeling of slippage, of gaining on reality momentarily, then losing my grip. It was as if I lay there staring into space with my eyes closed, unable to move, knowing that whatever was happening in my brain/psyche had to happen. I wasn't afraid. It is beyond what can be described. That is the nature of it."

"Radical singularity." That was what Arles called it.

I am tripped up. Destabilized, suggestible in the harmonics of seizure and memory. It is about sex. All of this opening will be about sex. It was pornography. I became the pornographer and the child star. My secret life as a child. I called the bits of personality that kept demanding my attention and, to some degree, his, "the 10-year-old construction." Here, I am as reclusive and solitary as the Unabomber. I'd said nothing to Bob. In his hands, it is only my body that speaks. He laughed a little self-consciously, "It's almost, not too explicitly, but I keep seeing girlie magazines. I usually don't get images, but this keeps occurring." Today I feel the safety in my arched back. It is inherently, posturally, safe. That's why babies do it.

He will need to ask me these very difficult questions about sex. He will have to gently insist that I organize a vocabulary around this. Sex has to become like everything else; it has to become possible. We are not aware of the nerves in our teeth until they are exposed, and once they are, they organize everything. This morning, as I returned to this account, the intensity of all of this has passed. There is no empathy for the girl who must have suffered these degradations; there is actually no girl there at all. Only these grizzly body echoes that demand knowing, but that never lead me to the actual girl. Intense focus and arousal keep the girl who suffered this eclipsed. The events arise through bodywork flashes; what happened in this sense is known. The girl who is me is not. Arles has to be active, has to help me find her. I did imagine arousing him into a sexual frenzy; apart from that, I am mute about sex. Within it, I have a lot to say—cunt language, the exceptional power of the prostitute. I want to characterize it that way, but I don't experience it that way, or even as perversion, but through that language, we might find me, the child who endured it. It was perversion.

Yesterday I just wanted to shut the door. I considered stopping all the information flow, no longer seeing any of these therapists, gently closing the door and walking out the back. Finishing. It is endless, so I will declare it ended. The intense flash of rage, the pure hatred that came unbidden, that slipped out between the cracks, that it can still happen given just the right set of circumstances, that makes quitting not possible. It was amazing, actually, to feel that I could walk away; that I would be ok. I have never been closer.

I went to him, trapped, trapped by my mind, trapped by the therapy.

"You are free, you can leave." He may have been tempted, but he didn't say "but." There were no foreclosures, no threat worse than the leaving itself. I went there wanting to forfeit. I was the panther, taunted, terrorized, pacing. There were no words. It was sensate, essential. The mind of one caught in the chamber that had been her home. It was not Iraq; it was not Auschwitz; it was home. It wasn't "I can't do it;" it wasn't "I don't want this anymore," although this is the kind of thing I said, and it was true. I wasn't exhausted, I was "Exhaustion." I was "Trapped." I was at the very core. I couldn't contain this. I stood up. He came to me in the corner. He put his hand behind my neck. I heard him respond to my protest, "I don't want this!"

"I know. I know." He answered softly. His hand passed gently across my cheek as he went to lock the door against the intruder that these states beckoned.

Words couldn't free me. I had used them all up. That alchemy was over. Somewhere, it began to clear. He took me to the sanctuary of his couch, and he sat in his chair for a long time, silently.

"Have you ever been to the Jardins du Plants?" I asked.

"Yes, I have."

"I wouldn't go to the zoo." It is as if the panther has outlived Rilke and is still pacing there. I knew what I'd see, and it was awful. Cramped spaces, rusty bars. "You freed me from that foul pen. I am walking freely, weaving in and out of the crowds on the Rue Saint-Germain. If they see me at all, they are not afraid. But it is not over for me. I am bruised to the bone from captivity, and it's in my walk. You can see it. The panther is here with a red collar, but no one seems to notice me on the streets of Paris." He took a quiet drink of tea from his artisan mug. "There is an account of a Holocaust survivor. His worst year, much to his shame, was the year after his liberation. It is like that for me. That is what these last two years of therapy have been, post-liberation. More trapped."

There are no words to say what it was that I experienced in the psychotic mind I shared with Johnny. I try to define it by saying what it was not.

"I think the analogy to homeopathy is right," he said. Spike had told me that the idea of homeopathy is to see what a substance does and dilute it until all that was left was its frequency, the vibration of the substance. Chemically, it isn't there. It is only its memory, its vibration.

"Is this the experience that was once, let's say, arsenic that is now an antidote to poison? Is this time the diluted version of the time before?" He nodded. This was not an analogy. "I wish it wasn't true, Arles, but this requires containment."

"I know. Of course. It's all right."

I know nothing of the windows or the thin walls on Friday. He'd noted it at the time. I felt his hand holding my wrist, and I relaxed a little, even remembering it. I have the image of the English Patient, then the beds in so many of my dreams; a bed, in the midst of the ruins of war, a beautiful old house, the patient without a face, without a history. Memory that slowly unwinds, nursing care, sadness everywhere, the diffusing of bombs, the room and the tender care, the white sheets, the proof of bandages... I would have to go to a hospital. I paused.

"If I told someone that I had been in a hospital for a physical illness for nearly 5 years, they would be horrified."

"Yes, they would."

"But it's all I could have wanted. The core of it – the image is of me in bed, and white sheets with Maddie sitting next to me." I paused again to find the image. I could hear his steady breathing.

"Memory like this is like a loved one being assumed dead because there has been some terrible event and they haven't been seen—not like the Twin Towers, we see that, more like Molly Bish, disappeared. You never really know they are dead. It's all shadow. Known and unknown. Out of reach. It's harder than if you knew they were dead. It's like that."

He sighed. "Yes, Sebern, exactly."

"Beds were my only solace. They came to represent safety. The attic had no bed for me. I am on the floor. Beds are safety and oblivion."

He asked me to describe the scene as I needed it to be.

"It is a farmhouse in France, thick stone walls with painted plaster, cracked around the ceiling, a flowering tree outside the window, a single white metal bed with white sheets and a white coverlet, a fan, a bedside stand with flowers and a pitcher in a bowl, a dresser with another vase of flowers, lilacs. You would sit with me even though I was in a coma." I started to cry.

"I will picture that. I will hold that image too in my mind," he said as he helped me on with my raincoat.

I was a long way into describing a new level of opening before I realized how intricately it linked to Arles. When I began, the otherness that existed was not otherness at all; it was projection. I didn't even register those closest to me. I cared for them or failed to, worried about them or tried to escape worrying for them; needed them, but fundamentally I needed them mostly to circumscribe the space around me. I did not understand that they had lives apart from their interface with me. It was rare when I saw this. It is how high arousal builds a web around us, and in it, we circle. It has taken years for me to discover Arles as an "other." I came to see the reality of people on the street as I got less and less scared. They are all suffering, and I am, for the most part, not. They are without consciousness, which is to say that they live out their arousal curve, as I have. Everything is occluded by arousal, and we are isolated within it. People on TV, all of them captive, most innocent, suffering war, revenge, genocide, which for some reason we have come to call "ethnic cleansing," adopting without thought the language of the Orwellian Serbs. One day, the family was living at home, tending their goats. The very next they are on the road, strafed and coming down with cholera. And just why is this? We are all stray cats picked up or kicked to the side, or scrapping in the alley or euthanized. Lucy, flea bitten, pregnant, bewildered, very young, is scooped up by my niece, cleaned, fed and loved. Her counterpart was hit by a car a week later and taken away by the sanitation crew. I am seeing the reality of these lives, most lived in grueling poverty, uncertain harvest and ethnic fear, these men in the back of the truck, these women who would be stoned to death for daring to free their faces. The sad whore in Saigon. It all challenges me. It does not exactly diminish awareness of my own suffering, but it contextualizes it in a very large world of very large suffering. I wonder if any science-fiction writer has speculated on this kind of advancement, the one that is made available by the lack of fear. Our planet, overtaken by an as yet to be imagined group of aliens who could teach us fearlessness, if we didn't kill them first.

Arles' new office will be spacious. I felt an electrical field of concern on my skin. I have been contained by the walls in his long, narrow office. When the horror grabs hold, I turn away from him, from Lee, from anyone and turn to the wall. In the new office, it will be too far away. I will need to learn to "turn to him."

I tried to describe it.

"Are you being choked?"

"Not from the outside."

"Do you know this is oral sex?" I felt the rupture of the question. There must always be another to have memory. It is a stupid question. Why does he ask it? It isn't sex.

"I don't know anything, Arles. I have no doubt, but I don't know anything. There is a chalk line around the form on the sidewalk, but the body is missing. There is no proof; there is an absence of proof. This reality in itself is very difficult to negotiate... Well, I don't negotiate it, I just live in it. No doubt; no knowing."

There in my body, the wave of memory builds and ebbs. It rarely breaks the surface into anything like emotion. When I cry, it is the same waveform. It doesn't go away; it will never go away. John helped me identify it as we drove to the Wolfram conference in Waltham. Waves of diminishing oscillations, like an echo.

States moved through Arles and through me. At the end, I was absently stroking my chest and crying softly.

"I didn't hate him. I loved him. Don't torment him." On the down slope of the wave, I said, "This must be Moses. How did I love Moses? I hardly knew him." I see King Kong.

I watched a movie about a march from Leverett down the East Coast, stopping at historical markers of the slave trade. Their pilgrimage ended at Goree Island in Senegal. They suffered the anguish of this place. That's where I was going before 9/11. Theirs has become a parallel journey to mine, up the stairs in Bronxville. He said on Wednesday that he wouldn't make me go up the stairs. But we are there for a purpose. He would hold me, now four but now prescient, twisting to run. He would soothe me with his deep voice and remind me of the year. Then he would hold me by the wrist, and we would share each step until the top.

At Goree Island, the Black Buddhist made a sacred space within the slave building with candles, incense and Kenté cloth. She described looking out at the ocean, the ocean with memory of all this horror, at her own daughter and the other pilgrims standing on the rocks with native people and her daughter described looking up at the doorway and seeing her mother. How would they understand that Goree Island has so much meaning for me? I am part of that. Images of shackles and irons flash in my right hemisphere. Scenes of attempted escape, shielding myself from blows, my utter helplessness. Much worse things have happened to others than have happened to me and will happen to me. No one will know more helplessness than I.

What if we get to the top of the stairs and the walls are brightly painted? There were stains on the sink. There is bad energy in this bathroom. Don't you feel the energy of what happened here 55 years ago? Perhaps there is a skylight. What would I do with whatever I felt? Talk to him about it in the car? Tear at my clothes? Go out to lunch? What would I do? What would he do? What if you'd traveled all the way to Goree Island and they'd made it into condos?

The shifts, the waves begin after this, and I didn't speak for close to an hour. I think I should, but no words form and I look up at him, and he too is in-state, in shifting states. Waves move through him, and I return to mine, rising and falling, separate from my breath. I ran my hand over my chest and down. Moses was leaving. He would go unharmed. The others were not in me. They, sometimes, when I didn't notice, had already gone. I have been sheltering Moses in this house of ribs along the underground railway. He will go to Toronto, and he will be safe.

I got him across the border, but then it ran into complications. He is not just King Kong. He was capable of terrible things. What have I released into the world? I thought about this for a moment as if I were responsible for the ruin of some child's life.

"Are you afraid he will be reincorporated?" I shook my head. I wasn't. He was gone. But when he asked this, I felt my heart burn. It hurt until the end of the session. I felt branded. I feel my life entwined, like DNA, around the history of Black people in America. I told him that I had always been afraid to write about what happened because of any bad racial consequences. I do not want to fuel racial fear or hatred. But I didn't know any of this. I didn't recognize that it began for me too at Goree Island.

No doubt; no certainty. Would anything change within that balance if I made this pilgrimage? I would have to make it to know. At this moment, I have the sense I am beyond it, that part of my life is over. Moses is gone.

I am at ease throughout the training I am doing in Genoa for Davide Dettore at the Miller Institute, and I notice this, surprised. Luca and I became friends quickly. Driving to Bergamo, we talked about the field of mind, the co-creation of the unconscious, that the unconscious is an interpersonal development and doesn't exist without attachment, how all of our capacities ride the waves of arousal and regulation in our brains. Tullio, his mentor and therapist, joined this conversation last night at dinner. Luca said at one point that Tullio became angry with him and said, "Somehow we must learn how to cut these wires that keep producing these thoughts!" Tullio may have begun to see that circuitry is more than metaphor. He asked me if I agreed with Bowlby that we needed attachment objects throughout our lives. I am accustomed to agreeing with Bowlby, so I said yes. When he explained further that Bowlby meant that there is always a child needing and forming parents in another, I did not agree. The journey from the transference need to the desire for a companion of the soul may be the ultimate journey of regulation—from healthy attachment to healthy, empathic non-attachment. Luca, Tullio, Nicoletta, John and I talked of such rich things that night in the church square in the dinner hour of 100 bells. I was in the company of a genius. Arles has been at every table, and I talk about our work freely. How could I, of all people, disagree with Bowlby? But I do.

I saw Bob two days after my return. He held my shoulder in his hands. "This shoulder is so deep, it is weeping. I heard myself screaming—my shoulder was separated. Bob put it back in place at that time and in this. Then he was on my right cheekbone. I started to cry as he found his way deep into the crevice of feelings beneath my eye. I apologized. "I don't know why you haven't been crying all along, given the depths and horror of this internal landscape." Then he held the back of my head. I dropped, absolutely still, into his hands. "Thank you," he said, "There is tingling all through me."

I have made a false distinction between my mind and my body, but they do remember quite differently. My body has not yet released what my mind has almost forgotten. I am learning the directionality of transcendence. I assumed it was up, away from the body, away from memory, away from traumatic resolution. I realize that it could be, maybe has to be, through the body. The commentator's androgynous voice never leaves. As Arles and I talked about all of this, about going into the body down to my vagina, my voice changed. I began to cry and pull away. I am within, not outside, the little child's experience.

"It was too bad. These men are in my body. But I am not in the teeth of this or thrown against the wall." The experience had its own containment, like a bubble. I always knew where I was, that Arles was there. I didn't have to climb through sedimentary layers of time. I was not shaken. But I am sadder. Perhaps more in touch with this new level of my body's experience without the takeover or amplification of the mind. Trauma. Fundamental reorganization. I imagine curling up in the cradle of his arms before I remember "that is over." This office can harbor my sadness as the first did my torment and the second, my suffering. And it will harbor my transcendence, too.

I woke this morning with this dream. *There was darkness, blackness surrounded by a police crime scene tape, except instead of being yellow, it was pink. I was saying insistently to the police, you need to solve this crime this time.*

We got the new EEGer software, and John installed it. I can hear him beeping. Chelsea is here, and she loves it when I lie on the floor with her, my neck over hers like we were puppies. Her tail, my heart, swap, swap. I am OK. Isness.

Arles did something I've never seen him do.

"When you were little, did you comfort yourself with a blanket?" He looked a little quizzical but not defended.

"I did."

"Did you rub it over your face?"

"I don't remember specifically, but it would make sense that I did. Why are you asking, right now?" He'd been lifting the collar of his white shirt and gently rubbing it over the corner of his mouth as we talked about the somatic unconscious.

I am sitting on the steps in the country. The sun is drying the dew. The crickets fill up every cranny of silence, becoming in their own loud way the peace of the country, the silence that is teaming with sound. I still feel odd, more odd and more sad after Alpha-Theta. Sleep isn't so good. My body hurts today... my untraumatized body that remembers it all.

John and I are preparing our talks for ISNR. I will begin mine with Freud's formula of health— work and love—and then offer mine, fearlessness and love and then talk about FPO2, the discovery that burdens me as it liberates others.

"I have two large black bells," I tell Arles, "cast-iron bells that are ringing in my temporal lobes. Far away, not loud but, you know, they are loud." As I talk, my fear dissolves. I return without force to the present world with all of its sorrows unshadowed by mine.

On September 11, I left my appointment with Bob, wanting to quit. At the corner of the busy intersection, I fell at the curb. It was as if I had been thrown down. It took me a long moment to recognize that I was in the street and that someone in a car might not see me lying there. I scuttled back up onto the sidewalk. When I finally crossed the street, there was a woman, I assume now from the DMH respite center, who wanted to reassure me. This had happened to her, too. She had just collapsed out of nowhere, for no reason, and no one believed her. "I do," I said as I turned to begin the three-mile walk home, cradling my hand. I lay on my couch. It was my patient that afternoon who insisted that she take me to the hospital. After X-rays and five hours in the crowded ER, they sent me home with codeine and my arm in a brace. Nothing was broken.

Sam could see me. He'd set up a table in his living room. He carefully unstrapped the brace and held my arm, feeling tenderly for the injury. He lay my arm across my chest as if it were still in the sling, put a blanket over me and took my ankle in his hands. I began to shiver and then shake, everywhere but that arm. It stayed still as if it lay protected in an entirely different field. I shook like this for over an hour with Sam's hands containing me and his voice soothing me, reminding me to have faith in the wisdom of the body, that this too would be over, that he would not leave me.

The next morning, someone called from the hospital. The orthopedic hand specialist saw the fracture at the base of my thumb. I would need a lobster-claw cast for three months. If this tiny bone didn't heal, I would lose the use of my left hand.

By the nature of the blood supply, this bone is slow to heal. Seven weeks in a cast is the minimum. He expects 12. I was grateful I had learned the meaning of being freed before recapture. I know the disturbing narrative that could be grafted to this simple here-and-now orthopedic decision. I didn't react except in the slow deep streams of the unconscious: I woke this morning at five, twisting and pulling, fighting against the cast.

"Perhaps yours is a baptism by fire," Arles said, "you don't often get to choose these things."

"Once you decide there are no accidents, how far back does that go?"

"Billions of years."

"That doesn't help me, Arles."

"Psychotherapy is a process of making sense, of making meaning. 'No accident' is part of that. It often implies a hidden intentionality to be discovered, and in finding that, you find its meaning. But it doesn't have to be that."

"I am exhausted by the force and power of meaning. Why was I the one chosen? Why did the soldiers rape one girl and the other escape because they were too drunk or didn't see her under the car? Is there meaning in that? No, there is randomness. So, the event of my torture was overly determined by huge forces of history as they played in the psyches of these specific men and my specific parents and perhaps even in some chaotic superordinate pattern that we cannot discern that brought us together. And I was white, privileged, unrecognized by my parents and the most available victim. This way it has inevitability, not meaning."

But the question I asked him was, why was I plucked from all of humanity for this particular brutal episode? I kept going.

"The only answer to this is randomness. Or I guess what most people decide, but doesn't occur to me, singular badness. Not even karma could justify, explain or justify or explain such events. Randomness is close to meaninglessness. And neither meaning nor meaninglessness suffice."

"Do you have any other choice?"

"It must be Is-ness." But "just is" is a vast territory; there is no continent. "This is because that is." Thầy's Buddhism, in a nutshell, is close to the overly-determined view that drives our therapeutic endeavor for meaning, and there is no containment in it. "I just want one beautiful statement that goes beyond all I know and speaks to what cannot be known. I want to get the experience taken out of me and transcribed onto a broad expanse of paper that rolls out like sky. It is about representation and dispersal simultaneously."

I got this letter today from Joey, my thirteen-year-old patient with cerebral palsy, as dictated to his mother. He has been given the diagnosis of childhood schizophrenia, which was understandable but not accurate. He told me that he was born on a different planet in a distant galaxy, and thousands, perhaps millions of people came into his head at night for training and then dispersed across the globe to help people. Every night. He was married, and he ran a private boarding school. He hears voices. On this planet in the daytime, Joey found it awkward to live in his body. His left arm moved with his left leg, and it threw off his balance; he couldn't read, his memory and motivation were poor, and he didn't understand jokes. He was also one of the sweetest human beings inhabiting this planet, sincere, well-liked by his teachers and well-loved by his parents and his older brother. He ran up my stairs for training. His memory improved. I asked him each time what F.O.R.D stood for, and over time, he got it. He remembered the joke: Found On the Roadside Dead. He exploded in excitement when he told me that he'd skied the double black diamond. It was the bottom of that trail, but he skied it. The trainers were reduced in number each night, down from thousands to two or three, and they were now learning to teach neurofeedback. At times, he told me, he put the answering machine on so it would stay quiet in his head. Things were also waking up with HBOT.

As he came into his body, he became increasingly self-aware. It wasn't easy to join the common human dilemma, and I often wondered if he would have chosen this path had he been able to choose. Never more so than when I got this letter.

"My old body left me.

It's not coming back.

My old body was good and bad together.

I was mean and nice together.

It is the first time my body has felt sad. I never felt sad before. Yes, this is the first time I felt sad.

My body had the world record of not feeling sad.

My new body broke the promise. I was going to be the first person not to feel sad. I wanted to be the first person to live to 102 and not be sad.

I broke my old promise… When I am very old, I should feel sad. Now I am broken… I feel sadness now. I do not like my new body now.

I have mostly sadness now. My new body does not understand me now. My new body does not want to listen to me now. It is my boss now, and it tells me what to do and to listen to my new body only.

There are no voices. These are scary feelings. These are feelings, not voices. My body is confused. Big time confused."

His mother asked, "Do you think the medicine is changing your body?" and he answered, "Maybe it is the medicine, neurofeedback and hyperbaric. Maybe hyperbaric is waking up good things and bad things. I do not know what part of my body should be awake or dead."

❧

"The energy moving through me is like a night flood in flood lights. The carcass of a cow, the roof, the heirloom table—it's all here—held by my foot, dislocated shoulder, banged up against the wall, the sexual winnings in the game of poker, held in the lap of Moses weeping, my parents never coming home, they see nothing. The footsteps overhead, the car crash, the rapes, the knife at my throat, seclusion rooms, injections..." I could have kept adding to the string, but he stopped me.

"Terrible history," he said. I was only trying to answer his question.

"It isn't water, though, not that kind of flood. It is streams of electrical particles and waves, intense energy through my whole body. It is the gathering up of all of it, known and unknown, and moving out. There will be no debris when this is done, but it is a passage kind of like how the Tibetan monks describe death—it's not either good or bad, it's both good and bad, but more so it just is."

But here it was. The strange burn on my hip, almost perfectly round, smaller than a quarter, which Sam too thinks is a traumatic eruption.

Arles received all of this squeezed through tears into words on the phone call, but I could not settle. My heart felt hollow and all around it, cold, the temperature of shock. I wrapped the red quilt around me. I wore double socks. I didn't recognize it at first, my obvious need.

"I know what's missing, your hands on my head."

"Yes," he said.

"Will you be there?"

"Yes." His voice turned toward me. I filled up on it.

Thursday morning, *I dreamt that I was looking out into the clear night sky and saw myself as far back as stardust, and as I woke up, there was a great sound, a woosh of energy, and I knew then that my body was a point in time, perhaps between stardust then and stardust to come.*

I asked Arles to look at the burn. It put him in a difficult position because to say no had to be possible, but it wasn't. He agreed.

"No, this is not a burn from a heating pad."

"From my view, it looks like a burn from a cigar."

"Do you think they burned you?"

I sat silent. It could be they did. There was a security guard threatening to burn me with a cigarette. Both Lee and Sam felt heat radiating off of it, and it could suddenly turn ice cold. I cannot penetrate the mystery of my body.

"It could be."

He broke the prolonged silence.

"The cigar is true, but don't hold it only in that field of trauma, or you can get stuck there. That can become all that is. And you know that there is a much bigger All. The All of your dreams. The All of the light that is greater than the All of the repetitious dark."

He asked me about meditation, and I tried to understand why I didn't sit. There is some opposition in my head, in my brain, actually. There is some tickling sense that I shouldn't be meditating, but I don't know why. I think it would be good, but I feel I need to comply with this opposition in my brain. I know the accounts of great yogis. They heal wounds. They prove the power of the mind. But how are they in their relationships? Do they dissolve delusion? Are they free of it? Is Thầy? Is the Dalai Lama? Arles had wondered aloud whether anyone lived outside these realms of delusion. The Buddha. This is Buddha nature. Affect regulation is the path. Perhaps it is that I can't quite find where meditation will amplify or deepen this. It should be so, but I can't find it. I don't see this regulation in most meditators. Of course, I don't see it in most neurofeedback practitioners either, but they aren't, for the most part, trained.

"When I was four, and my parents would go out, I threw myself down at their feet, then down the stairs. This went on until they settled on having me sleep in my father's bed. My room was under their living room in the attic. My parents' room was under the attic, where we stored the Christmas ornaments. In my father's bed, I couldn't hear them overhead; in mine, every footfall. When my parents went out, they were leaving me with them."

Memories come through my body like the early stage of a negative developing, with only the beginning of a hint at an outline, and then it stops.

It's emerging, but it doesn't emerge into pictures. I know about Moses holding me, his tears falling on my face and my chest, through my body. But I don't know what he looks like.

Bob pushed deep enough into my cheek that he went through time. I stayed in the present while experiencing the past. The only image that came was the face of Saddam, confused, tormented, childlike, an image that at that moment made it impossible to see all his victims. He was a brutal tick. I am confused by my response to this video of his being examined for lice and his docile compliance, his unguarded hunger for touch. His disorientation. I saw his face, not Moses. I said 'they have captured him!' over and over. Bob moved my thumb, and I yelped, but it was a response to the next moment, the moment that never materialized, the anticipated, unendurable pain. At the end, I sat up and fell back on the table like a tree cut down. I couldn't get my balance. I staggered. The rest of the night I listened to Mozart, drank some chocolate milk, and softly dispersed all that had just happened—57 years ago.

Chapter 14

Last night was the winter solstice and the mass of reconciliation. It is a powerful service of forgiveness. Brother Mark listed all of the groups that are hated as he asked for forgiveness from the Church. I want to remind us all of the first sin of hatred, misogyny. It is so deeply embedded in every culture that we don't see it for what it is, a template for all hatred and all oppression. It is even more fundamental than race. Anorexia is misogyny internalized. Self-mutilation is misogyny. Very few girls escape. There are more people in bondage today than at the height of the slave trade, most—not all, but most—women.

I trained too much left temporal, and it has edged me onto thin ice. Arles feels despair. He thinks he despairs of me, but he actually despairs of my left hemisphere overtaking my right, the non-relational overtaking the need for love. He bypasses the brain to get to the mind; he has no language for this.

Putting these events into words is vital to transforming them. It may begin the lift out of the limbic battle zone, or signal the transfer of early non-verbal memory to verbal, from right to left. It's almost as if one runs the risk of reabsorbing these events if they are not spoken and then received. Arles sits peacefully. My recitations sink into what seems an "affect-less void." There is a risk of my not knowing that he registers, even that he hears. Perhaps it is the case that not only is that the only thing to do, but it is exactly what is right to do. Maybe he is just done.

"I was not seeking this lost memory. My body formed into it, and then I could not escape the field. I wasn't thinking about anything else; I was drawn away, as if magnets were pulling my brain into different pathways. It is harder to walk. I took the hotel elevator one floor up to make my presentation on trauma, and it was, the talk itself, a difficult performance. Before the memory of two weeks ago, I could imagine giving a spontaneous presentation; after it, only a written speech. My ears are ringing. It is a very long post-ictal event. I finally trained on Thursday, and my slow wave at T4 was at 68 microvolts; it should be under 10. My memory is bad. I am vulnerable to gaslighting and humiliation. It takes a long time to find a stable surface. This is not abreaction. It feels as if there are capsules of energy in the body that either disperse this way through knowing or they contaminate the body, infect the organs and then finish the killing." I couldn't tell if Arles was in this with me. I tried to explain, "I think this could be traumatic recall, without kindling. This is what I mean when I say I don't believe it. I feel badly; I am in a state, it is both from and about what happened, but maybe now I am literally not exciting the amygdala – that this is the difference between release and kindling. The release is diffusion in the body just as the explosion of memory is out through the body." He wasn't responding. I gave in. "Words do not have enough substance to carry memory."

"Yes, Sebern, I do understand that, but all we have are words."

"I am still not at ease calling the person who experienced this, 'I,' but I use 'she' now mostly by habit. I believe this happened, but there is still some veil between me and believing. Or it could be that this is the original experience, remembered the way it is, at such a distance from the cortex, that believing is irrelevant, a stripped-down, bare neurological event that is seizure-like but that doesn't kindle fear. It takes its toll physically, but it doesn't land me back in the trauma. I am not retraumatized by remembering. It twists and ripples in my brain; it thickens my body; in the acute stage, I act like someone afraid. I must've seemed to Lee like someone being tortured, but maybe she, too, can feel, even at its most intense, the thin membrane between knowing and reliving. When she held her hands on my chest with a lot of weight, it was over. I knew I had to get to that position, but didn't know why."

"It sounds a little like resuscitation," Arles said. I had just thought the same thing.

"I was both the observer and what was being observed. I still can't get my brain to settle down between my ears. There is energy that has to move through my body." I tailed off

"Tell me more of this knowing."

"It is as if the atom of memory is fused at the edge with the atom of dissociation, and knowing is pushing a dull knife between them, loosening the bond. It is like waking a little more from the coma, learning a little more."

I try to turn my brain face toward all that happened, the whole of the time of the attic or the entire experience of my mother's not being, and I can't. It is as if my head pulls away from the hands that try to hold it, as if the only possibility is to squint and then fully close my eyes. It used to be that I got glimpses and couldn't stand the glare and turned away. This is different. There is no reactivity in it; it is just an acknowledgment of what's possible, what can fit in the frame.

"Knowing is an emergent property. It used to recreate the same energy field and the beliefs inherent in it. We have extracted the nucleus of fear from this cellular memory. I still can access fear as it is embedded in the memory, integral to it, but I am no longer afraid. No fields are replicated. Bob had said, 'This is not endless; there was a finite number of experiences.' But a finite number of events of this order produce infinite field replications both at the time and multiple times afterward in all the replays."

"Yes, I agree. There is nothing finite in this."

I might have expected despair. It will never be over. But it was a little like when I told him if I ever started the cry, I would never stop, and he'd said, 'Yes, it is true, you <u>will</u> cry forever', the bad news turned to affirmation. And it wasn't news. It is no longer lodged in me. It isn't of me. It is historically about me, but the critical issue is that now, no new fields are set up when I find myself in the old ones. I do not react. During the retreat on Sunday, Larry reminded us that there is no past and no future. Fear is the axis on which the false universe of past and present spins. When Lee hits a spot on my chest that is just over where the fascia was torn, I react to the pain almost as if it were today's injury—the ripples go only into the room, into the present moment, and then they are absorbed, or they have so little fear propelling them they just drop. And they don't seem to be attracting this energy toward me from others. Memory that does not give rise to pattern replication, fields that do not give birth to new fields. This is only possible when fear is extracted. It will never be over. That is the nature of it. Now, though, as fear subsides, it has less and less capacity to reignite. Replication is no longer a field requirement.

It was a kindergarten version of what can happen, but after the movie, I could not orient myself to the mall and the people in it in the same way I had when I arrived. I didn't like the movie Big Fish. In my brain, it's like furniture in a doll house, the way reality is moved around: the poster bed neurons firing in the kitchen. This experience lives at the edge of the very worst thing you can do to a person—to make it impossible for them to know what is real.

This morning, I can still feel some of that. I am rearranged. It's physical, beneath my skull. I don't remember this happening to me, but it would not be easily remembered, by its nature. Reality was replaced without comment. Of course, this happened to me! It was what happened when my parents came home. I was, the world was, the house was, the people were all rearranged in every molecule, and no one said anything. There is a way that I saw everything more accurately when I was leaving the mall, the fictions and the play acting, the frenzied and vacated beings.

It was difficult to get my body to Bob. He held my head and said that it was as if I were in a coma. He asked, with my head still in his hands, if I had ever been resuscitated. His voice echoed. I had lapsed into a coma, in my bed in my fifth-floor apartment on the Upper West Side. 25 Tuinal. What happened to my body? Who came for me? How did they get me into the ambulance? Were people watching the red light swinging through the dark? Were the medics angry or disgusted, sad or confused, bored? Did they try to resuscitate me? I'm sure they slammed the ER doors open, the very drama I yearned for but until this moment never imagined. Teams over me. It was, I was told later, too late for lavage. What else was there to do? What did they do? I think I woke up. I remember vaguely hearing voices a long way away. I think someone, a woman, was saying that I was coming to. I think it was four days later. I woke up anxious and fearful. "I have to call to tell them I am not at work." The nurse was annoyed. "They know you're not at work."

I came into this relationship with the dramatic narrative, vacant of me, intended to recruit. I brought him the lacquered pick-up sticks. I dropped to the elemental, to the particulate, the nuclear level. I was not. Before self, in no self, managing disembodied terror when I was not in his presence and often even then. We endured the hellfire of my creation, the explosion of new stars, the sudden formation of his body, the way you can kind of see what the primitive peoples saw when they looked at the stars and saw Pegasus. The star that was his elbow is the one this morning that I most remember. He parented me from no self to him to self. Neurofeedback sped the process, in psychic time at the speed of light. Amidst protest, I arrived in "No-self," and this is the default position now. I engage in the life of the person I am, throughout which is the reality of No-self and the episodic vibrations of absence and trauma. With body work, I am stabilizing myself within the events that were lived in dissociation or unconsciousness. It is the more typical ground of therapy, but I am not searching for memory—that could come, I suppose. I am evidently in need of reinhabitation or a first inhabitation of the events that are called my life.

"It is like the frames that flicker past at the end of home movies." These memories are white, and they stand outside the frame. Each frame is a girl child of intermittent age, and it's dim particularly next to the glare of the empty frame. I had started to cross this out; I meant to write "indeterminate" age, but it is both intermittent and indeterminate.

Arles and I have talked about inhabiting memory, but memory was a particulate fog about an arm's-length away from me. I didn't walk forward into the memory of the coma. It was a sudden burst of particles under Bob's hands that overtook me. I recalled the voices that I think I remember hearing, the siren and the slamming of doors, the violent heart-racing presence of others, their anger and urgency, clothes cut off and exposed, the void of unconsciousness, the continuous emptiness and distance of dissociation. When the tubes are removed, and I am taken to the psychiatric ward and the heavy oak door closes, I am trapped in all that preceded the overdose and all that has now happened because of it, the terror, the 7g of sodium amytal, the pacing until the next shot. It was boundless.

Sometime last week, I had the smell of the sweatband of my father's hat. It was a wonderful, reassuring smell laced with trains and bourbon and cigarette smoke. I don't have a direct memory like this of my mother. The closest I come is the smell of Nivea, which was the fragrance of her. But it is mostly the texture of it in my mouth as I ate it. I have the sense that most people feel closer to their memories, even identify with them. They have memory; they don't infer it.

I dreamt that I was returning home to Elizabeth Street and went in the door that my patients use, the front door. There was a dark, dusty charcoal gray cat with many nursing kittens. At first, I was charmed to see them right inside my door. But a little like those strange little flies they kept proliferating, these kittens increased rapidly, their numbers filling the stairwell, making it difficult for me to get to the door. They were very small and mewing, trying to get in the door. I had to be careful not to step on them. The situation was making me anxious, really and a little desperate. I had to push some away to be able to finally close the door to keep them out.

I dreamt that I was alternately the mother and the young girl about four. The girl was about to be sent away to a rehab hospital for major reconstructive surgery. Grafts were represented as different patterns of wallpaper, and limbs would be broken and repositioned. The grief and fear were equally the child's and the mother's, and they were surrounded by a community of women caring for them, watching over the scene between them. There was nothing to do but cry. It had to happen. They would be separated. The child would be a year in the rehab hospital, far from home.

I think we were Black Africans. And this was our community. I woke up crying.

Black cadence is embedded in my own. We watched the documentary on Rwanda. Mary Shelly, the spokesperson for the State Department, refused to use the word genocide. If she had used the word, the US and the international community would have had to take action. If the word is not used, we can watch the same horror and do nothing at all. That twists my mind.

Many of my patients endure these histories without any buffer. They were naked in their poverty; humiliated by their clothes, reviled as white trash or nigger or spic. These seem to be the most enduring wounds. The door shut in their face at age eight. They were not invited into homes like mine. Merrit, who was homeless at nine, walked four miles from her 'shelter' to the wealthy side of her town, cased the houses from their hedges and, when she knew the patterns, broke into them to play with the toys and to eat toast with peanut butter and jam. She told me this when I asked her if she had any happy memories. Her eyes lit up. "And there was the time my uncle—he wasn't my real uncle—bought me cotton candy!"

I was buffered by skin, class and privilege. My traumatized patients hope that they will be delivered from their madness into the benign world that everyone else seems to live in, but instead, they are delivered out of their own madness into the madness of the world. "I thought," Reggie said, almost shocked, "that it would be Disneyland, that everyone else lived in Disneyland and that when I got well, I'd be in Disneyland too. There's no Disneyland. People out here are suffering worse than me." This can happen quickly with training, always in some way partially, and outside any process that is recognized. They don't know where they are. I am still experiencing this. I am free of fear but not yet of all that fear has given rise to. I don't know where I am. I can't find myself on the map of trauma.

We talked about the black hole that forms in me in his prolonged absence, the hole that he is sucked into and how quickly that changes when I see him.

"Perhaps," he said, "I have not been attending to the orphan." There is truth in this, and I am also not orphaned. Both are now true. I have no urgency to inform me which way to lean, toward or away.

Yesterday, I had the thought that it is not just the mind, but the brain too, that is interested in dreams. Maybe beyond or beneath the unconscious, dreaming satisfies the organizational needs of the brain. The truth of things is ineptly disguised if not obscured altogether. My mother doesn't look like my mother, but I know it is my mother. There is economy in a pun. What is this midnight conspiracy of brain and mind?

I dreamt of Austin Riggs. This is about Arles. He is to psychoanalysis as Thầy is to Zen. *All there was to eat was bread and cake. We didn't talk about this or about the bacon that I found covered with a cloth and ate without greed and with great appreciation, but also with confusion that in this opulent place there wasn't more of this, enough for everyone, out in the open.*

Hospital dreams are back.

Body and mind are coupled but distinct fields with different capacities for memory, memory release and working through. When Sam triggered a memory in my left foot at the end of the session a month ago, my body almost shut down. I was constipated for three weeks. I had bowel movements like this when I was a kid, big, hard balls. Hypotonic. Sam had worked on that foot a hundred times. This time it triggers. What is the mechanism? If I weren't doing body work, I would weave these events into some other narrative, something regular, something I ate or something I could ignore.

Bob's hand jumped up from deep around my left rib cage, and I looked up—I rarely do. I asked him if it was the deepest we'd ever gone. He was hesitant to continue.

"What else?"

"It was when you were four, I think. It was as if I were holding a near-dead child."

"Yes," a few tears welled up and rolled down my face, "that is the way it was for me too."

The language of the body is Pali, once the only language, now lost to us and only hinted at by Sanskrit. "It must've sounded like this;" "this is what that could mean." The pictograph of the trembling response from my toe, or trying to drag my body to turn over. It's more like my body is trying to draw me a picture, then it presents a picture that I must decipher. But it's all the same; whatever is happening requires a translation from the body to the mind. They are separated by language and culture but drawn together by common interest, need and even, more rarely, love. They have a shared history, but the body knows more of it than the mind.

Madeleine screamed when they ran into Rennie's brother, her mother's primary abuser. Rennie felt strangely unaffected by seeing him there in the aisle in Walmart, but she had to take her baby not only out of the stroller and into her arms but out of the store before she could reassure and quiet her. Madeleine had never seen him before. She was 10 months old. Is this cellular memory, the body's registry not only of her own experience but of her mother's?

Madeleine is a presence. She is solid, playful, and in all senses, strong. She knows the game I was proposing, "Trot, Trot." She bounced herself on my knee. She was proposing it too. She sits on my lap in the center of her being. (Her balance is remarkable; she is balancing on a skateboard!) Two times during the game, she leaned forward and hugged me, a joyful, spontaneous expression of love. She tried sherbet last time and made the appropriate face, registering how cold it was and then her wish, without any urgency, for more. She is a child who has enough. She also wants the spoon, but when I say, "Let Sebern do it," she does. After four spoonfuls, I decided enough, and that's fine with her. She makes the transition without difficulty. She sees no need to protest; life suffices. I asked her if she wanted to take my hand to go down the stairs—she goes up on her own now, but not down. She came to the edge like one would go to the edge of a cliff and turned around to her mom.

"It's a long way down, isn't it?" Rennie said, "Would you like me to pick you up?" Madeleine turned back to me and took my hand. One step down left her other leg on the stair above, but she did it. About halfway down, she launched herself, both feet, which left her swinging from my hand. She'd decided it would be easier to jump. She waits for her mother and then waves goodbye, happy to be here, happy to go on to the next thing.

I trained Rennie when she was pregnant with Madeleine. When fetal movement began, it was all heels and elbows. Rennie had said that if she didn't know better, she would think that her baby was aggressing on her. She asked for training at FPO2, a site that always relaxed her, and when she trained there, Madeleine trained there too. "The baby just laid down and went to sleep!" It just got better between them from then on.

THE CRASH

Today begins my 40th reunion at Smith. Carol, one of the ten people I remember from college, is here asleep. Last night, as we walked home from a meal devoted to a conversation typical of such events, "What has your life been like?" I felt the distinct visceral sensation of my big story becoming small. She'd asked me what happened after I dropped out; I'd asked her how she'd proceeded with her life. As we got to the door, I said, "We all have lives that must be led," and suddenly any lingering investment in the importance of all that happened, the inherent specialness of it, shriveled up, a dried fruit. Along with this, strangely, came a greater clarity that I should write this journal out. The first years laid silent siege to my mind; my youth howled. By the time my friends were ending their graduate studies, I was being discharged from mine. I am married, I raised children, I found work and returned to school; the quiet years of gardens and a lover and the needs of unquiet children. 10 years ago, I entered this relationship with Arles. I had reasons for therapy, but they weren't the reason. I made discoveries. I was rent by discovery. And this is part of an account of that decade. So, it has not become insignificant, but it has just become small, perhaps even containable, something I can write about.

I probably have emails from some of these college friends that I can't get to on my computer upstairs. My leg is broken.

The first hour had been peaceful, even sublime, over the farms and forests of Conway and Deerfield, charting our way imperfectly along the river. We could watch the chase vehicle down there, keeping track. Allison, my friend and my neurologist, who'd organized this trip, called Kate, our pilot, to say that the winds on the ground were picking up. It was so quiet where we were in between the bursts of fire. The trees were quiet too. Kate and Jakob spit over the edge to look for currents. None. But as we began to descend, we were caught in a windshear. She took the balloon into the woods, using the tops of the trees as brakes—we couldn't land at that speed. When she tried to get up and out, the sheer pulled us back down into the trees. One of them caught on fire. Hunched over in the wicker basket, we broke through the forest canopy; branches and ash from the fire fell on us. Kate saw the only possible clearing and dropped us into it, rainbow, fire and ash. The rigging caught on an oak limb dangling us, for a moment, fifteen feet above the ground before the branch snapped and fell on us as we hit the ground. No one else is hurt. Jakob is fine, with a bruise on his knee, and the best ending possible for any 13-year-old boy, celebrating his birthday. I am in a blue cast from my toes to my knee for 4 to 6 weeks. I will once again be in rehab.

"If I were absolutely honest," I said to Allison, "I wouldn't ask for the insurance money. I caused this accident. We were forced down by the field in me." She didn't take this up.

"Just? Just!" he yelled. He couldn't believe I was saying this. Just a broken hand, a broken leg and a burn in the last nine months. I couldn't quite believe I said it either. He became quieter. "Do you mean 'just' by comparison?" I was crying, and after a moment, nodded.

"I think that this all started with the parking garage, my shoulder, my hand, the abscess, and the EFT-induced or remembered rectal pain." He nodded. He is relying on the idea that this arises from the unconscious. When I disagreed, he asked me how it felt to me to be in the thrall of forces beyond the unconscious.

I live in a field, and the particles coalesce, or the strings begin to vibrate under cue. I don't know what will constitute the conditions. Arles asked me how many events there have been. That's when I said "just." On the list I wrote today, I'd forgotten the sudden onset of the malicious HPV virus. My body manifests the absences and the assaults. My mind doesn't anymore, and this adds another layer of confusion. The body's emotions are mute and wild: Helen Keller. I don't have the language for this or, in a sense, the mind. I can't raise it up from my body to my mind, or maybe from my right hemisphere to my left. Unlike Helen Keller, it is quiet, offering itself up to the crash, dumbly, unable to do anything but comply with the field.

"I haven't been able to organize myself. It is as if I have fragmented somewhere with four sentries, one at each corner of my experience, to watch out. Somewhere within this, I am not only mute, but I am still. Like an animal injured in the woods, making no noise, attracting no attention."

"Not," he said, "the stillness of equanimity, although that may be also true, but the stillness of the freeze."

I am feeling different kinds of stillness, the shock and horror of hanging; the frozen, the dissociated sympathetic withdrawal; and now the fearlessness and equanimity that encounters this history. I have wondered about this leg, though. Did it hang helplessly in space? Did he hold this one first, along with the left? Was it the first to be dropped?

It felt like Bob's hands descended deeper into flesh memory, to the muscles, to the organs, to the four-year-old child who left this body, who was knocked unconscious and who felt every assault and knew every bewildering, terrifying intention, even playing dead or being half dead or almost dead. I still feel broken in the deep interior body that he pulled out of the rubble, and he couldn't help but hurt me if he touched it at all. I reminded myself of this when I wanted to scream Stop. Fragments of bone and psyche strewn across the table as the storm formed and raged outside his open window. I knew where I was, and I knew he would stop; that was what made it possible. He didn't stop. It seemed to be the memory of torture, now in his hands. All I wanted was to go through it and have it be over. I knew he would stretch my legs, and that would be the end. I wanted to be in the Smith infirmary in the room at the end of the hall that had once been a solarium, overlooking the Mill River. The room was in the trees. It was October. My first known concussion. Bed rest. The firm almost sternly Dr. Lewy. The World Series on the bedside radio. The possibility that I could drop Spanish. A white bed with white sheets, ginger ale with a straw. Complete bed rest and occasional friends. That's where I wanted to be. In the silence, there with a kind nurse and a forgiving doctor until everything healed.

I arranged my bed here carefully. I bought white sheets. John read to me. I woke up bruised and tired, brushed my teeth, ate breakfast and went to work.

I had noticed the case of pick-up sticks I keep on the lower shelf in my office. Several times. When Arles arrived Friday morning with his paper mug of jasmine tea, they were sitting on the photo album. A ritual was emerging in the service of a field change.

I open the album to the portrait of me at four months old, already passing away. I gripped the wooden bundle of brightly colored sticks up on their ends. The black one slipped out of their midst to the floor. No one else fell. I picked it up.

He broke the silence.

"What do you make of that?"

"The black has to be a part of all this. It's in everything." He nodded, "Yes, it is."

"Perhaps it is separate from me; perhaps it has its own gravitational field; maybe it will fall away."

Then another slipped out – this one the color of the cast. I gathered it back up and held the bundle tightly. I made a head motion toward the photo.

"We have both seen that; this is where I first shattered."

"Yes."

I dropped the bundle, and it scattered across the floor.

Pick-up sticks were my first gift to Arles. I gave it no thought. I am enduringly grateful that he withheld interpretation and just received the gift. It made the unfolding mine; it made the treatment possible. I'd taken such care in presenting them, shellacking every piece. I didn't ask him if he still had them. He has endured so many eruptions. They are only symbols, only the fragments. He helped me collect them. I held them again in a bundle. I talked about Moses. I read what I had written and my discovery that I was not just nearly killed as in a natural disaster, but I was nearly murdered. It felt important to use the word. He took this on slowly, and after quiet consideration, he breathed out. "Yes, that is right."

I dropped the sticks again.

"What are you feeling?"

"Bewildered."

"Bewildered? Tell me how you feel this."

My recording mind goes blank here. I can't remember what I felt then, that was yesterday, or the then that was then. I felt fear and disgust and helplessness and hopelessness in Bob's office, but with Arles in this ritual to allow me passage, I don't remember feeling anything but shame. Thoughts are impossible without words. There were no words. These are impressions, not descriptions. The state is one of unconsciousness, of dissociation. We gathered the sticks again.

"Necessary." That was all I could think to say. I felt inhibited, but he gave his permission, and I put my mouth around them all and held them there. "Comforting, actually," I added.

I dropped them again. "This is when my parents came home and didn't know."

I talked about my fall over the rocks at Tassajara, the nakedness, the shame of being so injured, my long hard climb back over the same rocks naked and bleeding, awash equally in blood and in shame, terrified of being discovered, getting myself dressed with a possible broken elbow, lacing up my boots tight and walking a mile or so up the hill to the first aid station. I kept the others on the trail at bay, shut out, until shock took over in the kind arms of the Tassajara nurse.

"That was this, Arles," I said, pointing at this baby portrait. He knew, of course. It has all been what it was.

I dropped the sticks again. All that lawyer, Larry, did I think was French kiss me, but he did it with such desperation, such voraciousness, it scared me. I was eight and nine. "I know," my mother said when I told her in her kitchen on the Cape, "He was after me all the time." It was all she said when I told her, and all that I said too.

I picked the red sticks up from all the others and dropped them. And I broke open crying, "This is my father's kiss on the lips and his heart attack and my terrible fear that I had broken his heart. I fiercely rejected his goodnight kiss, and he didn't understand it." I talked about visiting him weeks later in the hospital with the white iron bed and looking out over the exercise yard of Sing Sing at the mostly Black prisoners, mostly just walking or sitting in the shade of the high walls. I learned that some of these men, called trustees—that's how I saw what I heard, not trustees—were allowed out unattended to care for the gardens at the entrance of the prison and perhaps even those around the hospital. It made me watchful. I was surprised at how much I felt about my father's heart attack. I gathered the bundle up again and held them under my nose long ways and then against my forehead. I leaned on them. I told the story of Alma's car crash that woke me the morning I chose to skip school, the horn that didn't stop, pillows under her head that turned pink, the ambulance and the next day, when I chose to go to school, getting the news of my father's death. I didn't drop the sticks. I leaned against them. These were not somehow shattering events. I was already shards.

Then I held the black stick up. It was Moses, it was the stairs, and I moved it to one slant, then another. I held it between my fingertips.

"It is the space this all happened in." He nodded. "It is the darkness of his skin; the blackness of no mother. What should I do with this stick?" I didn't know. Then I broke it. It splintered into three pieces, three black kittens; the three of us. I realized I would bury them with the dying peonies. I'd given Arles the others, piece by piece, in twos or threes, and he bundled them. Then I gave him the case. He slipped them in and replaced the cap.

"And what about these?"

"They are OK." They are, I thought, my bones. "I will just keep them here. They are what they are."

"And what about her?" he said, moving his hand to take up the photograph.

"She will always be with me. I don't hate her anymore. I would pick that baby up and hold her. I can, Arles, I have, and I will."

He responded quietly when I thanked him for being there throughout.

"It is a privilege to be here with you."

After he left, I drank the remainder of his sweet jasmine tea, more honey than spice, warming it with a bit of my water. The ritual was completed this morning. John dug the hole, and I buried the three black fragments and covered them with petals and the remains of the flowers that died with me in the long days of nearly unbearable grief. Unlike the days when any of my family was buried, today was blue and filled with bright, warm sun.

On Tuesday night, I did an Alpha-Theta session with my long-time patient, Nan. I was—I checked—feeling OK. She felt quiet as she slipped in. She heard herself ask, "Are you alright?" in the midst of the gentle surf of Theta. She didn't say anything but told me later that it disturbed her. I would've answered that I was fine. That night, she had a nightmare, the contents of which, she said, shouldn't be a nightmare and woke up screaming. It was hard for her to get back to sleep. She has been extremely tired all week, sleeping a lot on the couch, watching movies on TV, getting to work late, leaving early, needing to nap before her late class, exhausted. When she arrived, she told me it was hard for her to hold her head up with her neck, that the frame of her body was hardly strong enough to keep her upright.

"It doesn't make sense at all, but it feels like it comes from a tremendous expenditure of energy, of giving to and taking care of," I asked her to tell me her dream. "*I was in a house like my old house, in the room in which I'd felt psychic energy and my sister, my friend/former lover, and you were in combination, all one, and in the other bed. There had been some kind of disruption between this occupant and me, but I was turning toward the bed as if to address it. I saw a figure in the hall, although I never turned toward it. I have no idea why this figure would scare me so much. It was a small child. She called out for help from me in different manifestations and got no response. Every time she screamed, the child just got more scared and ran back and forth in the hall as if there was no escape.* I woke up screaming, although in the dream it had been silent or muffled."

"Can you describe the dream house, Nan?"

"It was the second floor. There are two rooms and an attic." She filled in more details of the attic configuration.

I worked to quiet my accelerating heartbeat. "How old was this child?"

"She was four."

I considered my next question carefully.

"Could this be my dream more than yours, Nan?"

She nodded without hesitation. "It's a strange thing to say, but I don't think this is my dream."

"How big a door do you think you opened to my psyche?" She paused only briefly and said,

"I think a very big door." And after a brief hush between us, she said, "I am so grateful to you, Sebern. This could have been so easily missed, and you didn't."

She seemed unperturbed by my disclosure, I think because at that moment it felt more like a confirmation of her experience, an understanding and a validation. She told me of a hypnagogic image she'd had as she fell asleep. She was laying hands on my cast, and it broke open; then she thought, "Now what do we do?" She'd wanted to heal me.

"I wonder if your exhaustion was about caring for me all this time?"

"I think it has been."

"Well, you are off duty, Nan. Perhaps you won't be so tired now."

She laughed, "I think this is already true." We sat together awed with this event, awed with Alpha-Theta—no her, no me.

I told Rae about this, and she said that in the future, I must learn to wrap myself and teach my patients to wrap themselves in a bubble of white light out of respect for the power of this transfer; to assume it is always happening or at least always could.

THE CRASH

Johnny and I chatted about the balloon festival going on in Greenfield and his desire, if it weren't so expensive, to go skydiving, now that he is no longer afraid of dying. I said something like, "Then he'd be broken and have to stay." He came to drive for me after I plummeted out of the sky to the forest floor. I have loved him as much as this, but never felt this close to him. He, too, is tired of all that childhood trauma has heaped on him. He takes comfort in his relationship with Jesus, and he wants to study archaeology and to learn anatomy. He is, after years of death, stirring towards life.

Johnny took his dive. I couldn't save him from taking the wrong turn in the night and stepping into the air. He fell down the stairs at Molly's, banged his head through the wallboard, fractured his right wrist, fractured a vertebra, and bruised his legs and his face. I can't get a hold of this, but his tumble into the dark, his stark vulnerability, his tenderness, his mother's horror, all of his trauma field—it's not separate from me. I was pulled into an empty hole inside my head. I could not orient. My bowel erupted, and my head turned to the left. It wasn't as if I were someplace else. It was that I was nowhere at all, with no energy to look for myself. How many children's bodies hold what mine has? Billions. Johnny does, and he doesn't know this. He is with the orthopedist now. He tells me that he may avoid surgery, that it will only need to be set. I will be cut out of my cast as he is bound in his. He is taking this in stride; I feel the gravitational pull.

I don't want to sink here even for another day. I want to swim the river of sadness through all its swells and eddies and out to the green living sea to ride the backs of whales, instead of them swallowing me whole.

Arles told me about a book called God is Trauma.

"You had an encounter with God, the primitive God, and it is true that no one sees the face of God and lives. This is most often spoken about in reference to Moses."

I could feel wild neuronal scrambling. "An encounter with God?" I was incredulous.

"Yes. It was just that." I censored what kept coming to me about Moses and then said it softly,

"He was beautiful to me." He was beautiful in his brown skin and his arms. The "he" that was beautiful is not really so clear as the pronoun "he," but the skin is specific, and it is different from the not-beautiful Moses, whose skin is black and shines with sweat. "It feels as if I were electrocuted and all my circuits conformed to the singular shock and continue to emanate wave after wave of discharge." Behind the shades, the sun came out. "It wasn't psychological, Arles."

"No," he said, "it wasn't, and you have to embrace this."

"I am." I paused. "I will." He picked up my metaphor and gave it back to me as fact.

"You were electrocuted. That's exactly what happened. And the discharge which seems repetitive to you is a new wave that ignites a new charge."

"It is dispersing. I can feel that. I am devoted to dispersing it."

He suggested that I address the circuitry held in that leg with meditation. "There will be further discharge when the cast comes off. Prepare yourself, as best you can."

There are spaces, almost rings of air and light, the breaking open of the density, the field changing its nature.

I felt an odd sense of otherness as I watched Jake and his friend playing in the water and the people reading books in their beach chairs. The woman slipped off her cover-up and snuggled into her chair. She was close to my age and wore a straw hat. I knew by the way they each moved that she was innocent of the life I have lived, that Jakob was and his friend probably not. So many live on this side of the trauma divide. Once your innocence is lost, traumatically lost at the time that needs innocence, like young trees need water, life is not only never the same, you don't live the same life as others. I may have been assessing them with a soft envy. It was not possible that it would have been otherwise.

Good memories are drifting back on the sea breeze. The smell of the salt air and of tanning lotion; the giddiness of wet sand pulling away under my feet, learning to swim, daring to jump into my father's arms from the dock, smelling my mother's soft skin, Mary's brown skin. I am tired and light. It felt like I'd opened to sun and ocean air and beach plum blossoms.

Johnny's field and mine are conjoined. I contributed, somehow, to his fall and his injury. The doctor warned him, as mine did me, that he may never have full use of his hand. He broke his wrist, his elbow and the T2 vertebra. Bob worked for weeks to release the memory lodged at T2 in my spine. Some in their traditions believe that trauma lodges in the spine. I asked my friend, the energy healer, to tell me if my field and his were as intertwined as I felt.

"Johnny and your mother," she said. "No one else is there but John and your mother."

We spent the weekend together. There is no barrier between us.

And still fear continues. It is looping back into history, one loop setting off another loop, like dancing strings, like vibrational pools.

My acupuncturist is using a new energy approach. NMT (NeuroModulation Technique), I said to John, is a powerful medicine, and I could have added, indiscriminate. It perturbs and assumes it can control the perturbations, channel them the way the body has hoped and agreed to. I am not sharing that assumption. I have felt the original horror, and I have felt it originally. I hadn't known the prey animal character of this before, not like I know it now. I had never felt that I was both in and anticipating a terrorist assault. It was, though, a micro, not a macro experience. I am not afraid of terrorism—it is in my consciousness, but my view of the sky and the trees is not warped by the plane flying over. But it is by this early horror. I walked out onto my steps, and as if rediscovering this, I said, "Oh, this is not evil, this is my neighborhood."

Johnny and I have been doing NMT often in different rooms at the same time. We walked out of that first hour energetically fused and delighted with each other's company. We took ourselves out to Judy's for lunch.

It took me a while to understand the new terror engulfing me.

"Arles, this is not mine. This is Johnny's." I was nearly breathless. "It is so much worse than anything I have felt. So much worse. He's not feeling this, though. He is actually feeling light. I have absorbed what he has felt. I'm carrying it now."

Then and again, with more urgency after Johnny's fall, Arles told me to stop NMT. "They don't understand the forces they are letting loose, and it's dangerous for both of you."

I stopped.

❧

John and I, there at the Hyatt, waiting for Marsha, sharing the window table, watching bolts of lightning moving toward us from across the harbor, sharing the glass of Pinot Grigio, sharing the narrative of the present, were having entirely different experiences. I was deeply stressed by the fear that is of my history and Johnny's, the inescapability, the being hunted down, tortured, nearly drowned, and nearly killed. In the attic, in the ghetto, his mother watched dazed as he slipped beneath the bathwater. I am alone. No one can protect me from this. It is as it is.

The next morning, Marsha and I were having our coffee at the edge of the harbor. She started to cry at the thought of meeting a man and becoming a couple.

"It would be tragic to have that now when I don't need it anymore, always reminding me of how lonely I've been; what I always wanted and needed and didn't have." She looked down and then took a large swallow of her tepid latte. "You always had John and knew he loved you."

This is absolutely true. Our loneliness was different: hers starkly alone; mine obliquely shadowed by absence. My family filled me in. Each one that I loved and that loved me helped to staunch the wound and distract me from the ever-present, bewildering absence. They siphoned off my rage. How did they love me through that? How did they withstand the assaults? I did my best from the beginning to shield my kids, my mother, my friends and John. I told the detached dry narrative of utter madness until its bones bleached and cracked. Marsha was guessed at and diagnosed in rumors.

We had just pulled off of Route 3 to put the top up. We could hear each other now.

"The difference between your book and mine will be that yours will be a journey of the mind. I don't really have an interior life. I have made all of my life decisions through external goals." It was hard for me to think about what would be important about a book that didn't track the mind in a state of disorder.

"What are your goals in writing this memoir?"

"To provide hope." She was earnest and emphatic.

"I don't know if you can do this, really. People find a way to wrap your narrative in old newspaper and make it meaningless for them. They are just more worthless because you could 'make it' and they could not. You can't escape that without a narrative of mind, and even then, it is likely to provide hope mostly to the hopeful."

"My story makes my graduate students feel hopeful," she said, looking over at me, much too long as she narrowly passed a car on my side. I didn't ask how it made her patients feel. "I just don't want it to look self-serving or grandiose. I don't want a reviewer at the Times to ask why I even wrote it." For this, she needs a passionate biographer who writes well and who probes the quality of her mind. It would be well worth the effort.

"I feel you still, but at the outermost perimeter of my experience, as if in a large circle, me in the innermost middle, alone. My life is mine alone. If you faded into the wider embrace and abandon of the universe, I would hardly notice it. It wouldn't register."

"I know that's what it feels like to you right now, but it isn't true."

"There is a nuclear explosion going on in there. I am alone in it, that's the 'isness' of it. There is no one doing this to me. It isn't the attic. The NMT. It isn't Moses or any of the holographs of Moses that have visited themselves on me since. It was the essence of prey energy, of no escape, of no protector."

"Why did you place me at the perimeter?"

"I didn't." I felt for even the slightest withdrawal. He didn't leave. "This is energetic. Existential. It just is. I don't feel abandoned."

"How did I end up at the perimeter?" he asked again, as he talked about my reinstatement of motherlessness.

"I have a mother. It is you. That didn't collapse. It is something else. Something new. And I still feel that if you/the perimeter dissolved into the universe, it would be ok. Somehow the circle of light remains." We both went quiet.

"It is a nucleus," I said, stopping to really look at what I'd drawn. Arles had opened a door when he stopped insisting on these former analytic paradigms. "Arles, this is a cell. The place of the nuclear explosion is the nucleus, and you are the cell membrane." I described the cell again and used 'cell wall' instead of membrane.

"This changes the meaning," he said. "A wall is different from a membrane. Walls keep one of us out."

"It is a cell, and you were the membrane that kept dark matter out. Do you remember when you said I had experienced a tear in the fabric of the universe?" He nodded. "This is the tear in the other universe, the internal universe. This is the original cell. This is cellular memory."

I feel the cascade of neurons, left to right, the momentum of the fall. Mice have a single neuron that fires when their heads are pointed in the direction of the signal they are programmed to detect. Its firing slows when it turns to the side and stops when it turns away from the signal. Cells are the material form of memory. Everything is memory. The cell does not come into being without memory. I can't step out of this cascade. The neurons are all pointing downwards; they have me in the arc of the dive.

"If I were convinced that memory did not cross the synapse of death..." I didn't complete the unnecessary sentence. I have no desire to die. It is not at all about that. It is trying to imagine myself free of falling. "I fall across into eternity. In whatever incarnation, I am falling. I don't know how to free myself of this."

"Before you were hung..." He must have asked if I already felt I was falling, but what followed was white noise.

"No," he said, correcting me, "I asked if you'd ever had the experience of 'feeling on your feet'?"

"This is my task, to change the neuronal charge from downward in the stairwell at four to on my feet at 62." I changed this. "No, it is to be on my feet then. Even to feel myself lying on the floor."

"Where are your parents right now?"

"It's a thin white layer of vapor that outlines me beneath my skin, over the muscle. It takes the shape of my internal body, a few layers in. A ghostly homunculus." This white line is like that on the sidewalk at the scene of a homicide. That seems obvious. But the line ends at mid-thigh on both sides. It doesn't include my feet or my lower legs.

Blood vessels are broken in my heels. Lee couldn't get the energy to close around them. My gait was odd. I had a toddler's footing, heading out into the rain for the long drive home.

I fell picking raspberries on Tuesday. One nanosecond you are upright and the next on your face in the grass. I didn't feel thrown down exactly, but there was no transition between up and down. I felt the seizures in my legs. I am now trying to feel the energy of lying on the floor, to find that body memory, to find myself landed. These memory neurons are muted. What is this intercept? What does it do to memory? Where is the body's memory within the mind's dissociation? At one time, I didn't remember hanging either. It came in a flood during an early training session with Kathy. We watched the great bloom of slow waves on the replay. There seems to be fewer neuronal resources devoted to the aftermath. It is less etched. I can't find my legs now, and I can't predict what it will mean if I finally do.

Neruda writes about himself as "mysteriously protected." This is the lot, I hope, of most children. It's part of Art Spiegelman's account of 9/11. His daughter was in school two blocks away from the World Trade Center, but the events she had witnessed only became 'real' when he arrived in her classroom. When he came, when she was seen, she could see. He took his son from his school and then, his family gathered around him back home, he wept: his tears, his parents' tears, his Maus tears, the tears that vaporize in the fires. This was harder for his children than the yellow bones of the building just before the toxic cloud of asbestos and human ash consumed them. They had lost their mysterious protection.

"When I came here that first day, I opened the door to a journey that I can never end. I am learning to know my experience at every level, every manifestation."

"It is a gift," he said. "A rare gift." He leaned his elbows on his knees. "Everyone who closes the door on their histories becomes a terrorist."

I bought Sabelle a pad of thick paper bound in the signs of the zodiac, the black and endless sky. It was her 25th birthday. It is another invitation to make her trashed life into art. Charlie was the first to say it to me. “Some people make their lives into their art. You have done this.”

When I went back Thursday night to pick raspberries, the field was bathed in September light. Every red berry shone like an ornament in the blues and the greens all the way to the river. I was unhurried. I felt no pressure against the inside of my ribs, the press that arises in the absence of mysterious protection.

I described my experience of the ‘other inhabitant’, my brain. As I spoke, it became clear to me that the brain has its own mind that is quite different or at least quite separable, from the mind that perceives its brain. The brain has its own consciousness, at the very least its own awareness of its state. Its aura shimmers around the physical brain, dancing with potential and an inherent joy at its own existence. This awareness now is the closest I’ve come to a visceral experience of joy. The mind of the brain is effervescent; a halo.

The Othmers dropped their useless lawsuit.

I have never heard thunder like I just heard. It began as regular thunder, deep and sonorous, but instead of quieting, it built into drums of explosions that I felt in the earth. I didn’t want to do this, but I did. I looked for a fireball, the registration of the terrorist attack, and the notification of the crater in the midst of this peaceful landscape.

Another night of nudgy, perseverative dreams. I woke fogged in by worry that dissipates slowly without effort. It is clear to me that I am the cause of Johnny’s fall. It is all linked to the NMT. When Johnny and I walked down that Amherst driveway that day in early June, we had become linked together. Each of us felt more connected to the other than we had ever been and perhaps more connected to each other than to anyone else. It was unmistakable. Investigating this today, it is as if in some way our molecules became powerful attractors and hooked up. We have been bound together in a way that no psychology explains. It is in this that I am the cause. He fell with me. No one even tries to explain the mistake he made that night. This house is a second home. The bathroom is one door down and to the right. He went to the end of the hall and turned to the left. He had to fall with me. He was bound to it. His injury is much greater; his impairment might well endure. He called me first, but I didn't think to be the one, as I should have been, to call the ambulance. I got him to, I was in a cast, and he had the car. Molly, as she always does, took over the scene of domestic carnage and got the ambulance to him.

He said last night that I came through everything so well, in contrast to him. The difference in the extent and duration of injury is our mothers and the nature of our earliest trauma. NMT has given Johnny a mother for the first time. I am in and of and resonant with his field. But it has also locked our traumatic fields and field potentials. And I have taken on his field as well. This may be part of the prey feeling that I have fought with, the sense of being hunted. It does not fit into the geography of the attic. It's probably from him; him in me.

Lee held my calves and feet for a long time. I could feel them, lifeless and cool, submit to the embrace of her hands. I kept trying to get it, to know the present. I began to feel energy moving in my legs and even into the soles of my feet, and memory seemed to follow. As it had been with Bob, I twisted to grasp something overhead. I had become aware that with him, I didn't hang like Raggedy Ann in a child's hand; I swung like a pendulum. My hands fly up when I try to say it to Arles. This memory in itself is not as frightening as twisting to grab the rung of the banister. I cannot remember what I remember. It feels like something is tightening, being gripped and twisting in my brain, even as low as the brainstem. It doesn't feel bad at all. I am dizzy but more sure-footed.

❧

I was thinking out loud, "What are the conditions that allow the unremembered to become remembered? When I started to talk about twisting like strange fruit, when I felt this in my body, things stopped. It was a blank, putty-like space. It was more than neurons shut down than it was resistance. The neurons do not fire here. They have memory, and they are mute."

"Have you been doing Alpha-Theta?"

"The last time it threw me to the ground. There is always a demon."

"Perhaps it is an angel, not a demon, an angel who is throwing you down, who is giving you information. Maybe your transcendence, Sebern, will be down, not up."

I kept myself as close to the margin as I knew how to do, hardly knowing what this was. And then suddenly I felt sensation start up in my lower back. How would I get from hanging to being out of the stairwell, out of this terrible stasis of dissociation into this terrifying motility of knowing?

"Why do you think you can't enter the promised land?" That's when it happened. It was my back being dragged over the banister, then my shoulders and the back of my head. I am out of the stairwell. He saw this embodiment of memory. I wasn't really somewhere else; I was just out of the stairwell.

When he said, "You were a baby, just a baby when all this happened," it felt unbearable, cracking me open to blood and yolk, spinal fluid and sperm. I felt sick and dazed, and I pushed into the pillow for some relief. He asked me if I wanted him to, and he sat next to me and held the back of my head and my neck. I discovered him there.

"You are right here".

"Yes, I am right here," I said this a couple of times, and he assured me a couple of times more. He sat with his side against the fetal curve of my body. He was installing mysterious protection. He was returning me to time.

"Why do you try things like NMT?" He was challenging me, implying that it related to a quiescent engagement with self-destruction. Until last week, I was talking about making myself well, that trauma-seeded illness. And last week, I talked about freeing myself from death. Whatever this need is is subcortical. It was this part of my brain that was speaking its inchoate language. I want, before I die, to be free of it, to know what it is to live free of fear, absolutely free of fear.

Red Sox, down by 3, win four straight.

Bush will be president until 2008. What will the world do? What will I do but once again wrap myself in the Tao and in the psyches of those I love?

I have been crying for Moses. It is as if he pried open my body and deposited his ancestral sorrow, all the degradations and subjugation. I wish him no harm. It is not something done to me that registers—not the torn shoulder or the bruised head— it is the heart he left there when he disappeared, and Maddie stayed. It was dark, and it was deranged, but it was not evil. I was not left with evil deposited in me. This darkness in its lightest form is grief, and my tears slip down my face and drop onto his heart.

It is strange when I consider my identity—not quite an Episcopal, upper-middle-class older woman. I am a Jew, a black boy, a white woman of indiscernible heritage. The source of my name is yet to be discovered. I grew up in a country club with pink walls, but I was hardly there. I appeared to rebel, and perhaps I did, but more than that, I just didn't learn. The first four years significantly foreclosed the next 25. It grew like some silent strangling vine through my brain down my spinal cord. My sacrum was oscillating. He touched it, and I was gone, wishing only that I could get beneath this floor and go down to my bed; then I would know—simultaneously I would know—that this was a table in Bob's office. It brought me no comfort. I tried to plan my escape to my bed at the same moment that it occurred to me that this would never stop and that it was so intense I could have a stroke. Every time was that moment. I kicked away from his hands on my legs, but it was not about hanging. I was not back there. They were younger legs than mine, in black stockings (?) and slightly bowed. He said he'd discovered a new impact, a force coming down the right side of my face out of my left jaw. "Maybe this was the dive off the bed." Please, 'nothing new', a prayer I find myself saying. "Yes," he said and also "No." Of course, that's true to different degrees with everything I "know." I am burning it off, turning it to vapor. I felt small, frail, more bones than body, as if you could see through me with a flashlight, very young, very old, near death, at the very end of life. There is nothing I want to say about this night. I still feel it all shimmering in my body like an angel.

I have felt Arles back away. I asked him if he didn't want to know any more of what I was finding in my body, that I surely would be the last to blame him. He assures me. But, of course, who really wants to contend with such implanted horror? He is the mysterious protection. His understanding cradles my sanity. When he departs from the agreed-upon reality, I panic somewhere at the root. Salt is poured onto the soil. My reality will twist and disfigure. I won't know my way out of the mall. My kitchen will become a hall of mirrors. He seems to know that I am still subject to this descent. He did understand the madness that even madness could not protect me from. But I doubt he has ever felt this. I had never felt it.

Chapter 15

I am hesitant to begin a new journal. It has been, for the most part, a narrative of recovery, shameful and sacred. I read this to hear it, to collect it into one arc of knowing, to wrap it and tie it and then do what? There are too many blank pages after this one, and I don't want to fill them, not with this. I want to find the openings of light and pry them open even further. Trauma narrows the vision. I can feel this almost physically in my brain, in the field of vision. Like screws in the temples, a rigid halo of history. Turning the head is nearly impossible; it rivets you. I did, all that being said, end up bringing no GF bread, no rice milk and no toothpaste to this retreat, but seven pens. Weston Priory, December 2004.

I started to feel strange even before I got to Serio's. I put the package of sleeping pills in my pocket and decided to take the town route back home. Walking down the hill at the police station, I felt as if I wasn't weighted down enough. It was hard to walk. At the hotel and through the back alleys of Fitzwillies, I tried to think of the right food to fix this, but couldn't and didn't want to go in anywhere to get it. My brain is swirling in and out of strobes, and I feel the possibility of a seizure. I crossed against the light and went to Pops. I sat on the wall in front of Talbot's and ate the Milky Way. I looked for someone I knew in a passing car; perhaps they would drive me home. I ate the chocolate bar slowly, feeling the sugar getting into my blood and slowly reorienting my brain. Would I need another? Where was the next place I could sit down? I had a fourth of my walk left. I pushed ahead past the school and Duffy's; they would help, Sara would help or Harry or Michelle's parents. I needed to keep walking. I am drenched in sweat. Getting up the stairs to my apartment is an act of willfulness and faith. Half a sandwich left in the fridge. I ate it and some walnuts, then some ice cream with some more walnuts, desperately attempting to eat my way out of this. As the bright day turned into a moonless night, I fell into a post-glycemic swoon. It felt as if my memory body, my heavy memory body, had fallen through the crust of my present body and was lying like lead along my spine.

Arles does not say anything. I spoke from the original experience, the one that gave birth to this distant agony on the couch. A subdural panic stirs, and some voice yells at me to shut up. Is this a threat? Is this doubt? I don't lose his presence. He is there. He isn't stopping this. I need something more like a backboard than a mirror. This can't fall into his open vastness and disappear in there. It has to stay between us, these words, these awful memories of splaying bones, the new understanding of my sacrum torn apart in every direction, the new meaning of the pick-up sticks thrown to the floor.

"It comes like this in small movements, Sebern, any other course of memory would be false, 'as if'."

"What would it feel like if all of my cells released their memories at the same moment?"

"That would create its own toxic state. Such rapid depolarization would leave a toxic cloud. It would be the only air left to breathe."

"To me, it's more like the lifelessness of a helium balloon a week after the occasion, limp and sad. In some way, the cells of my body depend on this memory to live, to justify their own replication, to provide continuity. I feel like I will collapse on the sidewalk or into myself. It is a scramble to stay aligned, to remain alive." I stopped, and he seemed to be waiting.

"I didn't know if I was alive."

"There is an edge," he said. "It is as if your expanding patience has within it, or beneath it, a deeper impatience."

I recognize the edge that he spoke about, and it is like all the rest. It is no longer my own. It is "explicate order." Trauma, neglect and no mother are currents that run through the implicate order. They are always present, and when conditions are right, a memory, Alpha-Theta, bodywork, Bush, it becomes explicate. Our vocabulary has changed from that of psychology to that of physics to describe the same circumstances. In the presence of the nuclear explosion, even Bohm himself could not speak of the implicate/explicate order. He discovered this in the aftermath. The field is so filled with its own perturbation that subtlety is swamped; the nature of things is overwhelmed. It is a field of pure force, and the force itself decides or demands the new language.

I am sipping my peppermint tea in bed on the seventh floor of the Sheraton Old Town. The neighborhood streets are quiet, but trucks roll west toward Gallup and East to Texas without respite. Each time I look over, I see the same piece of footage. The old cowboy, getting in his truck below me, stopped to look at the sun coming up over a gap in the Sandia Mountains, light that was turning them pink. I fly home today with luck, threading the needle between snowstorms. I hope this trip is the beginning of handing off the many batons to the next generation. I am here to offer hope to 16 children who have had very little and to their endless number of successors. We savage our young.

Neuronal bundles that are meant to weave together begin to fly apart, and the function that depends on the weave feels precarious. I am doing something wrong, something toxic to my brain. This feels like a protest. It can make it hard even to take a walk.

"The future of this field is in the brain. We will not get better at psychotherapy as a field. There will not be breakthroughs of significance in dynamic, analytic or behavior therapies. This is beyond drugs. So young therapists must learn about the brain and how to appeal to it directly, and the best way we know to date to do this is neurofeedback. Here we have just begun." This was my lunch talk to the young staff of the residential center here.

Sabelle told me that she hardly remembers the visit to the Cape to meet Marsha. "Everything sparkled when I had DID, in a way that it doesn't now. Everything shone." I thought there might have been more shine since everything that weekend sparkled, the water, Cape light, long solo rides with me and the glitter of Marsha. She said she knew that she'd met Marsha in a condo somewhere, but that in her memory, it could have as easily been a boat.

I told Arles about the jolt of understanding when I retold the story of my wisdom tooth. "I have an 'electrical certainty' that a brain stores its atrocities in its neuronal pools. This one fired, my tooth being pulled, and then all the ones associated with it fired too because that's what they do."

I left the dentist's office on Elm St, perhaps impulsively—they said too soon—, and I took the stairs. A man coming up spoke to me, and it was then that I passed out and pitched over down the stairs, crumpling into the landing wall. The stranger came, told me to stay there, and he would call for help. I fled before they came. They were upset with me at the infirmary because I rode my bike. The compress was mostly blood. The next morning, they found me passed out in the bathroom. They admitted me to the infirmary for treatment of a concussion. So, there were all the elements of replication, of an attempt at communication and the necessity of confinement. Thirty years later, I went to another dentist on Elm Street. I woke up from the anesthesia crying. He had pulled the wrong tooth, a perfectly healthy one, a dog tooth, the one you bite with.

I had smelled cigar smoke for a few weeks. I had some mounting pressure in my back tooth. I had the taste of the pliers. "Electrical inevitability," that's what I called it. He didn't respond. He had nothing to add. What I was saying was plausible and complete.

"But this leaves me feeling...," and I stopped. I couldn't fill in the blank. "It's like the potholders I made as a kid. You pull the loops of fabric over the metal teeth; all different colors, making your pattern. It's like the yellow loop is left hanging, that you need to pick that up, that it isn't complete because it is entirely about our relationship, now, here, our consensual reality. I depend on this consensual reality." He knows this. He did pick up the loop, and he made the weave and stretched it over the last metal tooth.

"I don't understand these forces, but I do see them, and they are not nameable purely as trauma. Trauma is being hit by the bus."

"I know it is an inadequate word, a failed and increasingly empty concept."

"We don't move through life," he said, "life moves through us."

I told him yesterday that I needed him to enter me, to break the barrier of skin and energy, to reorganize my cellular/extracellular field with his. I could not change without this impingement, this overtaking of my disorganization by his organization. This is about fields, energetic capacities that we develop in each other. It is not about biography.

"If I am going to explore at these levels, if I am going to seek brutal knowing, I need to feel that I am touching you, that this registers not as a new construct but as pain in your heart. I can't find my heart without feeling yours."

"Yes," he said, "I know."

I shared my worries about Marsha with John.

"She's hurt her back repeatedly. She's in unrelenting pain. Her chiropractor said it had to come from a serious fall where she hit the top of her head. Well, right, of course. It would. It's like it's just a story that she took those dives off the bed. She's really never found treatment that helps her. She's gone to doctors. She takes Ibuprofen four or five times a day. She's overwhelmed her therapists. She's become famous. And she is becoming crippled. She has serious arthritis, osteoporosis, scoliosis and multiple disc problems. She has had many falls, like the one off the curb, with injuries to her knees and wrist. She is suffering from her evidence-based and insurance-reimbursed choices. I feel so sad for her. And I'm so mad at her. She's so fucking stubborn!"

"I've often wondered why you go to Bob and Sam, feel so terrible, but still keep going. Now I understand."

"I don't feel terrible," I corrected him. "I have some terrible experiences. But they are there, they are not inert. They must move on, or they deform."

"Trauma is being hit by the bus. Bones heal, you are wary of buses. You may overreact to buses. Every moment of that history is encoded so as not to be hit by a bus again. But what do we call what happened to most of my patients and to me? I cannot find a word with adequate power. There is no bus. Or every event threatens to materialize into a bus. It is a phantom of implicit memory that arises in the sensations of the dark. A phantom because so much of the injury— another wholly inadequate word—is about no mother. So much of what these neurons struggle to represent is not worthlessness but objectlessness."

An attractor or super attractor site is the place around which chaos gathers. There is some hint of magnetism here, of what gets gathered to us. What of all the elements of chaos are then selected? I actively perturbed these fields as they are represented in the firing of my brain, but I haven't yet dispersed the super attractor. Training the brain either enhances or lays bare the implicate order. I don't suffer what unfolds. I do not feel mortal despair when the implicate becomes, momentarily, explicate. I wonder in fact why now all that is still unknown believes it must stay unknown. There are cautions in the system that have nothing to do with fear. Perhaps it is just time.

"Johnny," I said to Arles, "doesn't exist outside of his states. He forms as the state, manifests as that, and when that dissipates, he becomes something else. There is no constituent self binding these fluctuations. He has not been able to string together an identity behind or through the states."

"And you?" he asked.

"I don't know who I am. This is factual, but it is not a statement of confusion, fragmentation or doubt. I don't know who I am. I am not fixed. I am coherent, but I am not 'I.'"

Allison and I were at the Mill River by seven. As soon as I wiggle free of land and I am floating down in the water, it feels like prayer. Birdsong and the tick-tocking of woodpeckers. I think, each time, about their brains. There are beaver and otters and a large white-bellied raptor that I tagged after for as long as she would let me. Even with the background hum of the interstate, it is peaceful here. As we pulled our boats up to the shore, she said, "I'm glad you broke your toe" (we can't play racquetball), only meaning, she'd rather be there than anywhere else.

I feel some pride and deep quiet pleasure when wild animals come close to me. The turtle who rose to greet me, the blue heron that lets me approach, these beings, unperturbed by me. My energy is becoming quiet, not yet quiet enough, but there are these little measures.

My patient Wally lives alone with his equally feral cat. They have shared the same house since she came to his yard 3 years ago. They have had nothing to do with each other except when he feeds her. After his first or second neurofeedback session, she raced to the door to greet him, rubbed against his legs and has since rarely left his side. I wrote about tracking changes with training and posted it on the Spectrum list-server titled, "Ask the cat."

I dreamt last week that *I was lying on a king bed in Arles' house, talking with him, deeply engaged, intimate—how we talk. I rolled toward him and felt the urge to kiss him. I knew the nature of the kiss. It would dissolve boundaries. I can feel it completely. He needed to change the bed, and I helped. I realized that we live in parallel and akin realities. We all have sheets, we change them, we climb over our beds. It then became the fact that the CIC was being held in his house and that everyone was staying in condos nearby. I'd moved my stuff into his guest room, awaiting John's arrival. I was told by the staff that we weren't granted the use of the bedrooms, only the large room, with French doors at the end. I stayed in the guest room, knowing it would be all right, almost certainly. I thought that perhaps we could move out of the guest room and use Arles' bed for the conference, but then thought better of it. It was asking too much.*

"We cannot leave Auschwitz behind. Not because we wouldn't wish to; it is not possible." Perhaps I am projecting my restlessness on him, my need to break through this ring into another reality. "I think you are impatient, too."

"No, not at all," he says.

Last night, John and I ate at Allison's before she, and I went kayaking in the night. Deep into the threads of the marsh, we found a plastic baby doll hanging from a low branch by its right foot. It wasn't debris from the flood. It had been put there. John said in a sloppy approximation of a Cajun accent, "No one goes into the bayou after dark." It was the solstice, it was the full moon, there was the doll, and I wasn't afraid. We watched the moon rise, and thousands of fireflies lit up the trees between the river and the meadow, thousands of stars fell and held on the leaves.

On Tuesday, Arles leaves to give a paper in Germany. During my recent trans-temporal episode, I felt myself to be a girl of about seven in a nice apartment in a city in either Germany or Austria. I was alone in a pretty dress in the middle of the living room with the chandelier. All the rooms were sparsely furnished with the few things left of personal meaning. I felt my way through sensations to a narrative. My father was in hiding. He was important politically and professionally. He was in a dark, small space, wearing dark clothes.

"Is there water in the scene?" Arles asked. I know if I go to him, he will be captured, and something bad will happen. This father may be Arles. He has not wanted to leave me, but he has had to. Both of us survive. He escapes to Holland on a boat, and I never see him again. I pass as Christian. I am taken in by a family.

Alan quotes Siegfried, "Neurofeedback is like therapy in the rearview mirror."

"I wouldn't," I say, "think of Siegfried as any expert in this, since there are few people on earth who need therapy more than Siegfried." He laughed. I told him a bit of Siegfried's history, and he understood how sincere I was. Alan was struggling to articulate his understanding/observation of what happens with trauma and feedback. He describes a purging and a return to the time before, to the one who existed before and apart from the trauma.

"For me, there is no 'before.' For most of my patients, there is no before. We are all rendered. There is no Garden of Eden. There are just all the big bangs, the endless propulsion of violent being."

Neurofeedback has introduced time into my traumatized mind. There is, most of the time, a "then" and "now." I do have days that are just the days that they are—lived only on this plane, and they feel like my memory of a summer day at six or seven, lived near the ocean, catching crabs, diving into the surf and then eating in the kitchen when we got home. I have these days, but they are still rare. I love them.

"Fear arising, is that the sign of this magnetized pull?" I asked.

"You will never be free of what happened to you. That's OK. That's how it should be. These are the circumstances of your identity. It's your history to honor." We had no disagreement.

"But there is shame that you're not getting free of it, Arles."

"I know. But that's just ego, Sebern, nothing more."

He asked me how I felt about his going to Germany. Until he asked, I really thought little of it, wondered what his paper was, how he would do on the flight, but I will do well; I will even miss him. When he asked, it was as if a body within my body retracted. That shape got cold and could have shrieked. "If you take me with you, I won't ever ever... I don't even want to presume... Don't leave me there."

"What would happen if you were left there?" Time in the room shifted back to the present.

"Something," I said, "in the grammar of your question." The vehicle for that smaller body, that shivering hologram, was the hospital in Munich after the car crash. But the holographic cellular body was not a memory of this. It was earlier, a memory that the hospital was a memory of. If it is true that there are no accidents in this psychic time and space, in our present lived history, could it also be the case that there are no accidents at all? That memory demands representation until it is known for what it is, no longer a disowned ghost haunting the landscape? Disembodied memory makes florid demands on me, but not just on me, on everyone, on nations. It makes the demand that we go to war.

He assures me, as we end, that he will be fine in Germany. He didn't need to. It occurred to me briefly to ask, "Will I?" but I know it is a false question because I am here now.

John wakes and says to me, "Your mind is like a cat. When you let it out at night, you don't know where it goes." The day here, beautiful, dry and warm, begins with blueberry pancakes.

A sparrow comes to visit. She taps on the window. She comes to all the windows and not just when I'm here. She visits Johnny, too. It's as if she wants to come in. John says it's as if one of our cats has returned as a bird. A right karma. We decided it was Mieka. A chipmunk came up to Johnny when he was out having a smoke. He called it brazen. I told him the experience of others with animals, those who have trained them. "Animals like what happens then."

I saw a bear, a young one, on the road to the pond. She watched briefly and, almost as if remembering what her mother told her, changed her mind and headed into the woods. I could follow her form a little way, mostly her silent paws, until she made the shadow darker and disappeared. The next morning, I swam in the fog. I would never have done that. I could feel how I could make it eerie, and my mind does not turn in there.

"It isn't about my mother or Moses anymore. My time with an unconscious, a personal, archival unconscious, has been brief." Arles agreed and added,

"The historical unconscious is much more vast than the personal."

We talked about my fear of obliteration if I dropped even more deeply into the mystery—the loss of all I know.

"Are you equating the mystery with motherlessness?"

"I don't think so. But I wonder if avatars who have no mother just burn up on entry." None of the avatars who came to mind, Christ, Buddha or Mohammed were orphans. I knew by account that two had good mothers. Mothering may be a prerequisite for entry. "But then I have you. I am not motherless."

I spent Friday night with Marsha in our annual sleepover at the Hyatt. We talked about Geraldine's wedding and Blake's. I could see that my lack of excitement confused her. She talked to me about celebration and spirituality and guiding Blake so that she wouldn't get lost in all the distractions that abound. "It is I who has gotten caught up in the distractions, Marsha. Thank you." Both of us slept unusually well. Marsha wakes up talking. She made coffee. I looked at her new stuff in shame, made comments and felt our differences. Her computer turned itself off. She came out of the shower with a towel pressed against her, sat down in her ample nakedness and rebooted the computer against the backdrop of a hazy Boston harbor.

❧

I told him about my dream of talking *with a woman at a peace rally. She is sitting next to me, and she pushed her finger up into me. She had a long finger that penetrated into my bowel.* After the dream, remembering it, the finger seemed like Pinocchio's nose.

"You mean it grew?" I realized what I was talking about, but when he said that, I was arrested, ashamed, almost sickened by a faint memory of pain there.

"I'd thought of the nose as more like the lie and the act, in the midst of a peace demonstration, a representation of the process I still go through. I feel at peace, very content, and then something takes me over from behind, and peace is, temporarily, shattered."

"Yes, that too."

Soft gray sadness wraps around me and seeps into my brain. I am sad for my skeletal son, 10 pounds less than when he was the stoic, suffering painter at our house a month ago. I started to weep when he said he was in end-stage AIDS and that he wanted to die with dignity and grace. Not doing it the way he was, lashing out, terrified, filled with humiliation and discharging it. In response to my angst and my anger and to his own private sorrow, John asked, "Would you rather there had been no Johnny?" and I couldn't answer. I wouldn't have known. I couldn't answer this.

"It is as if my brain is balanced on ball bearings, something happened, and it slipped off. I hear dissonant bells from different landscapes, different epochs all ring at once in my head. I can't reorganize myself."

I sat down later with Arles.

"I am in this place because you were away too long. I am here because I feel unprecedented grief. I am here to tank up on you." I am open to it. "It isn't the grief, it is what lies beneath it. Grief unifies. Grief makes known what is still not known in a dissociated space or disassociated space. Grief is born from real events, and it certifies them."

"Your mother couldn't feel a lot of things, but she wanted to kill grief." I think this is right, but it seems like it gives her an undue dimensionality. Except for the last nine months before she died, she didn't have that. With all I know and all the passionate and compassionate feelings I've had for her, I haven't been able to backfill, to give the therapeutic caricature flesh. Or heart or intentions. This felt like a failure of mine. I can't undo it for her or for me, with her. And when he is away and when he first gets back, he is "no mother and a father too far away."

They plead for their lives on rooftops so hot they need to dance. New Orleans after Katrina and Moses are not separable, the reality of entrapment, of torment, of race. Who was the trapped animal? The hurricane churned in my head; that terrible, irreducible, unresolvable confusion about Moses.

The Symmetron chair arrives today. I tried it at ISNR on September 10th, an hour or so after I'd done a Tomatis session. Larry, its inventor, told me that the motion of this chair activated the vestibular nucleus of the brainstem. I rocked for about half an hour with music playing in Bose headphones. I could feel that something was happening in my neck, but it felt sensitive throughout my body, most noticeably in my feet and legs. As I have with every approach, I looked for differences. I had to search for how I felt; getting a chocolate malt was atypical but not unheard of. My response to sugar can be catastrophic, and I couldn't quite trust my legs, so I went back to the hotel. Over the next hours and the next day, I noticed a new sense of inner balance. I wasn't struggling so hard to keep my head on straight. I managed the sugar but had no need for more. Written words were more fluid; maybe spoken as well. Sleep has been erratic; some mornings I have slept until eight, others I am awake at 3:30.

The morning after I arrived home, I felt something close to depression. The collision in my head began with trouble with balance. Bob sees it differently. To him, I am more on the ground, and when I am standing, I am in better alignment. He is able to release adhesions at C2, and energy begins coursing through this deadened zone. Sam agrees. Some channel has opened from that area to my right ear. Episodically, I have switched from my left to my right ear to speak on the phone, and I am able to keep my eyes open when I talk.

Saturday night, just home from the March in Washington, I fell asleep before John. When he came in, I was on his side of the bed.

"I need my seizure medicine."

"You are asleep."

"No, I am awake. I need this medication."

"You don't take that anymore." I got silent, grinding gears in my head thinking about this and finally decided he was right. I went through an inventory of night meds and couldn't find it, so I left the state—a bubble of wakefulness in the midst of sleep—and went back into the darkness of the night.

I dreamt about a boy named Kevin having a seizure and nearly dying from it. I was in a hospital, and I threw a canister of blood into the garbage. It was AIDS blood, and I was worried I had not taken the right precautions. I told the hospital people. I returned to Kevin, and his sister said he is not dead, but his pulse is very weak. I lifted the boy in my arms, helpless but no longer desperate. His breathing was faint. The next night, I dreamt of him again. *He was wandering into the forest and didn't seem to hear me calling him, and he just kept going. I lost him. All I saw as he disappeared was his back, his dark black hair, his white T and black shorts.*

Hospital dreams are back.

"What does it mean to integrate my history?" I asked him.

"People think of equanimity as rising above, no, floating above, but what it truly means is deep engagement without turmoil. You aren't floating above. You are cleansing. At times, that is all there is to do. It is the right thing to do."

It has rained for two weeks. It doesn't bother me. Just weather.

Tsunami, Katrina, Rita and Turkey are the sadnesses of the world. I am not sad. Floods here. Both houses are OK.

I rocked in the chair before I saw Bob, and he was able to move C6 and C7, and he went deep into the base of my skull. He had released the dura mater, which had been somewhat fixed at the bottom of my skull, and when it was freed, energy poured in and balanced my brainstem. Everything was different. There was no trauma in it. Just release and realignment.

Yesterday I felt my heart. It was like the shepherd boy coming upon the parchment rolls in the Palestinian caves. It felt like I stumbled upon it. And at other moments, as if there has been a shadow heart or a heart in wait. Every cell knows everything, every sorrow since the beginning of sorrow; everything of my own little and sad history. There are no places in the heart to shunt this off here or that away there. The mind can do that with its fierce agility, but the heart, this heart is soft and whole and gray and heavy. Remembering here doesn't seem to be factual or specific. Global historical knowing is not a singular capacity of my heart; it is the nature of all hearts. I was with Arles when this happened. I will know all of this in its entirety. I have no option but would not choose to choose differently. It is no more bearable, really, than it ever was, and of course it is entirely bearable.

This discovery requires 3 to 4 months of meditation in a white room with a small white bed and an altar. Someone would bring me soup. It needs that much quiet. I thought of Anne's recovery from terminal cancer, a year of meditation. No phone calls. This discovery needs that. Arles sat with me in my long, quiet, tearful silence before asking me what I was experiencing. I could only answer "Everything."

I am in silence today. No news of Bush's collapse or of the thousands who the world will let freeze to death in Pakistan. No requests for my assistance or input. Silence. Attending as best I know how to my new heart. It feels both very present and equally tentative.

"In the Kabbalah, the tree of life is at the heart," he teaches me. "One side of it is mercy, the other is knowing. All energy flows to this." There is, behind the gray, weighty heart, a radiant heart. I feel it. I see it like a child's drawing of the sun coming out from behind the clouds.

This all may have begun in the session with Bob. C5 has stayed free of C6, the dural tube slips freely at my neck, the dura mater moves separately from my skull, and on Wednesday, there was a freeing and movement of the whole frontal arachnoid layer that spreads over the cortex. Everything is rearranging, and there, in the midst, still in its cave, is my heart.

Arles put his hand on my shoulder. "The body is infinite".

Reggie feels wild and dark, "I can turn on every lamp in the house, light every candle, put Pachelbel's Canon on repeat and fill the tub with lavender, and it doesn't stop the ghosts of wild horses galloping through my veins instead of blood." She had gone to visit her mother.

The Monday before Thanksgiving, on the phone with John, Johnny threatened to kill himself, and then he hung up. Only for a moment, John had the terrible and inevitable thought, "OK." It's nearly impossible, inconceivable to have such a thought about him. We love him. He found the people to call. They busted his door down. He is in the hospital on Haldol by injection. He does, as Arles said, continue to drown.

"I have to find a way to get you into my scientific community, I just can't think how." Marsha and I were catching up. "I want to be on this neurofeedback train. I don't want it to leave the station without me."

I dreamt that I had a baby late in life. I loved her, but it was also difficult how much she demanded of me, how complete the giving over of self. I was ambivalent about having her with me. It may have been in a pub or a bookstore. I was in my apartment naked and realized I had forgotten her, and with terror in my throat, I started to run down the stairs. I realized that people might see me, and that would make everything worse, ran upstairs, put on a robe and ran down. I found her unharmed. She is still related to me. She was a beautiful and even-tempered child. She forgave me. We reconnected. Before this, I had the recognition, the horror of having forgotten her, and I woke up keening. My face was wet with tears. *At the end of the dream, I was sitting on the rug near a table leg. The baby came by with her nanny, walking now. I tried to get her attention to have her turn toward me, but she wouldn't. The nanny encouraged her, and she looked at me for a moment, but then both walked away.*

I'd watched the end of the Cream reunion concert on PBS. Without a pause, they followed it with a film on fractals and the Mandelbrot set. They showed all of these unfolding patterns in nature that can only be measured by fractal geometry. This pattern appears in all that seems apparently random. Then I think I got what Alan was trying to tell me. Stephen Wolfram has founded a new math in which the Mandelbrot set does not occur. The Mandelbrot set is a repeating occurrence, not necessarily anything as apparently comforting as order in the midst of chaos. It could be a repeating pattern that entraps. Alan told me he wasn't sure where fractal geometry was accommodated in Wolfram. He'd asked, but there were no clear answers. Wolfram is betting on the movement out of replication. There are four conditions. In the first, nothing changes, and the pattern dies, the second, the pattern endlessly repeats itself. In the third, you begin to see something new but can still recognize the old, and in the fourth condition, everything is new. Alan and I think that the Mandelbrot set could still be found in the Class 3 condition. The cluster of patterns within patterns. This feels fractal to me.

"Is Class 4," I asked, "when we give up our 'fractalness?'"

"Exactly!" He lit up, "This is having hit escape velocity!" This is for me not about speed and breaking free of all former facts, or even from the Mandelbrot set, or an escape from the apparent laws of the universe. Wolfram gave up on the EEG. There is too much complexity, but these conditions must somehow include the signal that constrains or liberates our consciousness, the EEG. In my experience with Wolfram's conditions, there is fluidity between Class 3 and Class 4. Mental illness is a Class 2 condition, repeating itself endlessly. We have to perturb this replication to change it. It can't be done with therapy; it can't be done without it. Perturbation of the most complex signal in the universe requires neurofeedback and the hands of another.

My father died. I saw him in a wheelchair with a cast around his torso, speeding aggressively toward someone else in a wheelchair. I was watching it from the stands. He fell back and may have been crushed by the cast. Someone comes to tell me he is dead. I felt the full weight of grief, the pressure it puts on your bones, the density of impossible aloneness that collapses inward between your ears, the heart-tearing sadness of it. I don't think I have ever felt loss so consciously or so fully. It was primal, animal. I could not comprehend it. I came out enough to remind myself that he died a long time ago, that I survived it, and then I slipped back under the water, and in the next dream, *my mother died. She wasn't old; she was slender in a long plum gown. She was laid out on a table, not in a coffin. The smallest personal world of the family disintegrated. I was alone.* It is still in my body.

This weight is the chair, the body, the bodywork; my handwriting is not so good. Tinnitus. Exhaustion. The chair.

"I have never been anxious or depressed, Arles." He hesitated and then nodded.

"You have lived either in purgatory or in hell. In a sense, you are Dante, not Beatrice, but Dante." I told him about the bedsheet with red lettering, "Abandon hope all you who enter here," that I hung across the ornate gates at Smith.

"I didn't understand Dante. I held onto the surface of everything I studied there, in fact, all through school, like I was at the edge of a glacier. I knew its gleaming, frozen surfaces, not its profound depths, and I was slipping. I took my junior year at the Institute. Charlie gave me constraints, but there was no context. I treaded air in some diaphanous supposition of Oedipal conflict. He was trained analytically. There were few drugs to learn about, there was yet to be any understanding, really, of 'pre-Oedipal' development, there was a professional rejection of attachment and no recognition of posttraumatic stress. Charlie knew my need for a father, and he provided that. He stood for that. It was his supervisor who recommended that he do sessions with me in cold packs. He may have considered this, but he knew I was afraid of them."

Arles said, playfully, "They were cold!"

"They were! The night staff would rattle ice when tensions were rising on Thompson II. But it wasn't that. I would be naked and bound. I would have been stripped or sedated. He told me, later, that he couldn't do this without certainty of therapeutic gain and the odds, he felt, were not good. So, I was never wrapped up except by his voice, his consequences, his fist on the desk frustration. But I needed to be. When he did not appear on the horizon three times a week, all I could do was echo around in all the tiresome looping distractions. He got tired of my being on report so many mornings, and he may have thought he was losing the battle. He may have understood that every skirmish was oxygen and proclamation: 'I am here, I exist, make walls around me.'"

"Charlie had the power of the state," he said, "At times, I have envied that."

My toss of the tennis ball knocked over the lamp, it crashed on the ground, the lightbulb popped, and Ester lit up. I had never seen anything like it. The moment before she was, as always, almost still, modest and grandmotherly, watching our base-running up and down the back hall. But then the light went out, the nursing staff rushed in, Ester shouted, swore and threatened. She made sexual gestures. I had thrown the ball that broke the lamp that turned Ester from Jekyll into Hyde.

I was like the boy walking along a country road in New Hampshire, dragging his stick over the utility poles. The grid went down. He was responsible for the blackout of the Northeast. Charlie was already mad at me over the way I'd treated a new and frightened staff member, and I had already started to slip. He didn't see how scared I was. I had sent Ester over some cliff I didn't even know was there by doing the things he had told me repeatedly not to do. I tried for a week to make a repair, but he was angry and would not hear it. I was a baby trying to elicit a smile, and when I couldn't, the last fraying thread of resilience tore. I smashed a glass with a towel and swallowed the shards. But it didn't work. And then the woman hung herself on Thompson One. The whole patient's body hung with her, oscillating in the pendulum of her death. I didn't know her, but she died in my room.

An old pipe came out of the wall over my bed. It held my weight. I made a noose out of my brother's red shirt. The bed slipped out from under my feet, and I landed in a ball on the floor between the bed and the wall, and started to sob. Alex, my roommate, found me. I pleaded with her, and she finally agreed not to tell anyone that night, but my appeal that she not say anything at all was impossible for her: "I could have discovered you hanging!"

Our appointments were at the same time in the morning. I blurted it out to him as soon as I sat, and I wept. All I clearly remember is that he picked up the phone when it rang and said, "Yes, thank you for calling, she has told me." I pleaded with him not to send me down. He agreed. The dam had burst. I was at no risk of doing this again; he was back. He had responded empathically. He wasn't annoyed with me. He wasn't angry.

An hour later, he came to the unit and reneged on his promise. I bunched up into the corner as far away from his words as I could get. He was sending me to Bellevue. I pleaded with him for 'a visit,' not a transfer. That, he said, was too short a time to assess. The consensus at the noon meeting was that the electric shock was wearing off! I pleaded for Thompson One. "No!" he was sharp, "I'm not sending you to that unit!" He said he would see me every day.

It was as bad on Thompson II as I'd always heard. It was Bellevue. Screaming, fecal smears, taunts. He did come, but I couldn't swallow the fear in my throat. I had gotten him back for an hour, and then he had put me there in the lowest circle of hell. I met Marsha here.

She has been trying to reach me for the last couple of days. I can't remember her ever being quite this insistent. I will call her tonight.

I am beginning to feel what I would've felt if the energy were not diffused into dissociation and redirected into the recruitment of the other. It wasn't "for attention;" Marsha used that unforgivable, vacuous concept about the noose when we talked late last night. She made a swift retraction, but she didn't understand this really. It was for mother, it was for skin, it was to make the nerves end, it was for the possibility of containment. It was for his hands. Dissociation was morphine. The recruitment was a hope. It was impossible to contain it. I needed walls. Human walls. I needed muscle and heartbeat. They all do, and they get skills training and Abilify and ceramic ashtrays. I needed the absolute presence of the other in my own muscle.

Bob put his hand on my sacrum, and my whole right hemisphere activated, filling up distinctly from the left. Then slowly it began, up my spine, and slowly I started to cry, and this time I talked, "It was sexual assault; my mouth, my throat, my jaws." I couldn't breathe, choking, coughing. Bones pulled apart in my sacrum. Black bats flew out from between my ribs. They lifted off my heart. I didn't stop crying. The release felt liquid. The sheer vibrating energy had liquefied me. If one could see the inner energy around me, it would've looked like melted wax.

Bob said something about what I do.

"I don't think I have a choice." He paused, thought and said, "I don't think you do either."

"Staying," Eva said. It is the title of Pema Chödrön's DVD. "Staying, it is the whole of the dharma."

I returned Sunday from Seattle. Marsha is tough. More so when she drinks, which she is doing more. There is little give and take. She is caught in data. But she is also trying to open the door for me, and she may. She introduces me as her best friend, and I dread that she will ask me to reciprocate that. I would say she's one of the people I most love, and that would be enough, and it would be true. I called her the morning I got home. She startled me. She said, "I am so in love with you."

UNRECOGNIZED, THE CHAIR

It's been over three weeks. As I wait for him, even as I turn my head toward our meeting, I feel demon voices pop up, embodied in me, say their furious, frenzied thoughts, invite others to join them, then a chorus that threatens to drown out love. They demand his recognition, his extreme health, his egolessness as the condition for love. And then what happens to me when I sweep them all off the table like a chess player frustrated with this game of war, what's left? An empty space, which I suppose is the space of potential. Self, as I know it, arrives only in these moments of fear and reactivity. And these seem to be about being forgotten, being obliterated in his mind, which, at least, at moments, his mind can do.

"Relationships are mysterious. You are particularly mysterious. I was born of the transference to you. I know or have slowly come to know the unelaborated essentials of your being." I know him, though only as the superordinate being who gave birth to me. My consciousness grew within him from a single-cell organism. It grew a brainstem, eyes and hands. All the limbs sprouted and developed, and now I stand, full-grown, apart, trying to see not only what happened and now what happens with him, but what all life was like that I apparently lived before I was born. And what do I, now in this stage of developing separateness, need to know of this ordinate and superordinate man named Arles Gabriel, the archangel. If I knew the nuanced dailiness of his consciousness, if I knew the context of his beliefs and his affections and his delusions, what would that provide me? No matter what more I know of the life he lives apart and outside of the penumbra of the life we live together, ultimately, I have nothing to say. He is a private person, and he does not welcome me into his sanctuary of self as I have let him into mine.

He said yesterday that my dreams of mental hospitals seem to arise when I feel I am not safe with him. That had not occurred to me. His willingness to see it and say it encourages me. Perhaps folded within this is his acknowledgment that he has contributed to my fragmenting. He has said, "I am so sorry that I made it unsafe for you. I know I did. I recognize this unreliable temperament, but stay with me because you can still reach me, and I can still reach you. There is still a great journey ahead for you and, in that, for us both." These would be the words that could ease my re-engagement as I stumble both toward and away from this outrageous angel.

"I have so completely thrown my lot in with yours, Arles".

"I know, Sebern." He was both understanding and sympathetic.

This is about knowing that my mind is truly enfolded in his, that he finds me beautiful as I slip away.

Blake is pregnant, and the baby will come before Christmas. I feel that rare feeling, joy. She will come.

Arles tolerates the body work. At times, when I talk about it yet again, he tries to understand it. "I thought that when I had run out all the secondary gain, when I had been understood and understood myself, when I'd been validated, when I knew, when I had been met and cared for, when I had been mothered and fathered, given cell walls and met with kindness, this would stop."

"Remember field effects," he said. "Whatever else they are, these are field effects."

Bob is long ago ready to be done, to have this one be the crowning catharsis. My psyche has been quiet for a long time. But the body is volcanic. The discharge erupts, and it is fully experienced; there is no decision involved. The body is off the table, the throat is burned.

"No, no, no!" I screamed. He asked me if this was a specific memory. I could only nod my head. He helped me sit up, but it wasn't stopping. He worked with my neck and head, and it quieted. By the time I got home, it was distant. It could be that these events, once held in dissociation, are now met with dissociation. It could also be that all memory is encoded in a specific location at a certain frequency, and that this is the nature of state dependence. I ate a cookie that night, and it felt like toxic shock. I tried to correct it with the Tibetan bell and then some F7 for terrible speech difficulties and P4 for balance, front to back, side to side in my brain. I woke up on Tuesday with my shoulder burning. I knew it was time. Low-hanging fruit.

Trauma creates a black hole, and too many treatments risk making this energy even more dense, more "attracting." All treatment should be toward dispersal. The episode with Bob is that, a breakup of energy, some of it released for good into the cosmos of suffering and light; some of it gathering back into and around itself, to form another weaker attractor site. I am mixing neurology and astrophysics, metaphor and synapse, but it is all in the realm of energy and information. We are all holograms, a micro-universe of strings and frequencies and their events. The valence of experience is set by early learning; there is Krakatoa, and there is an evening in early summer. There is matter and no mother. The universe is mind, and mind is the universe. But the whole brain never has access to its memory until we happen upon it at the right time, at the right place and at the right frequency. Neurofeedback may be searching this out or randomly discovering it, and now this site at these coordinates is quieted and always will be quieter. But a close neighbor isolated from the shocks by neurofeedback may well have discharging to do. I can't get all of this, but clearly trauma is both a local and a non-local phenomenon. Neurofeedback makes me less reactive; the event remains more localized in the brain and more manageable in the psyche. In a way, as best I can tell, it doesn't have to be managed at all. It is dispelled from the mind. It doesn't drive me. But I am afraid, or more accurately, my amygdala is clearly engaged during these episodes. My brainstem is activated. Bob was actually working on my neck. I don't have the cosmology yet or the rules, or even an accurate description of the chaotic nature of this. Metaphor is a trap as much as it is a map. I could, I imagine, diminish the power of the attractor sites, and when I do, this brain/body will slip into Class 4 space.

A round beaver-size muskrat posed for Allison at the end of a narrow log. Two herons erupted and flew over my head, almost close enough for me to touch one dangling foot. An Osprey glides up the river. Huge fish spray debris in their spawning rituals. The bright flash of a tanager, a cardinal and a yellow finch. The flooded life of the Mill River, rejoicing in the sun.

Neurofeedback is amazing. I forget that sometimes, not really in a state of humility but in a state of impossibility. How can it be that I wander about in a barely perceptible but nonetheless known state of agitation, finally recognize that I need to train T3-T4, do so for three minutes, and the fraught state, full of hidden meaning, is gone. Really, what is this? Kathy and I had dinner in an impossibly loud dining room made so by shrieking social work grad students delighted by their own company and impervious to the din they set up. I didn't see her, but Eleanor was one of these kids in the cacophony of celebration. We gave up after an hour of this with nothing to show for it but two mango lassis and got our meals as takeout.

"The symptoms," I said to her, "are never worse than the conditions that gave rise to them." She was shocked by the terrible implication that it was true. I had tears in my eyes; I was fine.

Sunrise spreads instantly over the desert, and the sacred rock Uluru awakens as I do. The desert floor is red, and now the rock is gold and red and filled with the shadows of its spirits. My encounter with Uluru reminds me most of my encounter with the elephant at the zoo, with her eye, with her sorrow and her beauty. There is a section which confirmed this, which looks just like the head of an elephant, as well as the head of a whale, the archivists of the Collective Soul.

Uluru is a place unto itself, beyond the country, beyond the continent. It feels more inhabited and perhaps of God even than the Godhead, the Grand Canyon. It is powerful, but its presence, like the people who live here, is not a presence that involves you. Whites are "ants," and we are kept at the surface of their beings; their spirituality and their myths are theirs alone. We are uninvited.

I write this looking out the window at the great presence in the great void. I watched the rock rise with the sun from an early dawn halo to golden red to rock. The rhythm of the day, the clock set more by Uluru than by the sun.

The conference is in Cairns, and I do my best to share what I am learning on PowerPoint slides.

I have returned to the geographical containment of New England and to my historical self. Peggy asked me where it had been when I was away, and it seems clear that it stayed in these hills, or in that attic, awaiting my reentry. Many people remarked on how refreshed I looked. One said, "10 years younger." It was a shedding. I fell asleep for a two-hour nap the afternoon I got home. This is unheard of. I slept until my session with Bob the next night.

I was naïve. I thought of him adjusting the quirks and kinks that travel leaves in any body. He said most of the pain was energetic and that the energy was diffuse and massive. He worked on my face, which led to pain in my left knee; work on my left knee led to emotional discharge and to the temporary pain of dislocation of my left toe. Very quickly, without intent or consciousness, I re-entered my trauma body, and here I am.

It feels as if I have lost the topography of my internal life. The mountains and the glaciers, deserts and oceans, the teeming wildlife that arise from and depend on the other. Arles is that other. And in a moment of homeopathic madness, he brought his god palm down and flattened it all.

He apologized again and again with sincerity and warmth, but as if for the event and not for himself. He was sorry that it happened. He did not say the words that I have perhaps been waiting to hear said, perhaps all my life, "I am sorry I did that." It becomes something that should not have happened, but more like a fragment of a comet breaking off and bursting through the walls of the office, killing off life as we knew it. The absence of him extends then even in the apology, and it goes on that no one has, and no one can take responsibility for what they inflicted on me. In this, I stay stunned, open-mouthed, bewildered. I dreamt of *trying to get somewhere on a treacherous, icy mountain road, and every time I went to grab the safety rail, it would collapse. It was an illusion. Patti and Howard, stand-ins for neurofeedback here, are talking me through this. After hours of slow, dangerous travel, they said I had only 1/3 left. I felt relief. I would be home and safe in only 1/3 of the time and terror I had already experienced. I was calm, calm even in the fear and knew I would make it there.*

Arles talked of the terrible episode as "burning off trauma." Clearly, my early demanding self was part of this, and it was fueled by crippling hip pain, a marriage coming apart his patient who committed suicide. I didn't want to presume. I called it "challenging."

"Challenging?! That's a WASP word for it! I would say it was a catastrophe!"

"I couldn't know, Arles. I expect I have no impact; that is my default position. All patients believe that they are the only patient."

I hadn't thought of my own life in those years as a catastrophe. During the same epoch I had four DID patients, all of whom threatened their own lives, one who threatened mine, the residence set on fire by one of my patients, the purge of me from my job, the death of my mother, my son turning from alcohol to psychosis and back to alcohol, threatening to bomb the mosque, threatening to torch his own home. AIDS. And Arles was pulling my psychic skin away as gently and as savagely as skin that's being burned. I was coming apart, down to the viscera. How would I be able to see his life as catastrophic? How would I see his life at all? He suffered deeply, though; he was depressed, and I am associated with it. On that day, he took revenge on his suffering, and there I was, innocent of it, bearing the fury and the humiliation.

He has lifted his palm. There is air and breath there. I have gone from no self ever being born to the particulate "non self" that the Buddha warns us of, at lightning speed because of him, because of neurofeedback, because of Sam, Bob, and Lee; their willingness to know what my body does. And even my own subcortical drive that is no longer a drive and is no longer about knowing. Knowing seems incidental, along the way. This has happened for the most part in the last 10 years. It is the span at least of a lifetime, perhaps of many. The writing in these journals is the only record of that warp speed change in consciousness. The account is not, as I had hoped, written in a beautiful script across the front of his mind.

I did find myself looking for him or at least suddenly attentive to someone of his general stature, hair or gait, particularly in Sydney.

He gathered me up at the end of our first session, "I think you need to be held." It was so. It is a memory of an old hunger.

"Non self," it seems, should require "no other," and perhaps on some plane this is true. I could live without that need; most people do. It's a common terrain, with wind and trees and weather that you dress for. But all my little miniature villages and train stations, hills and valleys, all the people of that earth are flat. It is not that they have never existed. It's not that they require suffering or pain to realize topographic dimensionality. They require—I don't know what else to say—a divine model maker, someone, Arles only, who is as interested in this topography as I am. Or perhaps it requires an entirely new orientation to all of this history, reality and metaphor that I just don't yet have.

He is going through something akin to what I am describing. It is for him, an empty self, like the state perhaps of non-self, I'd described before.

"It isn't a state, though, Arles; it is the default reality. In this no-self, I have no need of past or future, even of present, but I still want memory. I often just can't think of what to say. Nothing rises up as important, even very important and beautiful things, like Blake having a baby and Todd getting on the phone to say, 'I gave you your granddaughter.'"

I didn't want to be anywhere else. I was cold. I was wet. I was constipated. I was dirty. I was hungry. I was sick. I lived in a body. I did not suffer. The teaching of this trip is in the fusion of the wilderness, and the practice has no preference. Pure Is-ness. We were rafting the Sheenjek with our guides, Anne and Shannon.

This trip turned me inward. It was about endurance with tinges of reminders of survival. It was about the weather and a frail refuge. It was about the unadorned nature of life without distraction. Life of great beauty. Life of some hardship. Life of companionship. Living that was up to you to do. The first night, pushing into a crowded kitchen tent in the rain, I said, "What have I done?" It was met with laughter and acknowledgment, and by Shannon with dismay. It was for me the last moment of protest.

I was standing, arching my back over the pack, and Peggy was asking Shannon how long it would be until camp.

"Peggy," I said, interfering, "Have no preference."

"You wouldn't prefer to be there?" and I could honestly say no. This was the entire Buddhist truth of it: be here now. There is no other place to be. Who would forgo the opportunity of such a deep encounter with the disappearing wilderness, with the aging body, with the practice? In a certain way, it is easier to do this in the wilderness, particularly the wilderness that shrouds much of its extraordinary beauty in clouds, mist, hail and rain much of the time. My body required attention, my down sleeping bag required attention, my safety required attention, but no egregious self was ever required. There I was. There, no one.

Anne said, "Never meditate in the wind. You open yourself to too much." She and I stayed one night near the embers on the bank of the Sheenjek River. She had invoked noble silence, and everybody had gone to bed. It was probably late—who knows—and we talked about waves and frequencies. She told me about Irving Dardick, waves waving within waves, and I talked to her about what I saw when I appealed to waveforms in the brain or began moving them in the chair.

For a week or more after I returned here, my sleeping life to waking was in Alaska. I was either in the tent in the wind or at the hillside covered by seven rainbows. I wasn't really disoriented in these moments, just still oriented to Alaska. I fell out of bed one morning when I slept at its edge like I would on the ground on the Thermarest.

I am reading about setting up optimal cycling in the body, about heart rate variability and the coherence it creates in heart rhythm. Oscillations, chaotic and rhythmic, are the key. In this context, Arles questioned the wisdom of regularly evoking the waves of trauma. I have used two different paradigms: One of purging or release, and this new one, the development of optimal cycling. The first suggests going at it; the second suggests perturbation and rest. It may be analogous to under-training the relaxation phase of the heart—I may be pushing these waves, not allowing enough refractory time.

"You ride these waves incredibly," Arles said to me, not when I was drowning, really, but when I was still scared I could.

My feet pulled out of Bob's hands. It surprised me. When he was working on my throat, I pulled his hand away.

"Is this alright?" he asked.

"It depends on who you ask." I had to restrain my young body from biting him.

I felt like a wave. Bob "aged" the event, but not at age 4, which I had expected, because 4 is the tiny black hole that's threatening to absorb all other waves. Perhaps since it was such a large wave, it is difficult to discern all the others as distinct from it. A tsunami event that obscures all the lesser storms.

After my lunch with Blake, who is rounding out with Emily, that was after an important session with Arles, which had followed two hours of kayaking in the Oxbow, I talked to Patrick Harbinson. We talked about his episode on Law and Order: Special Victims Unit. He shared with me that he had paraphrased my thinking to friends, and they told him he was brilliant. I smiled at him on the phone. He is pleased with the episode and tells me some of the plot lines. He has permission from Ed Tronick, the attachment researcher and from the mother to use the Still Face video that shows how quickly a baby begins to fall apart when her mother's face becomes suddenly unresponsive. The Defense will use it to introduce what these abandoned kids endure and how it warps them. "Usually at this stage of production, I hate what I have written and want to kill myself. This one still needs work, but I think it does it." It airs on 11/21. We talked about whether he could write about neurofeedback for Law and Order, and how to dramatize it.

"What I see is often dramatic, but I don't see a way that it is easily dramatized. You may be ahead of your time in this, Patrick, and the Law and Order venue might not lend itself." He is evidently in debate with his boss, who is, he said, "a brain chemistry guy" and working to win him over. I love the idea that people on Law and Order are having the debate.

On my walk into town, a child was kneeling and screaming on the other side of Bridge Street. Her mother, furious, grabbed at her arm and tried to tug her. She made herself deadweight and screamed harder. Mother left her. She screamed even harder. Louder. The older self-possessed sister came to her and sat down next to her on the sidewalk. It seemed clear in her body that she, unlike her mother, knew not to insist, and before I was out of sight, the screaming stopped, and, at a distance, I watched the younger child follow her older sister to the van. It rumbles through me and lights up a neuronal pattern. I screamed like that. It was a visceral memory, though. I felt the interior of that screaming fleetingly. It is these moments of neuronal recognition, of pattern recognition, really, that are memory. These moments are all the memories that I will ever have of childhood. It is archived in my viscera and in some faded etching in my brain. There is no narrative and no film. My biography, I told Arles, would have a hole in every page where my mother's face should be. There is text around it, but you would pick up the book and see right through it to nothing.

As I waited for him in the late autumn light, I was thinking about memory and scanning to find a face and eyes. Memory is through the eyes of the other, and there are no eyes, not even his. There was an absence. I was motherless, again, but I can hardly recognize it because I feel no mother hunger. I have the nervous system of a well-mothered person, but my mother feels genetically immaterial; she is so not there. Arles has, like the boulder in the dream, filled in the chain of my DNA. He asked me what that felt like.

"You are not absorbed like a stitch," his metaphor to account for his absence in front of me. "It is much more elemental than that. It is as if you gave me stem cells back then in the dark room, in the night. I needed high-contact therapy, or I would not remember. You would disappear by the time I got to the bottom of the staircase, or as it often was, the fire escape."

I read a piece in the paper about a memorial bench for 800 people, most of them unknown, buried at the state hospital. It had rotted away. Someone thought to restore it with mahogany. I am horrified at the story. They were left there to die unclaimed. It made me think how really close I came to slipping through that crack and never returning. My mother would not have abandoned me entirely. I don't think she would have let me become nameless at Rockland State Hospital. But if Arles hadn't squared my shoulders a little each time, I might have slipped sideways into madness. It was a body orientation. He kept me physically present. As we talked about all this, we also talked about the millions of motherless children in the world and how my story aligns with their desperate stories.

"Mine is one of such privileges."

"You are privileged to be here, and I am privileged to be here." His inclusion in privilege surprised me, but we do share immense privilege: the privilege of our circumstances, the privilege of that room, the privilege of being born human. "It is," he said, "privilege that makes this book possible. And it is more important than ever that you write it."

When he doesn't ask about memory, the need for memory is eclipsed. Without his interest, without his eyes, my history is just a distraction. I have no ego to carry this; I have no need to write it; I have no capacity to remember it if I don't write it down. I showed him the pink striped nightgown I'd bought for Emily, and I wondered if I would remember this time. He said I would. I will know this baby in a way that I have never known a baby before, not even my own.

"Somewhere in this process, Arles, you became my therapist. At first, I could hardly see the sky around the edges of you. You were the stars. You didn't have a face or a reality, but you took up the entire room." He nodded. I had lost the harbor and the sanctity of him and me. I have it tonight. He bent down slightly as we parted, put his hand on my shoulder, and softly, like a whisper, kissed my forehead.

I woke up crying. *We were trying to escape the Nazis, and I couldn't get my family organized. My mother was wearing a coral pink suit with the tags still attached. There was a lake, and it was dark. I woke up as I drowned my mother or let her drown to escape. Sophie's choice. We all have to make it.*

Wednesday night, Bob held my hand and arm up next to him, and I started to cry. I'd been privately pleased with my lack of reactivity in our recent sessions. I tried to sit up, to be responsible for all the work, to my maturity, to my idea that I was done with this, but I had to call for him, "I am not coming out of this." I lay back down, apologizing, "This wasn't the plan." I was trapped, returning to a time that isn't a time, to a place that is only vaguely a place. He follows some wire from my thumb into an electrical storm, circuits popping, they don't find each other, it is not memory. It is fragmented like millions of live wires throwing themselves wildly around in the air, thrown by the power of the current, the memory in the thumb, in the hand, in the arm held just that way. I am caught there. Every once in a while, the space itself suggests a narrative or a face forms. It feels random. My memory of being held over the railing came the first time as an image or a flash of an image with neurofeedback. Many years later, it formed again with Arles, and I knew then that I had been hanging there for a lifetime, like the book Bob gave me, a book of optical illusions, where I try to find the pattern within the design that I can never fucking see. This is very much what it's like for me. If those designs were electrified dancing noise, that is how it is.

I woke up several times that night and each time found myself checking into my state—I wonder if I always do that without recognizing it—and noticed that something had changed, the lead sinker in my right heart had dropped away. It had been there, this tiny persistent depression, for weeks, hooked with a barb into the tissue, and it was gone.

I had come from Sam. There was no structural problem. Everything was inflamed, the brachial plexus, the solar plexus and the sacral plexus. He couldn't disperse the energy at the sacrum; he said he could be there all day because it wasn't the sacrum. He helped me turn over and rocked my brainstem gently in his hands. I had flooded it. Sam's touch opened me to the energy flowing between the finger of Moses and the finger of God. My soul was there. Arles reminds me of how profound these states are and how fragile we are in the experience of them to protect the vulnerability of the soul.

"Remember titration," he said as I left. Sam had said, "Stillness and gentle rocking. No chair!"

I dreamt several weeks ago of *going to Arles' office in a tall building. There was a glass door partially open, and he was sitting with an older man clearly bereft. Arles told me that he'd lost his dog and that we must help him find it. He lost his Newfoundland. Arles asked me to put my nose up to the nose of the dog. I felt the warm wetness of the nose so that I could find him. The lost Newfoundland was right under my nose.*

Chapter 16

May was removed again, not quite as far away, but away. She had wool to roll. On the third blue skein, she ran into tangles. She told me about some rough times.

"The spirits are asking me for the formula. I come close, but every formula fails. It makes me feel 'the pressure of will.'" I could feel the tension of her failure. The inevitable and imminent implosion of America into collective madness seized her, and she screamed in terror and unbearable grief.

"I am not good at this, this knowing." She pulled a strand into a knot as she tried to gather herself into a thought.

"I agree with you. You need to be surrounded by a community of wise women to help you through this, to learn the ropes."

"Yes, that is exactly what I need!" She kept focused on the blue yarn.

"But what you have is me, and our endeavor here is to stabilize your brain so that it, you, can manage this knowing. I don't want you to end up in an institution."

"Native peoples watch their children to see which side they would end up on, psychosis or shamanism."

"That is exactly it," I said, "and it is our covenant to keep you on the shaman side of that perilous divide."

"It is happening," she reflected to someone I didn't see, "I am in my therapist's office, and she doesn't think I'm crazy, she doesn't want to give me a diagnosis, she doesn't want me to end up in an institution!"

After this very difficult week and growing frustration with the wool, all she wanted to do was take a bath.

I went out into the sunshine and talked with her father, while she bathed in the claw-foot tub in the bathroom off the waiting room of my office. He told me that she'd felt poisoned and was moaning in the car on their long drive here.

When she finished her bath and got dressed, I took her by the hand into the office. The latest wave of intrusions of spirits seems to have been provoked by the massacre at Virginia Tech. She is flooded, and the spirits continue to arrive.

"They take advantage of you, May. They chose the wrong vessel. They ask too much of you." She smiled her odd smile, both looking at me and retreating from me. That may be the spirits' response to my naïveté. I don't know yet. Even when she tries to explain it, it can't be put into words.

She lay on the couch.

"I have experienced evil, Sebern," and I knew she had. When her formula failed once again, she felt as if her stomach was being eaten. She was thrown by the tangle of blue wool; unspooled. I talked with her at all levels about this, but to her, it was a terrible sign or a manifestation right there of chaos. I could not downsize it. When the tangle tangled more, she threw herself back on the couch and heaved in pain. I continued to work on the yarn, and it soothed her. But then something I said shifted her into gales of laughter that echoed in a sudden valley between us, angry and far away.

I slowly set the yarn down, as one who did not want to startle the small bird would.

"I think it is time to train," she took my hand, went to the chair, allowed the sensors at C4 and on her ears, and we trained. I took the large tangle away, put it in another room and closed the door. As she quieted with the training, I quietly challenged the "wisdom" she gave the spirits.

"I am not sure they are 'free.'" She seemed to accept that. I pushed a little further into her territory. "I am far from sure that they are 'wise.'"

"I am awed sometimes by what you understand, but there are also times I don't know what you're saying." From what I could tell, her understanding had failed when I challenged the wisdom of the spirits. During the time she was training, she was able to listen and understand.

"They are asking much too much of a novice, May. It is vital for you to learn how to let these energies flow through you. Don't stop them. Don't get caught in them or let them get caught in you." This is what she listened to. The room got quiet.

"Thank you," she said softly before pulling the office door open and returning to her father's waiting car.

I wanted to clear the tangle so I could let May know that order had been restored. She has a vision, a quite vivid one, that a new order will arise from the chaos, but that the chaos will be terrible. She told me that she knew she couldn't do anything about it, and then that she was worried that with the training she wouldn't be feeling it (!).

"I wanted to be a part of it, not just quiet on the sidelines," she'd been very unquiet and very much the harbinger just minutes before.

Sky arrived for her session, and I asked her if she would help me. We spent our time together working out the blue tangles as we talked. As we neared the end, I told her to be especially mindful because tangles only knew themselves as tangles. They would work hard to maintain this identity, just as they were at the edge of unraveling and taking a new, coherent shape. She and I worked within these mysterious parameters, and it may well have been one of our most profound sessions.

"You are psychic," she said. "This was exactly what I needed to do. For me!" We finished in the backyard, quietly, in the sun. She put the ball of yarn in my hand. I covered her hand with mine and smiled at her.

"I had a miscarriage Friday night."

"Oh, really. Oh. Did you want to be pregnant?"

"No, I didn't."

"Are you OK?"

"Yes, I am, particularly now."

I went in to my next patient. She talked to me about her brain changing and her fear that she could lose her fear. "Then who will I be?" Her voice quavered.

The time shift, the return to the attractor site, came after the chair. I wonder if histories like this contribute to brainstem strokes. Bob stayed with me. He got me water when I asked and Kleenex because I could hardly breathe. When it was over, he cradled my brainstem.

"Your feet aren't under you. They look like they are, but they're not," and I felt it. He brought my energetic body back into my standing body like stacking up blocks until my feet were actually under me, actually on the ground. He asked me what had happened.

"You saw it all. You saw what I saw. You saw everything. That's what it was," and when I got home, there was the long knife and the small piece of pink human tissue in the sink. It was some part of me nicked off. I wanted to faint.

May brought her spirits, the good ones and the bad.

"It is a long story. These are Black souls, slaves." She stopped when I said what was true: "I knew this." At times when I was trying to counsel her to close the door, she would smile and even laugh, and I'd ask her if they thought I was naïve. She said yes, and I had to agree.

Arles listened, empathetic to me and to May. Density, gravity, altered space and slippery time.

"You have an attraction to tortured souls. Don't invite them to stay." Then he changed the word to "love."

"Are you talking about Moses?"

"Once you accept that you love him, there will be nothing to cure."

I was astounded.

I felt awed.

My head was locked. I couldn't turn it to either side. There was no substance to the past. There was a long trail, but it was empty. I had no image of any continuity of myself going forward. After a long silence in which I tried to pull all of the particles back into a functional unit, he asked what had happened.

"It was like Chartres." This was the best image I had. "This explosion into emptiness happened within 'you and me.' The rose window is your pure heart with light pouring through it." What he'd said was true, and it took hold of my head, and it was over. All of the concerns I'd discussed had dissolved. "I am at peace. My back is just my back. It is a different universe." As I was leaving, I looked around to see if I was missing anything.

"Everything is in order."

"Yes, he said, "Everything is in order."

I feel I am in another world—in between—as if I've just been freed from a dark cell and the light hurts my eyes. I don't know what to make of it. I was not thinking then that it could be related to the movement in the Symmetron, the deep challenge to my brainstem. I am state-bound and stateless. I sleep as if it is no longer sleep. I've been left with tinnitus so severe that it can be hard to hear my patients. I trained, adding in 01-02, and that helped significantly. My brain feels tilted on its axis, and the trauma seems gone.

I have been in therapy most of my life. It is time to stop being a patient. Arles and I will always know each other. There is no one more able to travel here. We are done for now.

This, of course, could not be an easy conversation.

"What is 'a patient?'" he asked. I want to exit that context. I will live in the house we have built and cared for, but the door will also quietly be closed. There are some neuronal kicks when I write this, some demonic protest, and it exhausts me. I stumbled trying to describe this.

"I don't want to wait in the waiting room. I don't want to schedule time. If we met in a private garden under an umbrella, I would like that or if you rearrange the furniture or if we could draw a magnet over your head and erase your memory of me. I don't want to end our conversations; I want to radically alter the context for them."

"You are not the same person who came to consult me. You have changed dramatically. I have also changed." He paused. "Perhaps what you need to hear is that I know you over time."

I thought about this, but I don't believe I can escape the darkness that settles around me in his mind. I am not afraid of losing him. I know I will. It might just be enough to know that he registers the dramatic change.

I described my state to him as anhedonic. It is a pure state, related to training or brain rhythms alone, an accidental depression or worries about MS. I do have problems dropping things and at times with balance. It could be neurofeedback, or the chair, either or both, and it could be about him and me and my deep press for separation.

"I will help you if this is what you need to do, but I don't want you to leave."

"It feels developmental, Arles, it has that kind of integrity. I need to be new. New to myself and new to you. And you have to be new to me as well."

My relationship with Arles made meaning happen. It arose with him. He told me that the trauma memory that arises in bodywork doesn't resonate for him. I shook my head slowly, no.

"I understand. It is extra-mind. It does not generate from within my mind. If you saw it, though, it would break your heart."

I was crying as I left. “This is important, but it isn’t easy,” he responded with quiet reassurance, and then the door got away from him, and it slammed.

“I honor what you think you must do. But I don’t endorse this. I think you have chosen a relationship with these internal states, with the process of excavation over exploring relationships in your present life.” He stopped briefly. “You seem to be in a process of cellular purification.”

“Is that wrong?”

“Well, no, not wrong... just exclusive.”

“My relationships are not the concerns I would bring you. I’ve brought you epochs of being, of my interior that I can’t talk to anyone else about. What other mind could meet this mind?”

He leaned back in his worn leather chair, and it squealed softly.

“Yes. I understand.”

I have accomplished what I came for and more. It can’t even be spoken about in these terms, but they are the only ones that allow an ending to it. But it isn’t even that. He’s not been engaging with the narratives I bring him from my body. My work with him and neurofeedback has quieted my mind. My body holds the fragments of sharp metallic memory.

“Once you released me from Moses, I knew I would end, and I don’t want it to go badly. I want to end on pride and love.” I was crying, “I don’t want to disappoint you.”

“You aren’t disappointing me at all.” We softened together, “I want you to know you can always call me.” That will be harder if we botch this, and it may be that it will be my consciousness, his gift to me, that guides us. He will do the best he can, and so will I.

Emily is nine months old, and mostly she laughs. I miss her immediately after leaving her. She plays peek-a-boo with Todd and goes into gales of laughter each time. The joy sucked out of the universe by my childhood is replaced by her, in her. And Blake. What a gifted, attuned mother. When they are in sync, which is most often, I feel a kind of awe at what's possible not only between a mother and her baby and a baby and her mother, but what is possible between two emerging human beings. And Todd, too, has his own beauty with his baby, the Bears.

I love this child as I have loved no one else.

Bessel

I gave my workshop with Vicky Kelly at Attach. I noticed that van der Kolk's trauma stories were seeping in; they weren't glancing off. I was stung by a bee in mid-September, and my finger is still swollen and sore. It healed after the first bee and swelled again when I saw a second one had landed in the same place. I wasn't stung again. "Sequestered venom," the doctor said.

Johnny is here. He is doing better. He talks too much, but he stays open to challenge and maintains a light mesh around his own terrible history. When we are together, it is as if our fields fuse and intensify. He sprayed cologne on, for fun, at Macy's, and I got sick from the chemicals in the closed-in car. It's that. He has no awareness of this; he is so genuinely sorry about it and so genuinely unaware of how he engulfs me with all the horror and terror he cannot acknowledge. He would never want to inflict this on me, even when he does.

Vicky arranged for me to have lunch with Bessel to talk with him about neurofeedback. He took advantage of a pause I took to drink some iced tea, "You need to put the machine on your head!" I had been nervous. I smiled at him.

"You understand you are important in this. People will listen to you."

He invited me to come to the Trauma Center to give a lunchtime training in January.

I have been investigating the chair this past week. I think this challenged my immune system; its motion finds and exploits the gap. I'd been pretty well during the day, and my symptoms all returned after turning in the chair. I am lunging. I massaged my finger. I can feel little sacs of venom around the knuckle and get sick after that. We are left to infer so much about our bodies, almost as if we weren't living in them.

I will speak in Salzburg and then in Prague. Austria, Eva reminded me, is the most anti-Semitic country on the planet.

"Isn't it the task of this life to clear all this?" he asked me.

"It is. These energies have distilled in me. They have crossed the blood-brain barrier."

"I am sitting holding a bowl in a parallel universe. I am alone." The pronouns give me trouble.

"'I' and 'me' are necessary words," Arles said, "a designation of place or moment, not of Self. This image has nothing to do with 'Sebern'."

"There is a veil between me and all the rest. The field or overlapping fields that I finally get to participate in are passing by in another slip-stream of time. There is all the talk, all the brilliance, intentionality, purpose, and the talk is Babel. Spirit talk, therapy talk and all other talk. It is all tongues."

"What is the bowl?" he asked me. I have a sense of it in my hands and mistake, initially, substance for weight.

"It has weight," I just want to find a way to pierce or move through the veil into the world as it knows itself, and have the gift received. "Babel" and "tongues" are not derisive. They are all attempts "to speak of," "to get to." There is great meaning in all the words, but they are words. "I am sitting with the bowl, and no one wants it. No one will take it."

"That's right," he said, "everyone has to find it for themselves."

Oh, but the agony of the giver, the grief for the world, the needless suffering.

"But time, Arles".

"Don't," I think he said, "consider time. This is beyond time." He paused and asked again, "What is the bowl?"

I looked at it, felt for it. I knew first what it was not. It was neither glass nor ceramic. "It is love, Arles. It is divine. It is a ball of light." He nodded, and our silence filled the darkening room.

"You received the bowl through me, through a transmission. Not through neurofeedback." He said this quietly, smiling. I thought of the risk he took and that he was right. He was the mother, my mother, the domestication of God. It was a transmission through him, not through Thầy or even through Charlie. Most intentionally, personally and persistently through him. It isn't about neurofeedback—I hate the word neurofeedback—but it is absolutely about neurofeedback. Brain training made the transmission possible.

"The bowl is a vessel. A bowl of neurons and dendrites, a bowl overflowing, a bowl of light; a bowl of love." We both paused at the still point. "Neurofeedback makes it possible for humans to move beyond the limits of being human, beyond their unique suffering."

Arles is, of course, one of those who will not receive the gift. He will acknowledge it ambivalently, but he needs his own path. Everyone does. And this is not a path. I think of Julie's dream after her first neurofeedback session. She heard only a voice that said to her, "The path to the enigma is now clear." He sees it as no different from meditation or prayer, or perhaps less than those.

"What happens when the neurons stop firing?"

"The light joins the Numina."

My practice is my work with my brain. This work is the gift I have to give. I am sitting alone with this beautiful bowl in the quiet of my parallel place.

Chapter 17

The day begins with song and candlelight and will end that way as well. I have come to write more about this bowl. I have no interest in altered states, astral projection or past lives or future ones. I am far from a peak performer. If I search, perhaps I can find a goal—oh, of course—, to discover what it feels like to live without fear, every hour, every minute, every second. It is a miracle. Neurofeedback is not really a practice; it allows a practice. I do it; it allows me.

I didn't remember quite how much I love being here. I most like rising early, walking up the hill, the candles and the song and then a silent breakfast, all such sweetness. But nothing is better than climbing back into bed, still dark at 6:20 and beginning another deep practice working with levels of engagement and surrender; levels of consciousness, trance and sleep. This is the only place I seem to do this. It is a portal practice.

Brother Columba commented on my smile. "If we can't cry, we need smiles like that," he said. No one has ever commented on my smile.

I accept the gift given me, this chalice of neurons. I am neither afraid nor alone, although absolutely completely and uncomprehendingly alone. More alone than Galileo.

"Where are you, Sebern?"

"Way back there," the focal point was Moses, but Moses was just another door.

"Where are the Nazis?" Arles asked softly.

"Where are the Nazis?" I echoed his question. "It is the field, the sound of the footfalls, the cold room. You weren't here. It still sets up that way, an inevitable force field, innocent of itself. It isn't personal or persecutory. Everything that used to explode into a diffusion so terrible it exposed my nerve endings now settles into a point of stillness, at the very least of Isness."

I arrived at the beginning of this therapy without edges, without endings, no skin, no possibility of containment. He put his hands around that when I couldn't understand his words, and slowly, he gave me an outline, then, more slowly still, mass. They are opportunistic, beastly energies. Arles calls them out as they take form in my mind. Bob finds them in their hideouts in my body, and I think, really, there is nothing else to do but to seek them out.

I hadn't heard back from Bessel and talked to Vicky about protocol. She advised me to use the old fashion way, the phone. When I reached out to him to confirm the date, he made a reference to me as "the expert."

"You know what Mark Twain said about experts, right?"

"No, tell me."

"An expert is a fool a long way from home."

"Well, I have just come back from Perth, Australia. What does that make me?"

He greeted us warmly in the waiting room of the Trauma Center in Brookline. He said there would be 12 to 15 people there, his key staff. As we set up, the room filled up. There had been a notice on the website, and 40 people or so were there and open.

Bessel's introduction was gracious, "I am very much looking forward to this presentation, and it is way overdue." I showed the video of Ken, a young boy who was about to be sent to juvenile detention for repeated assaults, before neurofeedback and then after. A reporter asks his mother, "Do you have your little boy back?" and she says, "Well, look, I never had my little boy to begin with, but now I have my little boy." I gave them an outline of the theory and talked about fear as the core issue.

At lunch later, Bessel disagrees with this, or thinks he does.

"I have just spent time with my friend Sandy McFarlane, and he says it's about 'attentional systems in the brain.'" This is the common lore in neurofeedback circles.

"No, Bessel, it's even more importantly about affect regulation. Just like you have always said, 'the keys to the kingdom.'"

We came home to await Iowa returns. Obama wins. He is my candidate. A good and hopefully propitious day.

John and I took Bessel to the Eastside Grill. It was the second step in his introduction to neurofeedback. We spoke about 'rhythmical attunement,' I think, because that was what we were feeling. His arousal is high, which he doesn't altogether see, and that presents its challenges. But he is genuine, forthright, opinionated with the right opinions, and he gets it; he gets neurofeedback. He trained at the very top of the range that he will ultimately use and did some deep state training.

"How are you?" he asked sweetly as he opened his eyes.

"I'm good. You?"

"I am blissed out."

We talked politics, therapy and neurofeedback. He blocked my story. My need to tell it arises only to illustrate the profound nature of neurofeedback. I did show him my baby pictures. He put his hand on his heart.

"Oh my God, these are heartbreaking. They are hard to look at."

We were sitting at the kitchen table. I stood up and put my arms over his shoulders with my hand on his chest, spontaneously without thought.

"I'm glad they break your heart. It's right." He and I will work together. Arles was right. It's uncanny how often he is.

Bessel interviewed Sabelle. He was very impressed with her. She was nervous, but he helped her, and she spoke beautifully about how she had gone from walking from Amherst to Hadley because she didn't know how to take a bus to two years later flying to Japan on her own to join a peace walk. Her Japanese was impressive, and he commented on it.

"Do you think you could be where you are today without neurofeedback?"

"No," she answered, with the clarity of a glass bell. "If I were alive at all, it would be at the margins."

"You are extremely coherent, Sabelle."

After she left, he said, "That's not PTSD, right?" and I must have looked puzzled and likely, vigilant. "PTSD is the car accident. This is much earlier and more...," he searched for the word. "It affects everything, every function. We're proposing a new diagnosis to the DSM 5 committee, 'Developmental Trauma.'" I had never thought of it like this. This was right.

We were held back from our return by windstorms that closed Shipold airport, and ended up spending the night at a hotel outside Charles de Gaulle that could easily serve as a detention center. We ate with stranded strangers from all over the world at an all-you-can-eat buffet, of which all I could eat was radishes, couscous, fruit and chocolate mousse. I reflected on the disorientation I had dealt with when I was abroad because it was no longer there. It was travel; it was cultural adjustment and the vagaries of new languages, but it was not dissociation or ringing in my ears. It was another day lived in the world, probably pretty close to the way most people breathe in the morning air and set about planning their days. In Prague, walking on my own around Old Town Square, I saw an advert and climbed to the third floor of a Thai massage parlor. The mats were on the worn wooden floor with only tall canvas curtains separating each area in this ancient building in Stare Mesto. My feet were massaged by a Buddha. I am not one who would do that. I left Arles's cashmere scarf in the basement restaurant that had at one time been the lowest floor of a Masonic temple. I called the restaurant to try to retrieve it—I noticed, without anxiety—but that clearly was not going to happen. It is now on the neck of some young man as winter turns again in Prague. It was meant, I think, to be handed off there. Arles thought so, too.

I didn't feel overwhelmed by the energies of Prague, but I felt its density and its suffering. Juri, a neurofeedback practitioner I met there, was the embodiment. He smoked one blunt cigarette after another, he talked fast, he vibrated with his history. There is a memorial for the victims of communism in a small park in the Mala Strana. It begins at the first stair, a man whole but numb, arms out in front of him, almost beseeching. Each step up there is less of this figure until, at the end, there is merely a fragment. It is a memorial, Juri said, to every Czech who was killed or imprisoned or tortured and every Czech whose life was destroyed by communism. Juri counted himself. We talked about neurofeedback.

"It didn't work for me," he told me, pulling in hard on his cigarette.

"What did you train?" I asked him.

"Sterman told me to train SMR at C4. I did that for probably more than a hundred sessions. It didn't help."

"Oh, Juri, it might have made things worse for you! That reward is much too high for you." With some trepidation, but at his urging, I trained him at FPO2 at 3-6 Hz, about where I train myself. His staff looked on as he seemed to melt into the chair. They said they had never seen him look like this. He was quiet. The room was quiet. Juri sighed and slowly smiled.

I found my way to the Jewish cemetery. In Prague, it is still the Jews, the Germans and the Czechs. This cemetery is the ghetto, and depending on where I stood, I felt an enormous peace or an unending turmoil. There is no order. The headstones are tumbling into each other, in some cases huddled and miserable, in others just company in the crowded streets. I sat in the Franz Kafka Café, which seemed covered in historical dust and an inherited despair. I was sure the W/C was the same one Franz and Mr. K used. Most of the city streets spill over with high fashion and luxury goods, but I could buy fruit in the open market, which stood somewhere in the maze I navigated, trying, once again, to find Karlov Bridge. Prague wasn't all silver and gold, amber and gems, Juri's new oppression. There are fresh oranges.

A young man in Vienna hawking tickets in a Mozart costume mentioned my Obama pin.

I asked him if he'd like it.

"Really?" He pinned it to his Mozart lapel. During the performance that night, I thought, "I was never meant to die; I was meant for this work, the work that brought me to Europe." It felt like a revelation. In Prague or Vienna, I dreamt that *I was receiving refugees, and what they most wanted was to bathe and then to eat. I was working at a resettlement camp.*

CRASH

8:30 in the morning on March 28, Charlie hit a patch of black ice, lost control of his car, spun into another car and was killed instantly. The 80-year-old man in the other car was released from the hospital that morning. Unlike Charlie, he was wearing a seatbelt. I don't think the woman who called me said her name. She said she was calling for the Boren family. I'd just gotten off a wonderful unfolding conversation with Bessel. I didn't track at first, didn't quite hear the name.

Eva read the article to me from the Union Leader: 73-year-old man... Tied up traffic for two hours on Route 10. There hasn't yet been an obituary. I called the Institute that doesn't, in a way, exist anymore either. Voicemail.

I canceled my morning patients. Shock closes a pathway. It narrows the capacity for intake. I felt it in my brain. I felt the impact of the crash on the left frontal medial and not the moment of it, but repetitive, continuous impact. From left of center all to the right, I felt spacious, the Isness of my grief; the Isness of his death. And I feel so angry that his death was a careless one. He has become part of what he called my "crucible of loss." I called Arles and got his machine. I called Eva and got her machine. I called Blake, and she held me compassionately. I called Marsha and left messages. She called me back. She hadn't heard; she was calling to make plans. She wanted to help. She is practical, and with the details attended to and the advice received, she again compared our relationships with our therapists at the Institute, then disqualified them both. She lost track of the reality of the moment but regained it. It comforts me when she affirms that he is in the Bardo. She does her best, as she always does, but she hovers above connection like a hummingbird, distracted repeatedly in mid-sentence by some other thought that vibrates in her, pauses, but never comes to me.

Arles called. He took time for me. I felt that. I felt the velvet softness of his voice, but we derailed talking about my decision not to go to the funeral. He said something about the Oedipal drama, and we were not only not in the same conversation but not in the same reality, or the same century. He is sitting still in that slightly dingy café next to Berggasse 19. Charlie and I lived out a profound developmental story. He'd begun his work with me two days after his brother's funeral. His brother had died in a car crash. It ended on black ice. As we were finishing, Arles told me that he'd been to the bank and had said to himself, "Remember to put on your seatbelt." 10 minutes later, he got my call.

I felt punched in the heart. I am still feeling that blow, diffusing into a bruise. John's shock and grief were immediate. He came over, and in a way that felt almost entirely new, he held me. "This is huge," he said, and I fell into his arms and wept. I had been waiting for him to be able to cry. I, who have always been a solitary crier.

Bessel brought me orange tulips. And Peggy, so warm and patient, helped me open to new levels of this incomprehensible death, to any momentary anger at his carelessness.

I would've said that there was no netting in my brain to catch the fact of his death. I would hold little pieces of the reality, but the weight of it didn't settle. It fell through into space. I found his assistant, Ruth, on Monday.

"Sebern... Of course, I remember you. You are the person I have been searching for. The obituary is being written. It will come out by the end of the week."

My appointment with Arles ended with me crying.

"I am disappearing, you are the witness in the archive. I am disappearing in increments."

I lay on this bed deconstructing myself, gently disassembling everything that was/is important to me, all of the colorful building blocks of me are put tenderly aside in the playroom. As Emily constructs a self, I take one apart. I needed nothing that I thought I needed; and, more scary, no one either. I wasn't alone; I wasn't at all.

I can't quite get it that he is, in fact, dead. I don't know where he is in my psyche. There are moments that I look for him, to him, and the reminder is abrupt. "He isn't alive." My backstop is gone, and I am without forbearers. Charlie was proud of me. He watched me grow up. He was part of it.

John waited for me, sitting on the stairs up to the bedroom, while I finished with my patient. I opened the door to the kitchen, and he came to me, stricken. I knew immediately. I held him. I am OK. He is OK. "Is Johnny OK?"

Last night I finally wept, and it dispersed the weight collecting behind my heart. Nothing seemed to move except Sam's hands. I wished for grief to flow, but I felt thick, slow, numb. My heart is the gray of a ten-day-old kitten. Waking that morning, I couldn't raise my head off the pillow. We have just returned from Miami and all its hot sunny vacancy, the desultory scene of yachts and pink pants, the segregated eating of the Old Republicans. Sean's sweet vacancy, too; his life is manageable there, small enough. He says he is adjusting. He tells us his philosophy of life: a path with many bridges that you either cross or jump off, and he crosses them.

We are back in the welcome rain and cool, 2 AM, home with his ashes, which somewhere along the way have been named cremains. The Bain Range funeral home, across the street from the domino park, is as full on Tuesday as it had been on Sunday. Maurice Dixon, a large, sweet-faced Black man, gentle and practiced with it all but real. Another bigger Black man entered; credit cards apparently were not often used. We thought that as he came toward us, he was there to give a blessing, which he did, but he was there to learn how to use the credit machine. I expected a small room, private like my mother's viewing had been. But Johnny's body lay in front of row upon row of wooden folding chairs in a large, brightly lit room. It was not him, less him even than a wax statue. My knees buckled momentarily. John and Mr. Dixon held me up.

"Would you," I had yelled at him, implored him, after yet another dangerous binge of alcohol, "have me bury you too? Would you ask that of me?" I was angry then. He died probably as much from psychiatry as from his mother. Bob asked if he had done what he came here to do. When I told John, he too said yes. It will be easier for him in the next life. But yesterday morning I lay in the weight of impossible exhaustion as dumb as the mallet that kept whacking my head until I realized it was the day Hugh had been buried, it was Charlie's birthday and there on the bureau were Johnny's ashes. It was the day they killed Robert Kennedy and the day Barack Obama won the nomination. I meditated for Obama. I prayed that the angels flock around him.

I couldn't stand upright against the pull of gravity. Sam worked to release the grief. Nothing moved in me. At some moment, it came, "It is your fault," the oscillation my mother left in me. I saw John's body, the thinning hair and the pancake makeup, the hard set of his mouth and chin, the body he left behind, the body he feared would decay around him, the body he fled over and over, now a husking in this place at the edge of the ghetto, in the center of its own deep sadness, and I couldn't stay there, even long enough for the decency of it. I needed to go to the ocean. I needed the clear, cool brace of it. We went to Bill Boggs Park in Key Biscayne. It was Sunday, body-to-body Cuban music, picnics, all as it should be, fitting for a hot day off in early June. We sat on the seawall with the quiet fisherman who caught nothing, and looked out into the bay. My feet could not reach the water, and the rocks were razor sharp. After we picked up the urn, we went again, this time to Crandon Park. The water was as hot as the air. We ate our Fresh Market sandwiches that tasted like a vending machine at the splintering picnic table under the slight shade of the palm in the sweet, slight breeze off the sea.

Sean asked if I thought what had happened to Johnny as a baby was part of all this. My mother had asked such a question in the abstract about the kids I treated, "Dear God...!?"

John was caught where he died in the shuttered, almost drab place he had recently remodeled. Sean had been willing to live in the surroundings of John's former psyche, with urine-stained carpets, far too many cats making more strays because no one really had enough energy to get them to the vet. It was Johnny who designed and painted and pulled up the old carpet, who laid simple, clean tile, who bought, just last week, the bedspread to match the bedroom walls he'd just painted. He'd made these renovations within himself, too. We watched the changes take hold as he trained his brain. He tried to seal over his loneliness there with daytime TV, but it bore a hole into him. He died on that couch in front of the TV. When we went to the house to see Sean, the TV was on, and he kept it on until I asked him not to. In this sense, Johnny's death was seamless, from bottles of medicine, to doctors, to vodka, to TV, to early death. But he was ascending from his old age; he had glimpses of a possible life. He was, as Blake said, broken down in my arms, "just coming to us."

Sean had taken refuge at his sad little club during the worst of it. He tells us that John had begun to drink again. There were bottles of Antabuse unopened. This is crushing news at first, needless to know, but to the point. Few people recover from the brutality of child abuse. He did his best. Child abuse should always be listed as a cause of death.

The afternoon we first heard, Blake and Todd sat with us in the small kitchen at Elizabeth St. Emily was vigilant. Todd was a sheltering presence.

"We can grieve anywhere," I said. "Let's not stay here." We went to Look Park, where Emily practiced walking on yet another surface, loving the mastery, loving her body and all it can do and how deeply it is loved.

Blake and Molly will bury their brother tomorrow, and Sean, his partner, a man I don't think he knows. People have to ask me about how he is doing. They may mistake my not including him as homophobic, but it isn't. I forgot him. I wish I didn't, but I do.

Johnny captured me in his terrible innocent net, and some part of me fought it like a dying fish. Yesterday, it felt like I had been crushed by a wave and cradled in its curl all at the same time.

I had never been in the office of the Sleepy Hollow Cemetery. I was surprised to find it regular, sunny, functional, with a man, Andy, in a blue short-sleeve shirt and Janet with a painted rock on her desk, "Janet." I couldn't easily understand what they were telling me. My mother bought 12 plots thinking she was buying two the day after she'd brought my father's body back from Bermuda. Without this mistake, we could not have ever gathered together as a family. First my dad at 44, whose third heart attack, alcohol, cigarettes and Madison Avenue were the causes of death; then Kevy, 33, the baby of the family, the golden girl, who never looked happy, who died of motherlessness and aplastic anemia, a side effect of a drug after a failed surgery to fix her heart, my heart-broken little sister. Her headstone is beneath our father's. Then Hugh, beside her, who died at 45, mimicking our dad as he said he would. Cause of death: alcoholism. He bled to death. Then our mother, in her fashion at 81, was never really happy, never really unhappy, never available somehow for either, but contented enough until twilight and then she drank too. Hugh is buried beneath her; she is next to my dad; Hugh is next to his sister and mine. And now Johnny, who died most clearly of the primary causes, his abused 20-year-old mother and the horror that she inflicted on him. They were all heartbroken. Maybe most people are. But he had stopped smoking, he had renovated his home, he'd found homes for most of his cats; he and Sean were more harmonious if still not compatible.

The minister, Patrick, was an act of grace. He arrived in the office in shorts and his black shirt and collar. I thought, "This will be informal." Janet was surprised, too. But then he donned his white robes and joined us at the grave. After he said the ashes to ashes, John read the 23rd Psalm, Eva read a John O'Donohue poem on grieving, and we cracked our way through Amazing Grace. Gwen, Hugh's daughter, brought white irises, peonies and roses. I went and took a sliver of flower still in bud and laid it next to the urn. Each one followed.

It was over. We started to leave, but as soon as I started to turn my back, I could not. "We can't just leave him here," I cried, and everyone stopped. Patrick got the gravedigger's attention with a finger whistle and encouraged me. He handed each of us the spade. Jakob was hesitant, and Patrick put his hand on his shoulder, "This is important," and Jakob took the shovel, tipped it into the dirt and helped to cover his uncle's ashes.

In his last prayer, Steve thanked God for Emily, who walked up and down the aisles of the church, then to the front in her beautiful blue dress. She was living on after life had ended. "Hi! Hi, daddy, Hi, mommy," or just calling out "Mommy!" in sheer delight when she'd catch a glimpse of her again. After Catherine sang, Emily went to the stage and looked at her, wagging her head, encouraging her to sing again. The service was background to her joy in walking, to the joy of being a baby loved. She pointed at the pictures of Johnny and said, "Baby."

Sue Othmer wrote me a note, "John was a beautiful and tortured soul; we lose the ones we have fought the hardest to save."

After everyone left, I brought the singing bowl in for Emily. Again, she approaches it like a monk. She took the striker, turned it with her small hands deliberately, placed it soundlessly at the center of the bowl and then pulled it up toward her in a single stroke. She listened to the vibration until it disappeared. She did this several times and each time afterward said, "No." "No" what? She knew how to stop its vibration.

Yesterday, I returned to bed, weighted down particularly at the base of my skull. I never fell asleep and vaguely thought there was another agenda, another calling. It had no direction; it was a field, active but not specific. Then for a moment, perhaps his voice, him nonetheless, a vengeful presence, his old rage, envy, fury and scorn. It may have been some thought that flashed through his head, unforgivable, a thought that his new, open and fragile state had killed him. It was awful. It came from nowhere in me, it was demonic, and it tore through the base of my skull. When I recognized it, I talked with Johnny.

"Don't take this with you, John. We can all have these moments of dreadful envy and distorted desire when the other is getting what we want, what we need." He sent this to me to disperse into the universe. It dissolves back into particles, back into innocence. Johnny was innocent. But he and I are innocent in the lightness of our being, not in the density. It is this density that attracts demons, and they launch us down stairwells. It does, in its capriciousness, feel evil. Arles asked me to be careful. I clutched the railing on the stairs, leaving his office. I had to.

Johnny and I are still in this together. I'd come to join the rest of the family from my third-floor bedroom to leave for the service, lost my footing and was launched into those who had gathered at the bottom of the stairs. I think it was John who caught me as Nina cried out my name. I am trying to negotiate these fields. I told Bob last night that I felt like a Jedi Knight swiping at demons that still want to entrap Johnny, swatting them down, helping him to free himself of the evil his mother took from her father and laid in him.

This lightning strike in my lower brain might have been yet another, perhaps not the last, discharge of pure spite to allow him to make another step in his passage. Johnny loved, and he hated. To make his best reincarnation, he now has to discharge hatefulness, and I am his most reliable helper. I let him know I was there if more was needed. I got up clearer, and it was easy to lift my head.

Johnny and I are in it together; I am on his clock. I married John to raise Johnny, to provide for him. He was precious to me. I avoided him; his terror took me over; he was a pure tortured being, and he was mine. When I woke up this morning, I wanted to swim.

I ask John about his mind and heart, make the meals I can make, and initiate meditation.

"You help me," he said. "Thank god," I whisper to myself, "Thank god."

When Sam touched my sacrum, everything let loose, a flood from my earliest infancy, from Johnny's, from other lives. At first, terrified, crying, then sobbing, then some sound I've never heard—an animal sound. Then my son. I had told Sam that I was good except for the flashing in my right eye. There was a maelstrom there. I was reminded as much as I could bear to be reminded of what it had been for Johnny. I was an inadequate vessel. If he were too close, too proximate, I would flood and disorganize. He was often too proximate.

I went to the bar on Eastside to eat popcorn chicken and to drink a gin and tonic. The drink was like purple velvet. It felt exquisite to me and immediate. Then, when it registered in my stomach, it felt like poison. I was careful not to get drunk. I followed its course through my body. By the time I was home, my stomach wanted to expel it. There was only food, no taste of gin. "You wanted to feel what it did for him, Sebern." It was either Eva or Arles who said it, or it may have been both.

Johnny came to me several times, afraid he couldn't take the next step. I told him he had the right stuff, that he could do it, not to be afraid, everyone emerges, it is just what it is. He would be reassured and would turn again into the vital solitary journey of death. He is still in it. He has not been reborn, but his next life should be better, perhaps as exceptional as the light that was locked in him.

I feel Charlie's absence. I would have wanted to get his letter, hear his Hoosier accent—just that itself comforted me—and his true sadness for yet another terrible loss. Except I lost him first.

I dreamt *I was visiting a concrete quarry in a foreign country. It was beautiful, deep but not wide, like cut marble, with veins of gold through it. The workers' collective was built at the rim, floor to ceiling windows along the hallway, and bright sky-blue pole railings. A woman was singing an aria, standing at the far edge in the sun. I was taken by this and mentioned something to our guide. She said, "We have a wonderful tenor too," almost as if this were part of the collective Benedictine expectation. I asked if they would sing Ave Maria together. They did. I only heard it at a distance.*

I was going ahead to tell him of the next dream—*of finding where the golden bear lived or where they went to the river—Ice Drink Road, and the bear was named Flynn, so well known to the natives, so unknown to me.* He stopped me.

"Talk about the first dream. From the concrete to the divine."

I looked back into it.

"It's about carefully dissembling the energetic mosaic of Johnny and me and sending his with him without damaging either of us. We lived out the essential truth of our lives, together, alone and eternal."

"That is right. Yours is an eternal relationship. In this life, you saved him; in this, he was your son. In another, he saved you."

As I put myself together to leave, he instructed me. "Saturate yourself with the Ave Maria, Sebern. Bach's version, not Schubert's."

John and I talked about my feeling that he turns away from all the trauma of Johnny, and I am asked to participate again in a profound denial. He melted into tears.

"I don't want to forget how he laughed in my arms when I held him as a baby, even as all that was going on, or how well he was and happy at Blake's wedding." I went to hold him. He didn't quite trust me.

"Johnny was beautiful. I could not have lived my life without him. He needed to be born," and he did laugh in John's arms. He sought John's arms. And yet the photos in his apartment are of me; our tortured refuge in each other that I could not bear. Perhaps he couldn't either.

"I am not bouncing back from this as quickly as I want to," I told Eva.

"That is a lawful place," she answered, "Both parts." I rest in that.

"I feel as if I was crossing the road and was hit on the left side by a truck, managed somehow to get up and stagger across and was hit by another truck on the right. Two-ton phantom trucks." Eva's phone went dead.

"You have landed back in the early infant state of motherlessness." My body has. My feet still curl some. The arch is back. I asked him what it was like being with me, and Arles said quietly, "Wonderful." I have no protest to make; there are no interference patterns. There is no other place to be than where I am, as common and as vital as air.

I was watching a woman walking up a frozen river with her dog. I thought to go back and get boots and follow her because it would give me a new view of a familiar area. It was dusk. I wondered if the ice was thick enough—it wasn't that cold. I turned back to watch her and saw her falling slowly beneath the ice. She had a hat on and may have been wearing black. I realized that she was committing suicide. I was torn about what to do. Could I get to her? There were no branches or rope. Should I run and call for help? She would die. Should I let her just do what she wished to do? I watched her go under. It was almost dark.

It was early Sunday evening in mid-July, just getting dark. I was on the laptop, and John was standing in the living room. I saw him duck and swerve.

"There's a bat in here! This is not a hallucinatory bat!" In a minute or so, he dodged again, now looking for it. I didn't see it, but I went to Google, "How to capture a bat." Wikipedia advice was to open the door to a room you could close off, wait till it went in, close the door and turn the light on to make it sleepy. We did this and went to bed. The next morning, I had jury duty. John looked for the bat in the guest room, but there wasn't one. I said too casually, "Johnny comes to you when he is in trouble." This worried him. It made him feel sad and powerless. Then I realized this was Johnny being playful, reminding his father of the episode with Harry and Johnny's flying squirrel that he brought home over school vacation. It had gotten out of its cage and landed on his father's sleeping head. That night is family lore. John's shoulders dropped, and he smiled, "Yes, this is it. He came to laugh."

Arles called after me at the door, "Take care of your brainstem." The collapse happened on Monday. I was chilled, almost limp. I canceled with Arles. I didn't think. I used the chair because it felt as if some important front was moving through.

"This isn't me. Where have I arrived? I don't know this place. I am just privileging this room, Bob, over the mid-space or the other universe that I can touch if I thought to stretch out my arms and my fingers." Bob opened a ream of paper to show me what he saw. He walked his fingers along the top, and then suddenly he turned it up, and the leaves separated. "You fell down into the space between universes."

I looked at John and saw how valiantly he was trying to hold himself together. Johnny's death shattered him. It didn't shatter me; it stunned me. Arles asked where Johnny was. It is hard to write when the brainstem presses me in some insistent, unknown way; no sequence, no time, on the precipice of awe.

"Do you have a feeling where Johnny is, John?"

"I've sent out prayers, but I can't feel that they have landed anywhere." Grief has exhausted him. "Do you?"

"I feel he has been reborn. It was a quick passage." I searched around for where, "There is a wide horizon, very few trees, not Africa. Asia?... Mongolia."

"His life was beautiful," Arles said. "He lived the iconography of Christ. When you would say crisis, I would hear 'Christus.'" And I see it too, his agony in the emergency room, his nakedness, the ever-present possibility of humiliation. I wrapped him in the white sheet many times. I lay across his body. He went on, "John and Joseph need to disappear. It is about the mother and the son, and Johnny is reborn into the iconography of peace, surrounded by practice, not by beliefs." I can almost see his face peering out from bundles. I don't know that I can know this, but I know he is safe in the arms of his mother. He is a blessing. He will be a presence there; he is already. I asked John how he felt about what we were seeing.

"I feel that Johnny is even farther away. I miss him even more." We will take the morning to meditate with him and for him.

When I used the phrase "the tip of 1000 icebergs," Arles went to the DNA dream, the mountain ranges, the spinal column of a dinosaur, bleached white but retained.

Grief. We mostly stayed indoors with it, alone with it, gnawing through our dreams and our silent meals. It was impossible to face the humid, relentless days even inside the forlorn chapel of our home. In meditation, on a cool autumn morning, I asked myself what of this needed to be borne. What time did we need to give our grieving bodies? I thought about our dog, Fireworks, when she lost her litter. She could not be comforted or distracted. She ate very little and didn't walk with me. At the end of two weeks, her grief lifted, and she returned to us. It was organic and necessary. We could make this easier, but maybe not better, if we trained. John and I talked and, each month until we could no longer bear it, chose grief.

❧

Marsha is considering the possibility of an authorized biography, and she's uneasy about it. She has led an important life, but what in the end do these facts, strung together like her mother's pearls, really matter? She intends it as a message of hope. Marsha, though, cannot bear the toll of introspection; she makes no pretense. John has said it well. Marsha designed a therapy that protects her from knowing. It is an important therapy. So many people want this protection. She got lost in our disagreement and then found herself. She was arguing that there was a discrete thing, "borderline personality disorder," that I now dismiss, and when she saw what we were each arguing, she laughed and said, "And I am the behaviorist here!"

She'd called me when she got the news of Charlie's sudden death. She'd thought the news was about our friend Charlie Swenson and began to share her shock.

"No, Marsha, Charlie Boren." She turned her attention to me and tried to comfort me. She didn't really comprehend feelings of loss like this about a therapist. When she got the message about Johnny, she thought I was saying that John had died. At first, all she could tell me was her relief that it wasn't John. She cares for me. I care for her. We love each other on these different planets.

I struggle with these realities, that people would actually prefer to live sleepy and be blinded. I have to keep reminding myself, "But yes, they do, overwhelmingly." Why would she want to write this book or have it written if she doesn't want to learn from it? She drew away when I said she was still attached to the narrative. For her, this is an act of redemption for the discretion she has needed to take, discretion that was a lie, that this is an act of courage. And it is most definitely that. But it is thinly woven, a cloth that provides no comfort. She didn't want to betray her mother. I understand, and what else could a biography of madness do? As we talk, I see the photograph of her, professionally taken, at three or so, where she clings to a mother looking away from her. It hangs on the wall outside her bedroom. It is her favorite.

Marsha says I must write my book. "You are so much more eloquent than I; you think about all of this. You read literature. I read stories and spiritual books. Crime stories. That's the difference between you and me." I brace myself when she begins by saying "that's the difference" because we are almost all difference and when she begins that way, I am sure I will be the short straw. But that's rarely, if ever, how it turns out. She doesn't compare; she notes the difference. She's lonely. Bessel is lonely. I am not lonely and more and more settled with our shared aloneness.

It's hard to temper the ascendancy of the left hemisphere. It is hard to feel what we feel. This is no less true of Bessel than for most survivors. He makes theory and reputation through passionate commitment and through the terrible power of denial. He shames. He creates havoc and then rewrites his role to exonerate himself, his unbearable shame, the shadow of his tenderness. Arles asked what I found compelling about Bessel, and I answered his tenderness, his terrible hunger, his primary shame, the shadow of starvation and occupation, his motherlessness and his wish to do the right thing. I feel an affinity for him, but I am deeply disquieted by his willingness to do anything but feel the hunger and shame that churn in him. I can't help him with this.

The first Christmas for all of us. Blake broke down, and I held her, and she cried. I help her just to grieve her losses, not to worry about Emily or to anticipate our deaths. To grieve Johnny. We kept waiting for his call, much as I turned over every Christmas card looking for Charlie's handwriting. She was mourning her dog, Chelsea, equally and, in a way, unforgivably. I feel bad, too. It can't be that I mourn Charlie even more; this is not natural. But Johnny was hard for me even when he wasn't being hard. The space his death has left in my life is breathing room and uncomplicated love that his living could not allow. He made an important part of his journey here with me, and now he gets to live in the light that was always within him. I am sure of this. People see it in him already as an infant, in his smile, in his dark, clear eyes. He is not sleepy or fussy. He has serenity. And they will know him even more as he turns 12 and then 14. He will be wise, this old soul; this son of mine and John.

Dear John,

I am torn right from the beginning on how to address this letter. Perhaps dear Johnny is better. It's what Molly and Blake call you. It was 'Johnny' Blake who was waiting to hear from on Christmas Day. And 'Johnny', whose last news felt crushing to Molly. It was Johnny, really, who died again this week. Dad is on his way to Belize, torn apart, shattered again by the news of your death.

We learned that they'd finally released your death certificate, but once again, the papers didn't arrive. I asked John. He couldn't remember the thickness of the letter he'd shoved in his overflowing briefcase. He can't gather himself yet. He was afraid this would arrive when he was in Belize, and I'd be alone. He opened the papers, alone, at his office instead. His grief feels as dense as a black star.

We had all drifted into a different narrative of your death. But even if the heart attack had been true, it would've been the same. You died either way of a broken heart. But it was easier somehow to think of the physical heart giving out than the real heart, so we lived vaguely in that story until we got the autopsy.

I hated it too, but I did suspect you were drinking again. Sean told us you were, and your father couldn't bear to hear that from either of us. You and I fought, or perhaps it was more the case that I screamed at you, crying sometimes, "Will you have me bury my father, my brother, and my son all dead from alcohol?!" You never responded. When we were together, you just blinked. You may have even blinked out. You would have stopped if you could have. You wouldn't have put any of us through this.

You must've been exhausted. You took your comfort where you could find it, and you lived a heroic life battling the constant terror within you. It's a testimony to you that you lived as long as you did, fought as hard.

Who survives what you survived? How can the autopsy be a shock? It was how you were going to die, an accidental overdose of psychotropic medications and ethanol. Dad's impulse was not to tell your sisters. It is his impulse to save them from the sadness he so fears feeling. And perhaps he doesn't want them to be angry at you. Molly was, momentarily, the way she was always angry with you for what she feels is some kind of self-indulgence, some stubborn failure to shape up, to let us, her, save your life.

It would have been easier to write this on a computer. I could leave it then, leave you, and there is that impulse. My own anger. I don't want to leave you, but even in writing this, I am made slightly sick and anxious. It's hard to feel, and I always feel it. I felt it when I knew you were coming to visit and when you'd call. You never knew how I would respond. It was only in the last few years, maybe even the last two, that I wasn't swept into the vortex of your horror as you told me about a soap opera or trips to the doctor. You had begun to slur again, and I felt my ribs give out in the back behind my heart. I told your dad yesterday that if you had lived, which you couldn't, but if you had, that I could not have rescued you again. He didn't say anything. He could have said just 'Well, we don't have to,' but he kept silent so as not to betray you. We would've tried to rescue you again because, really, what else could we have ever done? Thank you, sweet boy, for releasing us. I don't know where either of us, any of us, would have gotten the strength.

That is the meaning of the autopsy, the blow of it. We didn't save you; not our love, not neurofeedback, not our love. Your mother, her father and her father's father claimed you. I am surprised that Sean didn't find you in a bathtub, but of course, you never took baths.

You finally surrendered. You couldn't do it any longer. You fought long enough. Lived long enough. You didn't fail, Johnny; your rebirth is evidence of that. None of us, even though we did, could ask more from you.

You were an avatar, you are an avatar, and now you are free and in the arms of your round-faced mother who beams at you, to shine out and help the suffering world. You know the depths of that—your suffering couldn't inform you in this incarnation—it was too great. It swallowed you. It kept you and me in a long and dangerous labor. But you are now again born. Be the gift you are. Your cells will know us, too: your dad, who always loved you, your sisters who went through it all with you and me.

I love you, Johnny, to the end of time.

Mom

Blake called to check on me out here in the welcomed snow. When I asked her, she said she was doing well with the news, and it was as I had said, "The way he would die, even if he didn't die that way." She was clearly peaceful.

"I think that the autopsy felt bad because it meant we couldn't save his life."

"That we could only save some of it, Mom. The last years were still the very real gift that they were."

On Friday, I did my first LENS session with Alan, who is now living in the apartment below that had been Johnny's. Friday night, I slept like an adolescent does, but through the day, I revisited epochs of symptoms—headache, sacral pain, difficulty engaging cortically, little desire to exert myself, shoulder pain, erratic eating. After the third LENS session—they last about three minutes—I can feel my brain rearranging its furniture. My body feels particularly stable related to PZ. There is ease in my legs. My appetite stabilizes, but I still get a metallic taste in my mouth. I'm detoxing. There is no animal cowering in me. All corners are airy. I think I will be able to work again. I have driven out here, into the ice storm, trees down, power out, limbs and live wires covered in fresh snow.

My kid is dead. "My kid is dead." I don't know why it sounded new to me when I said it that way. I don't lose track, but he isn't a constant point of reference. My kid is dead. That happened. The sudden wail of the Black mother who has, in every nightmare, expected the gunshot. He was doomed like that, my kid. Damned like that. I accept it. This is not a cry or a protest. Every word seems important, each standing alone for a moment before it joins the sentence. "My" is an intimate claim, and it surprises me that it sounds new, connected to "kid." And "kid" too is a deeper claim than "son," so he is more mine, not less anyone else's, but more mine. "Is" is always beautiful like breath; it affirms us; it opens me. "Dead" is a footfall, heavy on concrete slab.

I dreamt of Charlie. *I was in a mental hospital helping someone who did not want electric shock but was having it. It was a recovery room but a pit of suffering, dark, medieval. People were crying and talking about what the shock did to them. I was facilitating, and I said I can't know since I haven't... but stopped and admitted that what I was about to say was untrue. I have. I had 6 or 10. I do know what it's like. I saw Charlie enter, and he was wearing a red jacket that tied at the back and pants that were cut above the ankle (*what we do to people in dreams!). *A later glimpse of him, and he was in a straitjacket. He surveyed the scene, and he wasn't happy. There would be changes.*

The next day, my brain turned on me. The sewer men became my tormentors; "How," I thought to myself, "could you ever convince someone those demons were not real?" I was bad for days. It arose in work with Bob, and I felt the kind of disinterest that is attachment disorder. I miss Arles. The time seems very long. Had I been an inch closer to believing my own experience, I would have had to hear his voice to ask him where I was.

When Lee held the vertebrae where my ribs attach, it became a field of battle. I tried to breathe into it, but my head shook, "No," and I tried again, and the breath was spread out along the surface. It could not be borne. If the breath got deeper, I would go mad, and there was no way to convince myself otherwise. I am training now below the inion, near the brainstem.

Sam reported that since beginning training at the Inion Ridge, I have a "tranquil" nervous system. After the Beta reset protocol, symptoms gather in me like ghosts. I felt a yearning for protection; I drank a gin and tonic; I called Arles.

John just returned from taking a system to Ruth in London.

Writing all these journals was, at first, I thought, a tour de force. My mother could not form an image of me, any of us, but maybe particularly me and I write into that void. But it's hurled back, unheard and unknown. These are ghosts that I am writing about now, worn out, vapid and ordinary, that try to scare us, blowing around, making faces, insisting they still matter. John told me that when he came into the bedroom last night, I asked, "Who's there?" Not frightened, he thought, as much as curious, but later his snore came through my sleep like a gunshot, and I was awake guarding against the next incursion.

I am making neurofeedback-related organizational mistakes. Picking up the phone when I want the remote. Some moments of word hash. Going to the wrong drawer of the cabinet on the opposite side of the kitchen. There's a replay of many early problems, like not being able to clap in rhythm with the rest of the audience, but it's transitory.

Emily runs for the joy of her feet. She climbs to declare her balance. She makes faces that look like masks to make clear the discontent of the gods. I feel, at times, an unbearable and unknown desire to be with another human being. I can't be away from her too long.

"Who cares?" I was trying to describe the ephemera of emotional experience.

"That is an important question," Arles said.

"Looking back on it, it is two-dimensional, like tissue paper; ephemera."

"Yes, that is so, and it is also the reality of your early life."

It was as if none of it had happened. No mind. No reality. This is an unfolding experience all to be encountered, to be within. And I began to cry.

"How did a mind develop at all?"

"That too is a vital question," he said, "exactly the one we are examining."

My sacrum still flares, "Gentle body, it is over. You are safe. Be not afraid."

Bessel sent a letter to Senator Kaufman about developmental trauma disorder with no mention of neurofeedback.

"No matter what it is called, we address it with neurofeedback. Who cares about the DTD diagnosis if there's nothing we can do about it?" He knew he'd fucked up but was slow to admit it. "We were invited to meet with him because of neurofeedback! Now this looks like a bait and switch."

"You are right. Who can care about it if there is no way to treat it?" He gets calmer when he gets the reality of the presence of the other; he is safer.

"I love you anyway, Bessel." He laughs, warm and relieved, "I love Sebern."

We stepped into the red, white and blue hush of the Senate office of this reluctant senator, the seal, his name. He is a placeholder for Beau Biden. They brought us in early; he had a conference call he had to take. Ted Kaufman wasn't intimidating, nor really in the "corridor of power." What presses on you is what presses on him—no time, not enough money, too many children dying. This is the imperative, and this sliver of time squeezes you into form and into few words; too few words.

"Everything right now," he said, "is about healthcare."

"Child abuse and neglect costs 104 billion dollars a year. That's hardly a footnote in the healthcare crisis. One in every seven children is afflicted," I said.

The Senator agrees, "No, hardly a footnote."

There was no time to tell him about neurofeedback or the DTD diagnosis that was turned down by the DSM 5 committee. Vicky Kelly, who had gotten us the meeting, tried to underline neurofeedback, but the

Senator was being called to a floor vote, and really, he just wanted to retire from this job.

We sat together in the lobby of the Dupont, unsure of exactly what had happened. It seemed worth it, but no one could say how.

It was Sophie Freud's sixth birthday in Vienna before the war began. Hannah was her classmate, but she was new to this house and these children. They were served hot chocolate and tea with the cake. There was lemon for the tea and whipped cream for the hot chocolate. At home, she and her parents took their tea with milk, so she asked for whipped cream for her tea. The rest of the small clique laughed at her for such a wrong choice. She was, she told me as we sipped tea in her apartment on 112th Street, mortified until an old man who was leaning on the door jam to the dining room said, "Oh yes, that's exactly how I take my tea." I tried to write the story in the visitor's book in a somewhat neglected apartment/museum on 19 Berggasse, but I scrambled it because I so often do.

I felt compelled to tell this story of his empathy, his kindness and his willingness to rescue. His legacy, though, is neither kind nor true. He knew his patients were sexually assaulted, and he made it into a lie, a fantasy, an unconscious, seductive desire not for the absent mother but for the father who raped them. There are other parts of his legacy for which Freud should be honored. This one is a crime against humanity.

Madness takes the forms it does because words falsify it even as they form. There is nothing to do but demonstrate, you "act out" or your body bleeds, or you have organ failure at a young age, or wrinkle into bitter fruit. Recovery is not a word about this; even assault is too easy, too limited, too kind. "Regulation" is an ivory tower word not even close to sufficient. Then I remember to be thankful for the regulation that arose in the circuits of my brain, or that Arles's hands pressed on my head. It isn't like that anymore. I am not so available to dysregulation. Lee, though, asked me what I am holding today in my sacrum—as if there is a past tense. It is the trajectory that we change, which makes all the difference. The experience itself is ever with us, for everybody.

The morning air is stagnant and ominous. It holds the night's garbage, puke and skunk. A beer bottle on the lawn. The air is drenched in despair. Something is arising in me. It presses on the inside of my ribs. I can't walk easily; my head has a slight crook. It reminds me. I wonder, as I have been, about what happened in Irvington that night. The man was a predator. He sat at the short end of the L in the counter, a regular. I wore my white and turquoise uniform with ice cream and sweat stains and a fine mesh black hairnet. Among those women, I could have been any age, but I was 16. I doubt I recognized him any more than I recognized Leonard. I should have been an expert prey, but the smell of it did not alert me to flee; it moved me into fugue. Death feigning at HoJos on the turnpike. My friend Carol was there, it was her parents' car; I think we argued about this in the parking lot of the place—it was a tourist stop—that he interrupted. He soothes our fears, luring us deeper in, alarming me into deeper dissociation, weakening my legs. I was practiced at collapse, surrender, going out, and waking up, having survived. Everything is blank there.

❧

We struggled with Buzsaki's brilliant but obscure keynote. We all decided he should do a TED talk, that he could make it funny and simple, and he certainly has an idea that changes the world. Ed would follow with the neurofeedback talk. It was a time of community, odd, competitive, brilliant, new, unseen and shiny. The people here at ISNR could tear each other apart were it not for the reality that we are absolutely in this together, and the world must have this. Buzsaki said the next decade of neuroscience will be devoted to neurofeedback.

My interior life is quiet, and I can look around. I am never without a now more distant foreboding. It leans against my joints, always there, the genetic memory of an anonymous person born into war, the Holocaust and camps. This is my experience, that's all. I no longer suffer from it, but I will never be innocent of it. Resolution is ephemeral; acceptance quiets me.

I dreamt I went to my mother's house on the Cape. I looked in through the glass doors and saw her furniture as she left it, perhaps a red plush armchair and a white one as well, and there was a padlock on the door. I told myself that this was my house, and I sought out the realtor who agreed and let me in. Someone brought me news that the doctors in the nursing home were saying that their only choice was to decapitate her. I was horrified, but somehow, I also understood. She menaced, shamed and frightened others, and no matter what they did, it didn't change. I kept feeling I should go, but I talked to them so fully that I was able to see her in my mind's eye. I argued with them to help her die peacefully with drugs. They didn't seem to think it would work; they insisted on decapitation, I on lethal injection to end her suffering. I woke up in the midst of this argument with unseen doctors and the image of what they were proposing, the word echoing in my head. Arles will talk about the undead, and perhaps that's just it. But the dream jars me. Our last days together were our most peaceful ones. Where did this come from? Did I drag it here from the Cape?

"This is a powerful dream," he said. I felt a deep horror and betrayal of her and tried to throw the image out of my head.

"I would never have hurt her," I cried, remembering the yard man who dumped grass cuttings over her car. Her bewilderment made my heart break. He listened, he understood, and he changed the course entirely.

"Chor is a Tibetan word that describes the dismemberment of the body, limb from limb, the naked, dead heart left for birds and maggots. The reality, the metaphor of the decapitation of attachment." My mother is always at the core of my anguished arousal; her body that absently gave rise to mine, her emptiness and sorrow and rage. In the dream, the doctors could not contain her arousal, no matter what they did. They were doing what must be done to protect the body, detaching. It is a hard dream. The visuals are so distressing, but slowly his way of seeing is seeping into the bones of my consciousness. It isn't a dream of death or hostility. It is a dream of liberation. This death, this dismemberment allows Me. There is a different house, full of long windows, rooms filled with light, the red chair and this too, transitory.

"Dreams are proof of mind," Arles said. "The brain does not do this."

I want to find my way to the middle distance of my history, to drop into it at will and then return to normal commerce, to dailiness without dislocation. Like people go down to the Riverwalk to engage in the vitality of San Antonio, and then must ascend to a chaotic, broken little city where there is a building with this sign: Robt. E. Lee Hotel and above that a sign also once in neon "fully air-conditioned."

There is more predictability in my life. The dog who romps in the backyard across the street, and I live in the same frame of time. I double-check often still, when I walk into town, that the wheels of the cars move with them in the same direction and most of the time they do. When they don't, my stomach sinks. I live in the primary colors of my grandchildren, in my work and in my writing. This is all a meaningful life; it is Right Livelihood.

There are these moments, though, where I feel a former undercurrent, like cars in a flood with their headlights on and then a cow and a scream that seems to shatter through time, backward and forward, from the moment it lets out. At these moments, there is a different color to my life. I understand it better, I am not forgetting. But it is more than not forgetting, it is remembering anew without descending into the hall of mirrors. I am no longer just an inference, that legacy of her absence. There was no "there, there." I discovered it all through feel. I was never able to see, and when I did, I didn't know whether to believe or not to believe.

There are long stretches now when I don't see Arles. I was missing him yesterday and felt the feeling out to its edges, and it didn't explode or fizzle. It ended with him right there, in me.

I woke up depressed. I didn't understand it. I never feel like this. I couldn't talk on the way into town for breakfast.

"Are you tired?" John asked.

"Yes, are you?" I stumbled over a crack in the sidewalk, and he grabbed my arm to steady me.

I felt better in the shower. My mood felt like a betrayal. I couldn't walk that day either; my balance failed. I couldn't quite pay attention. My thoughts slipped sideways. I struggled to make sense in the group, not let go into a beckoning forgetting. I thought about training, but only the next day did I make sense of it.

We'd had a wonderful weekend in New York. Saturday, we were with Thầy at the Beacon for a day of mindfulness. A friend gifted us with third row seats, and Thầy seemed to be focusing on me as he spoke. I dismissed it. I knew everyone would feel that in themselves, too. It was the quality of his presence. After the talk was over, friends approached me, and they each said, "I think Thầy was talking to you." We had a nice room at the Empire, the weather was beautiful, and we went to a play. OK, the play, that was probably a piece of it. The powerful rock opera Next to Normal. We both felt buffeted. A day of mindfulness and a night of losing the mind. We checked out, walked up Broadway and ate breakfast at Niko's outside in the sun.

On our drive back, I asked John if we could go to Bronxville. I didn't know this, but we were approaching the Bronxville exit. As it turned out, we were six minutes from my house.

John asked me if I wanted to get out and walk around. I couldn't answer, but I stayed in the car, and I kept the window shut. We drove around the block to Eliot Avenue, where we sledded with the fathers and where my piano teacher lived, and where the boys threw rocks at me. I saw my school and the route I took home to avoid the hail of humiliation and bruises. The place where I repeated preschool. From there to Lawrence Hospital, where I had my tonsils out, to the remnants of the park where we'd go to feed the ducks, to the Dutch Reformed church. We got out there and looked around. We went from there to my school, Dobbs. The doors were locked, the kids away on a four-day break. The school is beautiful. I told John about waiting in the circle for my mother's friend, Mrs. Lundberg, who finally came to tell me in person what she'd already said over the phone, "Your father is dead," and wandering around looking for arms and feeling guilty about that, like stealing. They sent me to the infirmary. We went on and stopped at

Washington Irving's home and walked the grounds. He was there in 1847, the first American to make a living writing. And we drove past Lyndhurst. That's where that night happens—the night I can't remember. The Howard Johnson's is now a diner with blue chrome, through Tarrytown to the Sleepy Hollow cemetery. There were tourists there too.

"It comforts me," John said, "to visit Johnny's grave." He touched it with such tenderness. We stopped in Middletown for coffee. I was beginning to feel a pull downwards. We looked at Wesleyan and stopped in the store, Little Tibet. We liked the men there and bought a rug. Then to Plainfield. Todd, Blake and Emily came for lunch the next day, and we went out to explore the woods. It was all lovely. Maybe tomorrow, when I see Arles, I will understand why it was that after all of this, I could barely stand up.

"I sent my request to visit 44 Stewart Ave. There is no 44. It is 40 Stewart."

"Your ambivalence."

"Yes, that and it's not a random number. This all happened when I was four."

He nodded and then said, "You don't seem fully inhabited. There is some of your animal eye." I fell silent, trying to find the back of my head, to feel the disconnect from the front.

"Why do this?" I came out of my silence with that question. Arles responded slowly.

"Why would someone return to Auschwitz?" At first, I wanted to protest the comparison; nothing is as bad as Auschwitz. But the protest was a diversion, and it died. "Why do people go back? What happens to them? What are they looking for?" But he quickly turned away from the analogy, and we both saw what he saw. Auschwitz is known; it is affirmed. The suffering was unbearable, but it was shared. It was acknowledged, it was not alone, it was not your home, it was not denied. Holocaust deniers are so hated and feared because they twist reality. There is no reality for children who are abused. It is unacknowledged, denied, ignored, and yet still condoned. There are no markers, no memorials; the house is regular. People live there.

"You feel the fear in Anne Frank's house. It is unmistakable." Would 40 Stewart Ave feel the same after years of rehab? A red door. I think we had a red front door. You can't see that there is a third floor from the street, no windows to the front. "I didn't look around. It was a fixed moment within the bubble of the car, a fixed moment of present time. I wasn't curious."

Sometime this week, I began to experience original memory. I remembered the events at 40 Stewart as they were then, not through all of the harmonics they gave rise to. These aren't memories; these are vibrations, a tone poem without the words or the pictures that words can give rise to. It is challenging to live in this oscillation; it is more accurate than memory, and it dissembles me. I can't quite walk. It is, I came to understand, a cerebellar memory. I am kept off balance. I can't find my feet.

Last weekend, we watched Julia Sweeney: Letting Go of God. All through it, little hairline fractures opened, little shivers of light and disequilibrium. It was for me the breaking up of a belief I didn't know I had. Arles asked me if I felt that belief was like the cup, and only then could I find the sense of this. After that performance, talk or sermon, something had disappeared, best described as a thin translucent veil or skin. He said in Buddhism that this was called the dharmakaya, the primordial nature of mind. It unsettled me as much to realize that I still relied somehow on belief to enter this absolute spaciousness. It is as if I am lying out in the field, knowing but not really feeling the support of the earth, and then there's no earth, and I am amongst the stars I have been gazing at. I don't think the experience of this has diminished much since it began a week ago. John didn't feel it like this. He has the comfort of the ground, of the great intelligence, the harbor of belief. Who knows when these things come to us or how? Arles said again that I am doing this outside all tradition, but he taught me a meditation to support it. It's clear that he has experienced this and that he pursues it, which is, of course, no pursuit.

Chapter 18

I make the walk up and down the hill three times each day. It is Christmas Eve at the Priory.

I feel confined by the liturgy. I moved the Bible out of my room. There is nothing for me in Christ except for the moments he transcends Christ. Maybe this means the end of the Priory for me. But now I am embraced by the Brothers' kindness and beauty and goodness. I read Pocket Ken Wilbur.

I am not skeptical. I am not a theist. I am not an atheist. Not a Christian. Not a Buddhist, not an "I am" or an "I am not." And still, there is a lot of me and mine for someone who has disappeared. Habits. Reflexes like those that people can have even after they've died. I thought about Wilbur's belief that it was not darkness that was the enemy of enlightenment, but superficiality. Darkness is always part of enlightenment.

It is a sad thought that this may be my last Christmas here. My Christian self needed this place. It may be time to give it up to others. What had run clear for me last year has overflowed its banks. Its path isn't clear; it isn't bound.

Emily was playing doctor with me, putting Band-Aids on "ouchies." She put one over the scar on my arm, then she stopped, touched my face, looked at me with utmost compassion and said, "It's OK, Grammy." We then lay face to face on the deep couch, and I started to cry. How was I granted this child? The child of the wild blonde hair, who doesn't eat, who runs like a colt, who breaks through time and then restores the seam as if it had never happened.

It has begun to snow. I was thinking now of the separate chamber for children who fall into fugues. A chef on the radio spoke about getting cauliflower for soup, one with no brown spots. I can still feel the echo of this separate chamber as if I were so far away and in such a warp that information came to me in echoes. It's not that I haven't seen many cauliflowers with brown spots or that I don't avoid them. The news was that this was a universal problem, not solely mine.

If Johnny were alive, he'd be on his way here, moving slowly, unpredictably toward health or catastrophe, and I would feel the challenge of his presence in my viscera. At the reconciliation service, a marker service that focuses me on where I am, I felt a sudden blow to my chest and then tears—Johnny was there. I keep track of him. It's winter again, a challenging time for a mother with a newly walking and climbing baby in the small hut, yurt or tent.

The talk throughout the film Snow Falling on Cedars is about the worst snowstorm in decades. It doesn't stop snowing, and yet the snow somehow never builds up. It's like the memory of these awful events; it doesn't accumulate. It may be an artifact of the season and the filming schedule, but it makes the movie in a way that drifts and shoveled paths would have undone it. It's like the dream: the three-story boulder disappearing into the undersea mountain chain, completing it.

On the Sunday night after Christmas, someone set twelve fires in Northampton. Two are dead, and the arsonists are not yet captured. The fires happened all around us, but none on our street.

Arles and I talked about this, mostly about my initiative to have locks and deadbolts installed on the front doors. I am conflicted about the energy of locks. In a slightly challenging way, he said,

"Given your sensitivity and history around invasion, I am surprised you don't have locks already." An interesting point. And I've never thought of it. I have been vigilant about locks inside my house and made sure I could lock my door to the third floor, which I never do. It seemed to be that I was doing something unsafe or at least, normatively, odd.

"I grew up in a very small town," he continued, "and everyone locked their houses. It was your house. You locked it."

I hadn't thought the fires scared me until I was alone Thursday night with an idling truck outside my house. I called the police. They assured me that the whole town was jumpy and that they much preferred that I call. On Friday, they arrested the arsonist, at least one of them, a 25-year-old resident of Hawley Street, the street he first set ablaze. No one believed that one person could have set twelve fires. For me, there was still the question about the locks. I had to attend to this, and I bore down. The realization was sudden.

"All danger came from within my house."

"Yes, of course," he sighed.

"And there was size. It came down to size. No locks, no walls could keep this monster out."

"It came from within."

"Yes, it did. It comes from within." I stopped before adding, "I have lived all of my life in a volcano, Arles. I furnished it, commuted in it, worked in the white heat of it and over the past 10 years, I have been moving increasingly toward its cooler edges, and then one day, I am hurled out, and I land in paradise. It's an adjustment."

10 days ago, I tried a new protocol for the cerebellum, Inion ridge 1 - Inion ridge 2, before I used it with those patients who continue to struggle. I couldn't quite find the word, talking with Eva the next morning.

"I am empty. Empty in the Buddhist sense. More emptied of self. It doesn't feel dramatic, probably because, by its nature, it couldn't. Clearly different." Over time, I realized that I felt more balanced, physically and emotionally. A couple of hours later, I lay on Sam's table, and he put his hand over my brainstem.

"This is very different from how it's ever been. It's," and he searched briefly for a word, "empty. Empty of congestion, of noise, of stagnant energy that has always been there. Maybe a little jazzed, something as you'd feel after a cup of coffee." He let his hand rest there, picking up more information. "It could be energy attempting to clear stagnant pools." A few days later, Bob said, "It's clear all the way from your brainstem to your sacrum."

I should know this feeling by now. It's an aura. As I was going to sleep, I was struck. It wasn't fear, it was grief, deep grief over having had these experiences, having lived in such ambient fear that I was always at the tipping point into psychosis. The experience of memory and grief was hurtling out of deep space at the back of my head and struck me like a meteor or a piece of space junk. I didn't recognize the crying. Crying for some is like snow for Inuits, almost endless tones, registers, notes and phrases—once you pay attention.

"You located yourself in psychosis so as not to feel the grief."

"No, Arles. I know these books too, and I would gladly burn them all. This is grief, pure, unmuddled, about being psychotic, about ever feeling such density of confusion, uncertainty and fear. The moments when you are losing your mind. If I were floating out into black space, my tether broken, knowing I would never return, where is the time for grief? Where does it happen? Grief is a bubble in the amber. It was caught and held like the events themselves and polished with the stories into a beautiful gem."

"It's beautiful," he said, "but I don't understand you."

"What I want you to say is 'I understand you'. The bubble of grief was captured within the psychosis. I did not go mad to defend against grief."

"Yes," he said softly. "That is different."

"Will you burn these books with me?" He smiled and did not commit.

All therapists give the instruction to grieve. Or more benignly, perhaps, permission. I do. When my patient was telling me about the incestuous rape, I knew she would have been smaller than Emily is now. Subtly, I push that perception away... to keep her history from conflating with mine. All directions. I don't want hers to revivify mine in great part because I don't want mine to amplify or overrun hers.

"Therapists don't cry for their patients. You have never cried for me. I have never cried for any of my patients, even though I feel deeply for them. I grieve for the Hutiis not for my patients. It seems necessary not to. The one time I cried for Merrit, it scared her. I have cried when patients have left. But grief over their suffering must be sequestered or refused. So, as patients, we grieve alone. As therapists, we inevitably collude in not grieving."

I looked at my watch. It was impossible. It was noon. I did the impossible. I left his office.

I want to be done with recovery.

After the second double Beta-reset, I felt deeply quiet, settled in, and clear. I was telling the neurofeedback group about it and mentioned the episode of reflux. Rob, whose living room we were in, asked me if it could be body memory. I dismissed it. On Friday, yet again, I got a pill caught in my throat, and for five minutes I was choking and heaving and banging my back against the wall. My body is thrown around; it is trashed. Sam is alarmed. It registers as it was felt in the brainstem. Is this too a harmonic of rape? Are any of these things, these episodes, separable, unnested in the other?

It is March 19, and it would be a surprising day in April. Northampton is spilled out into the streets in all its oddness and desolation. The hedges are being trimmed. I don't like walking in town—too many kids sitting and, it seems, needlessly on the take. Sorry, guilty, sad, annoyed. Near the underpass, the guys leave a gooey mess that would attract flies if it were more convincingly their season. 1/2 quart of milk, orange peels and a smudge of grape. I am tired of them. I looked for my little private square in the sun to read my book. A young woman sat down, too close, with a baby whom she feeds bread and hummus. She's charming until she turns to ask the time that is showing on my large, round watch and displays her cheek smeared with avocado.

A young man takes shots at the trash barrel with his empty plastic bottle. He missed. He missed again.

"You can do this," I said, cheering him on, and he did. As he passed by, smiling a gap-tooth smile, he thanked me and asked what I was reading. I just bought "The Help."

"Is it good?"

"I don't know. I just started it."

"Oh."

"But I can tell you what it's about."

"What?"

"It's about White children being raised by Black women." My young conversationalist was Black. He got wide-eyed. "And that's my story," I added.

"Really?" He said this like I'd introduced him to an arcane but fascinating piece of foreign history.

"Really. Yes."

"I'm going to check in with you about that! I want to see how that turns out." We made the date to meet again randomly on the street.

I dreamt of a baby crawling happily out of her restraints and onto her head. She was a doll, my mother's term of affection or perhaps request, "Be a doll." *I just watched. Not helpless, not there.*

We visited my aunt in Morgan City. As my mother had, she told me tales of their wonderful childhood. Could this be? Could wonderful childhoods leave one uninhabited?

It is hard to describe, even to Arles, how it is to have no feelings about all of what happened that aren't themselves like bubbles that glisten with tears and then break and join the air or the tide. The past is no longer present; it isn't even past. I gained the past, I think mostly in training my brain, but even that has disappeared. And yet my body seems to archive it, insist on it. I am the slow student and the wise old lady. They arise together and ask something of me, but it's like a language I forgot long ago. Phrases come in, I recognize them, but I don't dream in that language anymore. I don't understand the question, and I don't know the answer.

A memory arose of the wet inside lips, the drunk kisses from their friend Barney—this one in my bed, his hand on my chest, slipping to my neck. It arises, and I must feel something—there is a trace of aversion—the helpless attempt to turn away, maybe even giving up to it. As I talked about it with Arles, I realized that it had gone on at their endless cocktail parties. This memory has too many settings, and my father's not there. They both let this happen.

"Of course," Arles said, as if we'd talked about this for years.

"This has no meaning to me either, but it is not meaningless to my body. Maybe this is 'Isness', itself, in the body."

"In Buddhism, there is a name for this, Sanbukaya. Memory without attachment, the 'just isness' of every moment, arising and floating away."

When I saw their parties at eight and ten, the remnant about their friend, the lawyer, the date rapes, it's like a flood that begins to rush in over the threshold, but then somehow never arrives. The rush of waves doesn't fill my ears. It is not that the levees have held or even that the storm veers or recedes. There is no storm. Like the boulder in my dream, it leaves no mark as it fills in the DNA, like the snow that never builds into drifts. It's held in that former time. I discover everything, usually the same thing, as if it has once again receded from knowing and is now new again.

The earth has been quiet; the volcano is dormant. My life just proceeds calmly. Since I watched The Girl with the Dragon Tattoo, there have been an increasing number of foreshocks, warning that tremors were again building. I don't keep a careful track. It just seems repetitive. The 'I' that is still 'I' is bored and done. I don't know what to make of it. Protest can begin, but it dies immediately. I don't really believe that it should or should not be happening; it is. My experience dissolves there in that lipid pool of Isness. This is the real nature of early childhood abuse, assault and neglect. It lives in you, and therapy is a combination of exorcism, containment and holding it all. My mind is empty of all that happened; my body not yet, and perhaps it never can be.

❧

The place was called Mantra. We had everything. A kitchen, laundry, jacuzzi tub, food, bath salts, gifts from Mirjana, our host from STARTTS, and a balcony overlooking the ocean on the Gold Coast of Australia. I walked on the beach at sunrise every morning. My class was wonderful, very bright people, including Richard Clarke and Leon Petchesky. When Leon introduced himself, he said, "There are two people I want to meet in the US, Barack Obama and Sebern Fisher." I was almost speechless, but said that I wished to meet Barack Obama, too. Pauline at the desk took on the challenge to find the origin of my name, thinking that it would be an easy task. She was an expert at ancestral searches. "Your name," she said, "just kinda disappears."

At dinner at his home, I told Leon about my patient's entirely auditory dream after her first neurofeedback session for intractable depression: "The path to the enigma is now clear." "This is," he said, "the voice of God." In the midst of all the brain map speculations, the technical fascination with the EEG, protocols and epilepsy, I talked about Non Self. It was a stretch for many there, but it is where neurofeedback has brought me.

We flew back to Sydney and its speed—buses, cars, motorbikes, taxis, the swirl and slam around Hyde Park. At the coffee shop near the hotel, there was a photo of the waitress taken with Thầy. We talked when I drank my coffee there every morning.

My colleague Evain bemoans the competition in neurofeedback and the lack of publication. "If you're in a business, you make money—not happening; if you're in a science, you publish—not happening."

"Until the paradigm shifts from mind to brain, we will have the 'salmon problem' and the pissing contest."

"I know what a pissing contest is. What is the salmon problem?"

"There is a lottery in Alaska that allows the winners to go on a hike to see grizzly bears up close. The guide carries a gun and all, but he has never needed to use it. The bears collect at a stream when the salmon are running. When there is enough salmon, there is no killing. Everyone who has invested their lives and mortgages in this is afraid of it dying, and so models become stakes, not just part of the conversation. Everyone lives in fear. I am trying to do something about that. It's my main interest in neurofeedback."

"Yes, we live in fear brains, we are wired for that. It's a game changer when you quiet fear." I feel a similar gratification that I feel when Bessel stops and listens. It's different from Arles. When he stops and aligns with me, I breathe my own breath. With Bessel, it's just good that he listens. I like to stop him. I had a brief moment with Sandy McFarlane, like that, too, as he listed off all the symptoms shared by PTSD and TBI. The only one not shared, he said, was dizziness. "It makes you wonder, doesn't it, Sandy, what is 'psychological?'" He smiled as if he might have agreed before being distracted by another person taking his elbow.

"Do you feel the energy?" she asked. Mirjana was giving me a tour of STARTTS in a suburb of Sydney.

"Oh yes, trauma like this thickens the air and permeates the walls, doesn't it?" We talked about opening windows with exhaust fans at the end of each day, playing Gregorian chants, and saging the building regularly. I learned this with Reggie.

"Most people here," she said, "don't seem to feel it. But that can't really be possible."

On the way home from the airport after the impossibly long trip, we stopped to see Emily. She was at the door, tall in her pink and white striped PJs. She danced in circles before she greeted us. She had told her mom, "I am so excited!"

I feel as if I am breathing differently. Bessel and Ruth have taken on neurofeedback. It will not die.

❧

One night here near Yosemite, I caught myself going into a dream. I was able to watch the images and stories in one mind slip into another consciousness, flipping over like the magician's playing cards. Then I was drawn back into the mind of the observer and then eased myself back into sleep, that whole magic show gone.

The deep soul, Yosemite.

It is Emily's fourth birthday. I argue with the rising apprehension that has such deep meaning somewhere in my brain and heart and none at all anywhere else. I can't make sense of it. It feels impossible. I broke down again over the men working in the kitchen and screamed, "I just want them out of here!" I couldn't miss the wild desperation, the feeling of being trapped in my own home. The terror flips to rage, then to tears. I think of the time that Arles guided me through the repainting of his office building. I insisted that there were three men just outside. When I failed to understand, he took me outside to see that in the present, there was only one. It is as if the memory of the attic recertifies itself, and there is no way out of there.

"Remember, Sebern, that you can call me if you need to." I was surprised, not stunned, but clearly surprised that this had not occurred to me at all. I don't validate the impact of terrible events when they don't threaten my sanity. I don't know, it's like learning that a loved one is missing and thought dead, but there is no body. Grieving depends on the body. It feels like a small furry animal, even cute, is chewing away beneath my ribs.

Were I to use the Hafiz sense of it, I feel "Near." There really is nothing to be said. I am following my body.

Chapter 19

I walked up the hill to the 5:30 vigil. It is the fourth day of Advent, and snow and wind. After the service is a silent breakfast: pouring Raisin Bran, the sectioning of grapefruit, the filling of the cup, the drip of the coffee, the toaster popping, and jam lids off and on. I am warmed by these preparations and the plenitude. I am warmed by the rustle of winter coats—Weather Tamer and Eddie Bauer's—there is no more wool, and the whine of zippers that seem sadder gliding down and happier going up. This is my community. Not my faith community, but my practice community. I am drawn here by their protection, by the gift of the morning when I return to my room and get back into bed, read briefly, and then turn toward the Theta opening. My mind unspools silver ribbon with gold flecks and unspools and unspools until the room is filled. I time-travel. I visit others who are strangers to me. I don't quite have the control yet to stop and ask who they are, and I don't remember where I go. But it seems to happen only here at Weston. It is this experience that feels so rich and so deep, and for that, my brothers shelter me. They may even, without knowing, cherish it. Monasteries, Arles tells me, are for exactly this: monks hold the place of "no-thing." And it takes the snow, the solitude of the mountain and the sacred time, today, when the light begins its return.

I am not on a journey or a path; that is too linear. I am not a seeker. There is nothing out there to be sought. There is no "I" except by convention. I rarely have desires, hopes or dreams and even more rarely disappointments. The dissolution of the I—the intimate fusion with all things—Weston harbors that. I come here because I am held here, because there is no other place like it and because there is no other place to go. It cannot be replicated. When it goes, it will be a terrible loss even to, maybe even mostly to, those who've never heard of it.

I had prepared myself as best I could for Emily turning four. But I am reminded that there is no talking to the subcortical drivers, no preparing —well, yes, preparing—but no stopping them. She came out to the house wearing a long blue down coat, open of course, and in response to my sense of seeing her as "new" each time, she said, "I am growing up." So it may be that this terrible clanging is just the fact that she is four.

Dawn is pale orange, a popsicle. It is so cold that everything is still. Even before I saw that it was 0° this morning, I would have known; the trees, the snow 3 feet, the wires, even the light seemed frozen, still. No children are out of their warm beds or birds out of their cold ones.

Peggy maintains that someone can be awakened—Trungpa—and it is an entirely separate condition from being emotionally well. I was raised by Thich Nhat Hanh, Arles Gabriel and neurofeedback, and I don't believe that. I told her about the book request from Andrea Dawson at Norton as if this were a piece of news to just jot down. She was delighted.

This young woman, who travels among spheres, came to me because of a lingering past-life fear. She understood it was irrational, not because it was from a past life but because it was. Knowing this, should she be afraid of death? But she was. She had been murdered; her throat slit by a man who was afraid of her healing powers. She did nothing to provoke it except to continue, and she knew it would happen. We came to the agreement that this was PTSD work. She is a stable and happy person, good parents, a satisfying career in medicine and a paranormal vision. We did the best we could with informed consent. We explored how she would feel if she lost some or all of her extra-sensory experiences. At first, she found it hard to imagine seeing the bedroom without the ghost. Will you miss it? Will it be a loss? This is always the deep question of informed consent with neurofeedback. Will you miss the terror, the OCD, the temper, the identity? The symptoms are easy, we think, to say goodbye to, but what of the person they are scripting? After the requisite twenty eyes-open sessions where we focused on her use of marijuana and sugar competing and complementary desires, she did her first Alpha-Theta session. She said that there was no separation between herself and the universe; the sun was on her chest, then the stars and the moon.

"Oh," she said, as an afterthought, "I met my slit-the-throat guy. He had dark curly hair. His knife turned into a lily, and he stroked the side of my face with it. Then we walked together on the beach."

I have turned away from my journal, disinterested, maybe because it has been propelled so much by need. It is a need that brings me back to it tonight. Bob was working on my brainstem, and I felt that a great darkness was just out of reach of his finger, that it was right there, the black heart of Moses. I saw this, the vast dark continent, me in the middle of his heart. It's in my pulse, beneath my pulse, thrumming, racing, trapped. I thought of Emily. If anyone touched her cockeyed, I would attack them, and my failed murder defense would be temporary insanity, which, mistakenly to Bob, I call "legal insanity." And my parents left me with him. They have left every night as I twisted in the stairwell until this day. Like a deep bruise on the brainstem, the airy white Westchester house is the second dark continent.

I was playing with Emily in her room while the others had dinner. I thought I heard John mention Arles. My mind fell through a crack, a tear in time. I was suddenly in some place where family members report on each other to the secret police. I felt the damp terror of it. No safety. It was a flashback of betrayal, beyond or aside of this lifetime, where I was not safe, no one is safe, even within their family.

Sabelle graduated from college, and she is talking about graduate school. I brought her flowers from Bessel. She was beaming with her accomplishment, and there we were together.

Whenever I head downstairs without my glasses, I am flooded by the memory of Emily. I slept with her during the night out for Blake and Todd to see the Celtics. She was grumpy when she woke up and protested some shift in the covers. I went to let the dogs out, and there she was as I turned around, handing me my glasses, holding them at the bridge. "Here, Grammy, you forgot your glasses." I am touched by her selflessness, flexibility and care. Last weekend, she noticed a scratch on my hand, and she covered it with a Disney Band-Aid. She knows how to apply them perfectly. Her mother's hands are in hers. As she was unwrapping the third one, I said,

"I don't want you to waste your Band-Aids, Ems."

She was clear with me. "I am not wasting them! They are for your cut."

"I should hear about the book this week. I have received so many gifts, I need to make a contribution." Arles looked genuinely surprised that I worried about that. I will look forward to writing the book, but I will not be crushed if it is not accepted.

Marsha's story came out in The New York Times on June 22, and there seems to have been no negative repercussions. I got a few calls and some emails thanking me. Arles disparaged it, "They haven't given that much coverage to Afghanistan," and compared this to other, more important acknowledgments of personal demons like Freud's or Margaret Little's. For her part, Marsha said, "I never used this to understand myself."

❧

"Would this be happening," he asked, "if I were doing neurofeedback?" I hadn't considered this. I was talking about the ending.

"Perhaps not," I realized, in thinking about the exchange, that he meant having adopted it with patients, and that didn't occur to me. We would have gone further and deeper together if he had pursued his interior in this way. Then he'd understand what I am trying to say when I say there is no inside and no outside, that the diffusion at my edges no longer exists because I no longer exist. He wants to think this is our therapy, but we have both said at different times that this is something new, in the process of definition, of being indefinable. If it is therapy, then it is over; a job well done, an endeavor he surely can be proud of, me a bit less so, as I gave in so totally to dysregulation, to infancy. If this were therapy, he would want it to be over, and I wouldn't. In this loss, I think he is at the mercy of what he knows, scared, at least with me, to discover something new. What I want in all of my relationships is to come awake, fully awake. I have noticed that time moves more slowly when I see him less, as if pages in my calendar turned in reference to him. Now they turn as they turn, in no hurry, no jumping ahead, no needing to be with him. I am not at that place where I don't want to see him, but I want the more awakened one that is not overtaken by the rip tides in his brain.

We celebrated Todd's birthday at a long table at the Eastside, his older daughters, his nephew, Blake, John, Emily and me. I only remember one bit of the conversation. We were celebrating the constancy of where we live in the western part of Massachusetts, each glad that blizzards were the worst weather event we had, and we knew how to manage those.

It was not predicted. Emily was with her half-sisters and their mother, Jackie, taking Sarah, the youngest of her three, to her senior prom. The sky yellowed, and the winds came up as they dropped her off at the MassMutual Center downtown in Springfield. They headed home and never made it. Trees, poles and wires were coming down. They passed a traffic control meter that was clocking the wind at 95 MPH. They took brief refuge in a nursing home until the wind and slashing rains died down. They got as far as a friend's house, a surgeon and his wife who sheltered them for the night. Todd tried every route to his daughters, and he had to turn back. It was dark now and devastated. Emily and Jackie went to sleep on a large bean bag chair in the basement. At one moment in the long motherless night, Emily woke briefly and said to Jackie, "I still love you." At dawn, Blake found her way around barricades and trees and live wires, to gather her child, still asleep on the beanbag chair, up into her arms.

In Lenox, two weeks later, we sat at the outdoor table for an early supper. The skies were getting darker. Emily slipped away, and I followed her inside. There was no prediction. I asked her if this was reminding her of the tornado. She nodded. "That was so scary, wasn't it?" She nodded. "Trees falling down and wires and rain and thunder and Mommy wasn't there. Very scary." Confirmed. "But now, Emily, we are all here," I named us, all, "right?"

She said, "Yes."

"And where is the tornado?"

"It's gone," she said. I sat with her and watched her take this in. In her time, she got up, took my hand and went back out to the stormy patio. It turned out that there was a tornado, and John went through another near miss in Plainfield.

I was with a patient when the building began to sway side to side. We both simultaneously said, "What's happening?" Once I decided that it was not my own vestibular event, we both realized that it was an earthquake.

Clesson Brook was flooded by Hurricane Irene, and they had to rescue residents in the next town over with helicopters. FEMA was sent here. Our road collected all the water pouring off the hillsides and down the driveways and became its own river. In Northampton, the Connecticut was as wide and muddy as the Mississippi, carrying full-length trees, barn doors, a blue Adirondack chair, a coffin, rushing downstream. The cornfields were flattened, and pumpkins floated.

It started with Bob, something had happened. As it came, I told him. "I was six or seven, and I was walking with my dog Teddy in the field like I always did, when a man came out of the woods and hit me on the head. I feel the injury this time, the swirling of unconsciousness and nausea, the slight memory of being carried to my father's arms. This was known, and the man was sought, but there is no story of this in my family. I don't know. There's a dent there. It comes and goes."

I felt the temporal lobe wonkiness, and I could feel my frontal cortex slipping off line. I am, moment by moment, herding my brain into the task at hand. It feels like something else is arising, and I am tired of it, disinterested and even in futile protest. Nothing seems to be happening, and Bob said, "I'll release here, at my temples, I think," and there was an explosion. I knew what was coming, unknown and unbidden. It was

Milici's voice fading, the end of the phone call, the possibility that I heard the phone ring as I slipped into a coma, the sense of commotion, my dying body taken to the hospital. There were no distinct or clear memories. I was remembering being unconscious. Somehow each period of losing consciousness was represented—the fall down the stairs at the dentist, the passing out in the bathroom at the Smith infirmary, the knock to my head when I was thrown from the tall bay on the trail, the coma, the black out in the Black Forest, in and out of that, even the dentist pulling my teeth—once the wrong one and from that I woke up crying. Twice, back with Bob, I thought I would throw up. Once I even started off the table, but he moved something, and the nausea was gone. I don't understand what happened in my brain or why my psyche took me there. It felt as if Bob had lifted a dark ancestral cap off the top of my head, and after the energy exploded and slowly dispersed in tears and discharge, I felt clear.

"It's over, Bob."

"You have thought that before," he said, as if to shield me against false hope, but then he said, "and I guess you've never really been wrong. I think this may be threshold work for a new level. The releases make it confusing where exactly I am."

"I just feel different. It feels as if there is no density, not even the slightest, that will pull these particles that are now out in far outer space, back into my field."

We celebrated my 70th birthday among friends at the Guest House Retreat in Chester, Connecticut: The Neurofeedback Mystery Tour. We had wanted to call it the Neurofeedback Magical Mystery Tour, but we were notified not to do this by the Beatles. It is a TED-style conference on neurofeedback at the edge of its potential. Ruth presented her amazing results on dissociation with 8 to 12 Hz down, and she'll get published. Larry Hirshberg talked about aging, David Kaiser about brain evolution and the social self, and Moshe Perl about the biography in the EEG. Emily was, for the most part, among the audience, either next to her mother or on her lap. Moshe asked the assembled community if they could see what he was pointing to at P6, and many answered yes. Her "Yes!" rang through the adult voices. Everyone laughed, and she was embarrassed, but she was quickly and easily soothed. People commented on her presence. Moshe called her "the second force, the balance to the first force of the rest of us." She was the child I expected her to be. She found her way to Mirjana's room. She took Rae's hand. She came to me several times to tell me she loved me. In a private moment, she looked at me and said, "Grammy, these people really love you!" It felt that way to me, too. Everyone was having a very good time, but it was Emily who made the party, who made the balance and may have set the tone. I have worried that I have never felt joy, but I do now, and for now, it is through her and in her.

Jay McMahon, a friend and professional magician, put on the show after dinner. He gave Emily a red ball and asked her to squeeze it hard. When she opened her hands, wide-eyed, she said, "Now there are two! I love this!"

It took me time to locate the feeling of being crushed, my bones at odd angles and muscles pulled. Then I got it. It was the way I felt after Johnny's death, run over twice. It helped to know. When I sat to meditate, I could see him and feel him in a space close to me. He was as he was with me, at a near distance and out of reach. I didn't actively miss him. I felt animal grief. Bob addressed what he described as "a ball of energy in the sacrum." He felt the powerful forces, engaging, integrating, working things out. He said when he got there, he expected a release, but was told, "We're talking!" Active inchoate processing. It has its own slow-moving integrity that doesn't involve me.

"My history doesn't matter. History and self disappeared in tidal stutter-steps; they washed away like yesterday's sandcastles. It has been that I could see no horizons, no place formed around me, almost like a fetus without a womb. It was that I was always scared. I am not scared anymore of being scared. And now there is a Nauset horizon, blues, pinks, silver, but I am not looking at it, I am within it. I am of it."

"Are you lonely, Sebern?" I nodded.

"Sometimes I am. But that doesn't matter either."

No form, no teachers and the best minds, his and Eva's, have turned away from this deep practice. They have their own. I have no company in this. At dinner at Bessel's club, Ed said, "You are the body and soul of neurofeedback." I have nobody to wear these mantels. The ego that has long awaited its acknowledgment looks around to find itself no longer there. Something in me feels the absence. I may even wish for its momentary return to have a bowl of this fruit. I tried to explain this to Arles yesterday. But the self can still form, and it's always the injured self.

"You know," Arles said, almost wistfully, "You are exceptional in your willingness to stay with something that is often very painful. You've always had that, and a few others do. It transcends phenomena. It is 'of the numina.'"

The summer is past. The soft dawn sky is as undecided as an infant's eyes. The sun is expected, and when it comes, I will watch it fill the grove with gold, lighting the top of the trees like candles before it drops down and fills the bowl of earth outside my window. The summer brought a drought after a slug-soaked spring. Where do they go when the rains dry up? The days are deep with sun and warm. I was again on the Vineyard. I can compare this experience for experience. There is always a trace body memory to compare now to then. It is so much easier to live in my skin. I move smoothly in the air, in the parking lot, on the deck of the freighter. I can tell that this island is comforting and welcoming to John because it is known. It is comforting and welcoming for me because it's not. I recognize everything as it was last year, but it is as if the friction disappeared. We went to The Black Dog for a sweat-shirt, bad coffee and a good cinnamon twist. I was doing as I so often do, managing my brain, trying to find the right food or drink with the right dose to settle it into a notch. Very wrong choice. I had another small but significant event. Thankfully, John cooked, and he and our friend San went off to Edgartown in the morning, leaving me to slip into Theta on my little bed in the back room. I moved through it, hovering in a suspended consciousness, riddled a bit with concerns that I wouldn't pull out. Finally, I could move and took myself to South

Beach to get my head underwater and be tossed around in the freezing surf. I swam as much as one does in the North Atlantic and then lay on the beach and talked to a woman sitting near me, an epidemiologist from Cambridge, about, of course, neurofeedback.

But the event didn't clear completely until after I saw Arles. He commented on my swagger. I went into the office with the monster shadow looming, and I am, when this happens, fundamentally ashamed and simultaneously incapacitated and impenetrable. I know how to train, but I can't. I lose agency. He stepped into that. That is what that state—disorganized, unseen, motherless—still needs. He had to organize me and nurture my awareness. He moved from his defensive position, and I moved from mine, and we found each other, and my brain settled down. I told him that I had states of bliss and then the shadow. He talked about the crushing descent. Not quite crushed because there is too little ego, but it confuses and shames me.

"I want," I said to him, "to be clear for Emily."

"Yes."

Yesterday, a 20-year-old kid dressed himself in black, murdered his mother in their home, drove to the school where she'd taught in Newtown, Connecticut and gunned down 20 first-grade children and six teachers and then of course himself. Last night I felt all of my organs rubbed raw. The horror is not in its incomprehensibility but in how comprehensible it seems. There is a tumor in Adam Lanza's brain, either by mass or by function, but the sadness and the slaughter in this world seem unrelenting. President Obama worked with himself not to weep when he spoke of the beautiful children, all of them really everywhere cut down by massacre, by gang, by holocaust, by rape, by madness, by gun. Senseless acts; there is no such thing. I can find no empathy for the madness of the shooter. I think only of Emily and the terrible suffering of the parents, grandparents and siblings of those Emilys in those families, all still bright lights, only one or two brewing their own terror, their own potential for murder. He shot his mother four times in the face and murdered those who took her away from him, whom she loved more. She is never counted among his victims.

Last night, when I couldn't sleep, I counted my patients who were better, like counting sheep. I worked at a cleft in my own energetic body between a collapse into sadness and misery and the beauty of life in all its human, wrought catastrophe. I love my children and my grandchildren. We live now in the wake of the mass murder of our children by a child.

Blake is working through a breast cancer scare. She broke my heart when she told me how much it meant to her when I said we would all be there, surrounding her with care and safety. In some place within her, she doesn't know this as a given. It is the awful hollow heritage passed down the maternal line. Emily was grinding her teeth when her mom was facing the threat that no one told her about.

I tried to sit up and attend to the manuscript, but I kept drifting from it, and no act of will could keep me in the chair. I mourn the children, but even more their brief moments of terror and the impossible grief of their parents. I wandered around in my own vacant mind, deep in the blood and sorrow of Sandy Hook. Women and children. Who can stand this? Blake was anxious about the weather, but she and Todd understood that they had to see Emily. After they left, I sat down again to write. I was getting headaches, my tailbone hurt, and my sacrum ached. I couldn't stay, and I couldn't go to Northampton. I couldn't concentrate. I drove the back roads to Yankee Candle to get some fire starters, hoping probably just to get warm, and the day closed in more. At some point, driving in the winter mix, I realized that I was cutting a wide swath around Northampton. I couldn't go into my attic room. I made up errands and took the longest and most dangerous roads. On Tuesday, I shook with chills. I stayed in bed, without a radio or TV. I couldn't bear to hear the endless replay.

If we are able to forgive in Newtown, who is it? This boy? His mother? His father? The NRA? The gun lobby? What total madness, a group that lobbies to make sure Adam Lanza could do this.

When I saw Bob the next day, I was calmer, but the curvature was there, the arched back of the orphan. "You could drive a truck through here," he said. I had no idea. I followed my body. I had no choice.

I am able to pick up the book again. This chapter is "somewhat of a brute," the term Andrea, my editor, used, but I think I see my way through it. I hope for power tomorrow, but that may be too much to ask in the midst of this nor'easter, this wild and sad beauty.

Emily learned a poem on her class trip to Emily Dickinson's house, and she was most sure of the first two lines that she recited to me: "I am nobody. Are you nobody too?"

"After a hard day of formlessness," I said to Arles, "it's good to come home to containment, to being seen and remembered in form." He smiled at me warmly. I want him to look clearly at me, see no one at all and know it is me.

I live in the sunshine of the present. It filters softly through the trees, cradling me in innocence and beauty and safety and peace. But every once in a while, a switch is thrown, and the light and the present disappear, and all that was good and nurturing just a moment before turns perverse and terrifying. The light changes, and I feel a slight convulsion in my belly. Those are the moments that I would turn on myself. I know it is a neurological event, I don't believe it, but I am it. Usually, now I know what sets it off. This afternoon, I was watching Top of the Lake, Jane Campion's working it out. I set off up the new gravel road along the high-tension wires, a steep, hard walk. I was pulled up the hill by adrenaline. It is terrible when the light changes and the very things and people that nurtured you just one minute ago now savage you. It means that it's time to train. It's still got its microchips in me. Bob discharged one in my mouth an hour after Emily asked me to pull her first loose tooth. She opted to wait for Grandad, whom I told her was "the expert," but it set up its trace, and he followed it to some unspeakable crime against my baby's body.

This book, which seems never-ending, disturbs my sleep further. I had two dreams in the last week, and in the dreams, I couldn't sleep.

During one day in the final press of the edits, I had states of awakening. I realized that in all mystical traditions, the encounter with the divine was made possible by or was the same as the loss of Self. Brain regulation was this path for me. I lost my Self as I lost fear. It was a simple but complex equation. Arles and I talked about Trungpa, and he asked me to look at the capacity of his practice to embrace the demons. Trungpa had a rainbow body. He was also very destructive. Arles sees this as the capacity of his practice; I see it as delusion alongside his practice. He stopped the debate.

"Let's bring this closer to home," Arles said, "Tell me about Moses."

I feel calm in this encounter with Moses. Now the most salient memory, deeply felt, is his cradling and rocking me and his tears dropping on my face. "Without him," I said, "I might never have existed."

HEG

We are both quite taken with the mountains when we can see them. John said it doesn't quite feel like the US, more like New Zealand. It is the landscape of the west more than the east, but not as far beyond our tiny human scale. We went to train in HEG with Jeff Carmen at his home near Lake Placid. Jeff had taken an infrared photo of my prefrontal cortex, and he could not restrain himself, "This is not good!" and he went on to compare it to a man he treated who had been blown up in a tank. We did five minutes of training there in Albany, and the next day, I didn't want coffee. There in Keene Valley, he took another series of infrared photos, and mine was better than it had been a month before and better yet, the next day.

The effects are both subtle and profound. Generally, I am a bit better organized, which is to say there is a reduction in the fluster factor. I am less bothered by the light at the dentist. I am more steady. A little more easy-going. Getting to things. More exercise. Headaches.

By Monday, the bones in my face ached. I felt muscles I didn't know were there under my cheeks and pressure on my palate.

"Your head is the size of a child's," Bob said calmly as if somehow he was not surprised. He pulled on a pair of thin blue latex gloves and worked in my mouth to open the suture of my upper palate, and when he did, my head expanded into its adult size and form! I felt it.

"What is this?!"

"I'm not sure. I've never seen this before. You tell me."

I shook my now adult-sized head, "I don't have a fucking clue."

That morning, while I was driving to the carwash, the subtle gray, slightly tragic background state I have inhabited shifted, suddenly, to an entirely different background: early spring, leaf green, and with it came a stream of light going through my left eye and out my left prefrontal cortex. I slipped into it. I spoke to myself: 'People are happy even with all the tragedy, even with Sandy Hook, and I can do that'. I fell into another slipstream. It was timeless; it felt before trauma, a time unknown before that morning. I became light where I'd always been dark. The axis in me had changed from dark/cool to dark/warm, and now to light/warm. I have never imagined this would be possible.

CHAPTER 20

My book arrived here yesterday, March 18, 2014. Bessel wrote, "Glory hallelujah! Nobody knows how much fucking work it is. Bookstores have become a totally different experience for me. Every one of those folks stayed up too late, shed tears, jeopardized relationships, and there it is, the fruit of your labor, the child of your mind and soul. Amazing! Love Bessel."

Andrea wrote, "I am so pleased that you are happy, Sebern. I have genuinely enjoyed getting to work with you and know you during this book-writing endeavor (not something I can always say, I admit). You taught me a great deal, and I know your readers feel the very same way. I hope we can get together to celebrate in person at some point. I would love to raise a glass to your accomplishment. We will be in touch, no doubt. I look forward to seeing it hit the shelves. All my best, Andrea."

And Ed, my friend and my reader, "I am so proud of you yet again, but this time for doing the writing you did to help bring such an important message of hope to the world. If anything I did made a contribution to the process, I am very pleased, but I also know it pales quickly in the light of what you did. I've been working on my own writing and know the struggles well. You persevered and poured yourself as well as your knowledge onto the pages you were writing. I will eagerly await my own copy and will press you for inscription and signature. It will be a prized member of my collection. Thanks, Sebern, for all you do and the person you are. With love and appreciation."

I myself don't know how to feel. Something like emerging from derealization into the shared reality. There it is, the real thing. I can't find my feet around the book. Other than the notable silence from Siegfried and Sue, of course, but others in the field as well, I have only received praise and gratitude. There isn't any place for this to land in me, much less to take hold. Many friends have said you must be excited, and I don't want to disappoint, but I feel neutral about it. And I am very glad it is out in the world and being received. A new way for people to think. And I was delighted yesterday when Eva said, unsolicited, "This is why I love your book."

I sat at the edge of Gaston Pond, the small lake near IMS, and meditated on the beetles, who were both frantic and organized, darting in brief spurts but circumscribed, it seemed, by the presence of their multitudes on the surface. They are at the service of their neurons and the embodiment of them. If it weren't for the five layers of cortical cells, approximately the thickness of Saran Wrap (crumpled and still this thin!), we would not be dealing with all these popping thoughts that seem as random as the beetles' jerks and squiggles, random and repetitive.

I don't experience the initial resistance that I often feel on retreats. I slip into the flow. I decided to fast on Sunday, and I awoke that morning, the fourth day of retreat, craving distraction. I was caught in this momentum and narrative until I pulled on my burnt orange fleece and slipped my hand into my pocket and onto the dharma beads my friend Barry made for me. I'd forgotten I'd brought them. I held them, and instantly it was over. I went to the hall to sit.

Larry spoke that night, and I laughed, and it broke something open in me, down to the particulate space of Non Self. Afterward, I was agitated, neither physically nor emotionally really, but perhaps foundationally, and I walked. I knew I could not sleep and might spend the night walking. Then I was crashing so fast that I might not make it to the 150 yards to my room. Then I didn't sleep. When I got out of bed, I wrote a note to Larry on a piece of scrap paper: "I got it! Thank you. I am left in many pieces, splayed out with no instructions. Perhaps an interview would help, or at least a hug before we leave." When I opened his note confirming a meeting at three, I felt an immense wave of grief. I tried to attach it to Arles or to Jakob or to the great grief of my life. It wasn't these.

Larry greeted me in his small office at the head of the stairs, "What does a guy have to do to get a hug around here?" We hugged like old friends, he closed the door, and I took a seat across from him. I tried to remain composed. It was hopeless.

"Why," I asked, crying in some new, very high pitch, "is this so emotional!"

"You have had an opening, they can be like that, don't get sidetracked. Just be with it." I told him about the particular self that is my default position and my confusion about why his teaching had been so big.

"It must've been confirmation."

"That's 'idea', Sebern."

"It was company, Larry. My Buddhist friends know what I am referring to, but haven't had the experience; others whom I love don't realize it at all. It was a kind of completion. It was the company."

"Do you think I have a lot of company? There aren't that many people even in this sphere..." he opened his arms, gesturing at the room, the building. "This is not Buddhist, you know that, right? This is every mystical tradition."

I sat enveloped and suddenly still.

"You mentioned grief. Tell me about that."

"I was happy to get your note and have looked forward to our meeting all day. This confuses me." I have loved Larry since I first met him at Plum Village over twenty years ago. He has been my very American Buddhist teacher. "What is this?"

"This grief is the ego's last stand. It does not want to die to itself."

When I stepped into the hallway, he popped out and wished me a good retreat. It was a "stay with it" message. I did. Engaged stillness. I was certain of my path.

I was introduced to the stim side of neurofeedback on the bank of the Saco River in Maine. It was more of a gathering than a conference, with people there using many different approaches to training the brain. With the encouragement of a colleague, I lay on a bed in an empty room on the second floor, and he pasted a flat flexible electrode to my forehead and one on each mastoid. I lay there expectant for forty minutes and a little apprehensive because this is my brain being fed high-frequency gamma. I chatted with my friends at first. Nothing much seemed to be happening except that I felt increasingly intrigued, which meant that something must be.

They lent me a system (which rents out at 2000 dollars a month!), and I'm running my own "clinical trials" with myself, John, Jakob, my friend Nina, and two of my patients. I may be making gains on sleep, but sleep aside, everything feels smoother. My balance seems better, my memory feels more reliable, and I feel better organized, more even. I have also had moments of all issues resurfacing—my heels hitting the back of the stairs, a jumble of fear and aversion toward the paper I was asked to write—familiar to me from episodes during the book. I've felt irritable, and I've needed caffeine and sugar. It is as if my brain is going through its Rolodex of reactions. Sam had some concerns last week. "This is a good, deep reorganization, but you're also a little toasted." I'd done two sessions the day before. I took three days off, and I've had four more sessions.

"Your brain is stable; your limbic brain is, well, 'placid.'"

"Have you ever seen this in me before?"

"I have never seen this in anyone."

It's unmistakable and still, with no regulation of sleep.

It is hard to believe that after 1000 sessions of neurofeedback, I could still experience something unique. Voids, unknown, become known as they fill with light. I feel clarified. The space between the particles of my being is even greater. People look like themselves in my dreams, and they are long, complex narratives.

I was in India. I was pulled back to the US, to Northampton, to my bed on the third floor, abruptly, as if grabbed by some force and yanked across continents and seas by waking up. I dreamt two dreams about Marsha, whom I haven't spoken to in months and who, of course, then called. *I was worried for her and described how she was trapped by DBT and had to get free of it, or she would die, and I expressed some concern for myself about being caught, trapped by neurofeedback.* The second dream was the night before she called me. *I had arranged for her to have an escort in our hotel suite. I wasn't watching, but could feel it as she experienced multiple orgasms. Then it was my turn, and I too.* I woke up fully aroused, but it was held somehow apart from the very body that felt it so completely, separately, in a dream state. When I told Marsha about this, she said, "These are the kind of dreams to have!" I dreamt of Johnny the night of his birthday, fully him. I couldn't hold the dream, but we were together that night and happily so.

Then this. *I was going down to the basement at Elizabeth Street. I stepped off the landing and into a spiderweb that stretched wall to wall. The basement was pitch black. There was sunlight behind me coming in from the window. I wasn't afraid of the dark, but recoiled when the web covered my face. In that sudden, primitive fear, I wiped hard at it to get free. When I did, I looked for the spider. It was the size of two fists and, only momentarily, a spider form. I tried to brush it off, afraid it would bite me, poison me, that I would die from it. It then became the Aztec sun, the legs of the spider were the sunbeams, and there was a hole in the center of the gold disc body, more two than three-dimensional. I could not get free of it. It clung to my leg, but it did not bite me. I realized as I was looking deeply into the unseeable or into the brainstem or both that it would always be with me, but it wouldn't kill me. I just sat on the stairs looking deeply into the absolute darkness of the basement, unafraid, the sunlight streaming in behind me.* Maybe this sense of being clarified is sunlight streaming into my brain/mind. It is almost true that my mind has dissolved into light.

I could not go to the Priory and hear the gospel again. I feel a secular emptiness. It's been my refuge from the unrelenting commercial drone of Christmas. I could not decorate the tree tonight; when I thought of putting candles out, I just couldn't. I will plug in the tree, but even that I feel a slight aversion to. The lights and the candles have always brought me happiness, and they don't. They feel more like a mandatory refrain, the thing to do because it is Christmas, but Christmas is hollow even at the Priory. Less so there but still so.

Thầy is in a hospital in Bordeaux. He had a brain hemorrhage on November 1. He came out of the coma in several days and now sleeps most of the time, either healing his brain or preparing to enter the bardo of death, or both. I am sitting here to join him in the field and focusing my meditation attention on my left prefrontal cortex. Earlier, I felt him awaken and then drift back into sleep. I feel this in my right temporal lobe and more widely through the right hemisphere. I find no turbulence and no refusal. He is OK doing what he must do, what he has practiced his whole life. He is peaceful. This field is peace.

I spoke with Arles about my moments with Thầy when I lived at the Lower Hamlet at Plum Village for almost three months. When I heard my name in the midst of the song of Vietnamese at the lunch table; when he asked where I was when the monks made dinner that night and I slipped off, sure of my anonymity, to take a bath a mile down the hill in the nuns' bathtub; when I fetched him from his library for lunch; when he took my hand and pulled me down to sit next to him as he reviewed his dharma talk on a tape deck in the gift shop at the Lower Hamlet. I commented on the violence in the phrase "killing time." He registered but did not respond. I'd written to him about John taking notes for me when he spoke at David Schoenbrun's class on Vietnam at Columbia. He asked to meet John at his Omega retreat. There is something between us, this teacher, this me. He opened a door, a wide French door to practice.

Chapter 21

The Buddha's Brain

Arles and I are doing as we do. We are renegotiating, more accurately, reunderstanding and recalibrating our relationship. I've been trying for a long time to get him to come on time; it never worked, and he had a way of making this my fault, "the time was too long, it was on Friday after a late night on Thursday, he'd made sacrifices."

"You are swaggering."

I felt only exhaustion and grief, "There is no swagger in me." He relented, and after 45 minutes, he let go. I resisted the word "sacrifice," but he held to this, and when I read what he did for me, it is, of course, true. I barely remember. The history that made his sacrifice necessary has evaporated.

"It isn't just not relevant anymore, it's just not there anymore. If I didn't have to write, it would not exist."

"I have been devoted to you," he said, his eyes filled with tears, "possibly more than to anyone else in my life."

We held each other for a long time before I left. I felt the strength of his body in stark contrast to his own feeling of exhaustion. The energy that kept us apart, that kept our particles separate, fell away, and we collapsed, grown body against grown body. There was nothing to say. He held me, and I held him, for minutes, one being. During our session, at the turning point, I took a tissue, recycled paper, the kind that can cut you. Blowing my nose, I said, "And this is shitty Kleenex! People have suffered enough. Get decent Kleenex!" He smiled warmly and nodded. "I will get better Kleenex."

Eckhart Tolle clearly has never heard the name Thich Nhat Hanh spoken. He mispronounces it the way people do when they take umbrage at the effort required to say a name right. The pain body he speaks of is the amygdala or the brainstem, less in a way, about the mind than the brain. I sit tonight, and I am swallowed whole by my history. I long for Arles. He and I lived in very different realities while we engaged passionately in this one. It wasn't possible to explore a trance within a trance or engage in the distance required for memory. He used the word "devoted." It is hardly adequate, but there is no better word.

I have been thinking about innocence. Arles never follows this line of inquiry. He embraced Catholicism for a long time and then psychoanalysis. He embraces original sin. Where is there a portal to innocence? I have been thinking of analysis as walking over sinkholes filled with vipers and CBT as walking in pools of concrete.

When Marsha and I talked recently, I said something like "the brain gives rise to behaviors," and she said reflexively and dogmatically, "No! Behaviors give rise to the brain." "Where," I thought as we said goodbye, "do we go with that?" She called a week later, perhaps forgetting this conversation entirely, to propose that we submit an R-34 to study neurofeedback for borderline personality.

I was called out of a neuroscience/neurofeedback meeting where I was struggling with the concept. It was a nurse at Saint Elizabeth's Hospital saying that I must come immediately to see my mother. I was in a cab with a stranger, and they were going to go to Brighton Beach. I asked if they would drop me off—it was on the way—but they were set on going first to Brighton Beach. I was told when I asked that it was 45 minutes out there and 45 minutes back. My pleas to be dropped off were, it seemed, falling on deaf ears. We were driving next to the ocean, and I said at least we are taking the beautiful way and then off on the right, across a field, I saw St Elizabeth's hospital. This time, he let me off, and I walked a ways across a field, then into the courtyard of the hospital. My mother was my mother in a gray suit, very well dressed and sitting at a table. Only when she rose to greet me did I realize that she didn't know me. She had advanced dementia even while looking pretty young and well put together. My breath left me, and then I felt compassion.

I have begun to step aside from the momentum of neurofeedback and turn my energy to saving my home. We live under an enormous threat here, the largest compressor station and longest gas pipeline in the US. Talented people have gathered in passionate opposition, but with a lack of focus –mine/ours included. So, I have begun to turn the huge ship of neurofeedback. I am faithful to it, but the demand is immense, and I can begin to offload the staggering burden. I have brought the gift, written the book, taken the shots, and made the trips. Neurofeedback saved my life. It can't take it now.

"It feels as if the whole history is etched in tiny script on this bone," I said to Arles, referring to my increasingly yielding sacrum.

"When bones are left of someone in a rainbow body, some of them have inscriptions of the Heart Sutra on the bone. Naturally occurring. Go to the Forest Refuge. You will find yourself there."

Blake and Emily came to visit on Sunday. Emily had been thinking on the way up, and she asked, "Grammy, you love the Buddha, don't you?"

"Yes, I do. Ems."

"I think you are the Buddha, Grammy." I gathered her up and then, holding her shoulders, I tilted her slightly away.

"We all have the Buddha within us. You have too."

"You are peaceful and calm, Grammy."

"I wasn't always so peaceful, sweetheart. I had to come to it."

Driving home from The Trauma Conference, I mistakenly dialed Marsha. She called back,

"Did you call me or did your phone call me?" She sounded exhausted, just back from a NIMH council meeting where they discussed neurofeedback. "They are very open to it," she assured me. Why do I have no sense of this? Why is Bessel turned away at the NIMH gates?

She'd sent me her manuscript, the Institute chapter. I wrote her what I hope she finds a helpful critique, but I said that she would not want this published. I left her a phone message too: "How can the most famous psychologist in the world say she doesn't understand why she was in the hospital? You can't say this, Marsha, even if it's true. And you know, I know why you were in the hospital." I haven't heard back. Poor Marsha, I love her, and this book is a curse.

In the quiet of an early holiday morning in Northampton, I saw a man dart across the street toward me, and I turned and saw a bird on her back, both wings fluttering. He scooped her up in his large, gentle hands.

"Was she hit?" I asked.

"I'm not sure. She may have stunned herself on the window." It was a cardinal, and he caressed her.

"She will heal in your energy," and he said, sweetly, a little afraid as we are in these hopeless, helpless, nothing else to do situations of unbearable innocence; "I hope so."

"She will".

But then I left. As I sat tonight, I wished I had this presence of mind, the gift of this stranger and of the bird, who I think is now flying.

At IMS, Jack brought his hands to his heart. "Wherever you are, take refuge in me." That is an astonishing prayer.

I walked to the pond to visit my beetle teachers, not as many as I'd remembered. Perhaps I conflated the memory with the activity of neurons that they came to represent. I waited for a while to see if I could discern a pattern, make a hypothesis or design a rule. This was what Darwin and Galileo did. I felt their company for a moment. I walked back feeling a bit more stiff than I care to be:

The annoyance of it,

barking dog of old age,

Living

interfering

with living.

❧

It's now late September. I am still wearing the red protection cord Jack gave us on the IMS retreat. I returned from San Francisco late on Friday, August 29, in an altered state, waves pushing through me, always left to right. I read *Whiskey and Charlie* and lay briefly in the sun. John took the calls, such as they were, and we kept the media off. I was overloaded. Solitude was the only solace. John protected me even from him. When I needed to eat, he fed me. On Saturday morning, I took a bit of Thầy's bread and ate it, and took the rest of the loaf to the compost at the end of the field. I was tired of managing the waves and just beginning to unfold into my home. On Sunday morning, I went out to the compost box. The bread was gone, only the bread. The tall grass was bent over about six feet away, toward the woods. There was a circle pressed into the grass where the bear sat to eat Thầy's bread. When I told Emily about this, she said, "Now the bear is blessed too."

3230 Jackson St. Thầy is trying to walk with the support of two young monks and is just turning in the hall away from the front door. I went upstairs with Phap Linh and tried to set up the system. "It can only be the cable," he said, and of course it is. I trained Phap Linh's brain initially as a proxy for Thầy's, exhausted and disoriented and stressed as he was by Thầy's moaning. They described Thầy's mood as erratic. At times, I'm told he's completely there, and others, gone, and then it's not clear if he understands. He will be doing this odd, foreign neurofeedback thing on trust and intuition—perhaps mostly from his Siddhic awareness.

Arles just taught me that word after my long weekend of solitude and quiet. No demand but the powerful waves of energy; taking in, holding, releasing, unfolding. All I could say was, "Oh my God, oh my God" or simply, "Now."

I dreamt that *I was in a squared off van, with other people who knew that we were about to have a very serious car accident. A moment later, out of nowhere, we were hit on the right side by another car I didn't see, and we rolled. No seatbelts. Serious injuries. Ambulances. At the ER, I was taken almost immediately for a course of Electroconvulsive Therapy. The doctor was insistent. I refused, "I have a concussion, I don't need ECT!" He tried again to persuade me. I told him that he was not a good doctor and left.* The dream had power that slips away in the telling. As it turned out, it was deeply accurate. I didn't realize this until after the day-long seizure on Tuesday.

I walked ahead of John to Jake's for a ritual breaking of the fast that begins at 7:30 on Sunday night and ends on Tuesday at 7:30 AM. I could only eat one egg. I felt queasy and nervous. I wondered if I was getting sick. By 10 or so, I was having a very hard time holding my head together. I know these neuronal meltdowns, and somehow, I'm able to organize thoughts and speech through them. My patient didn't seem to notice. I watch for this when I can't seem to keep my brain stable. At lunchtime, the hypoglycemic part kicked in, and I tried to find the right food, heavy in sugar and fat, measuring my reactivity, planning ahead for the next food, trying to balance. By now, the worst is over in my head. I am trying to quiet my stomach and my sacrum and tailbone. I felt kicked. My calves knotted up, and by that night, I felt pain in the arched soles and then the curved bones at the top of both feet. The only thing to call it would be a slow-moving seizure. I felt mostly clear of it the next morning, post-ictal and rearranged. Bob felt the impact of the event immediately. He leaned on my sternum and moved my teeth, which were also subtly displaced in the event. Cranio-sacral, palate, ears. I felt 100% better. On Friday, I saw Sam, and my body opened to a new level of revelation. There was the compression of my spine, broken ribs and concussion. The car is coming right at me. Brain bruise is memory, untouched in any work until that morning. Prepare to die, my head thrown toward and away, my back and ribs trapped by the seat, and Mary's sudden body thrown on top of mine. The Tuesday event didn't clear until late morning on Wednesday, when the heavy bowel movement itself felt sick.

I told all of this to Arles, who seemed to be looking mostly into the middle distance, claiming that space. It kept my story, the words like cartoon musical chords, dancing close to my mouth. He acknowledged a detail here and there to reassure me that he was in the room and at some point, he said, as if on a phone overseas,

"Do you think the field of Thầy's brain injury fused with the field of your brain injury?" I had been stammering about the flow of these events, but not at this level, and there it was. Multiplying fields, quantum fields of knowing each other, from my offer to go, to his greeting me and giving me all that he had to give, at first his bread and then his trust. We were in this unrelenting, relenting, forgiving and unforgiving field of injury together. I am clearer since the sessions, and my sleep is different. Driving home from Arles, I realized that the shape of the dream van, a detail that kept insinuating itself, was the shape of Thầy's wheelchair van that Phap Linh and Phap Huu used to pick me up at the airport.

Phap Linh looked at his watch. "Have you eaten?"

"A Kind Bar on the plane."

"Aren't you hungry?"

"Ahh, yes, I am. I hadn't quite noticed."

I followed him downstairs to the kitchen to find some leftovers from lunch. Thầy was there, his back to the door, eating a piece of bread from a round, freshly baked loaf. The nuns exclaimed, "Thầy, it is Sebern!" He turned toward me, and he lit up.

"Thầy recognizes you! He hadn't recognized your name. Wonderful!" Thầy offered me a piece of his bread. "Do you realize the honor of this?" the sister asked. I nodded. I felt overwhelmed by the honor, no sleep, hunger and the fact that gluten makes sores in my mouth. I bowed to Thầy. He gave me the loaf.

Thầy asked for neurofeedback that evening.

I had vetted this training with experts who use it for patients in their hospital the day after a stroke. They had never seen a secondary bleed or any other negative effects, with the exception of increased arousal if the protocol was wrong. Ed was backing me up. Phap Linh understood the technology and the premise of neurofeedback. Our goals were to help to decrease Thầy's pain and periods of agitation, to help his digestion and to increase the number of hours he could sleep.

I placed the silver sensors on the head of the Buddha. I have never felt more stressed. Everyone was friendly, everyone was hopeful, everyone was apprehensive, and everyone seemed to be in the room with us. He trained for six minutes before waving me off. I walked down the hill and up the hill to my Airbnb, put the loaf in the fridge, wrote my report to Ed and collapsed into a crumpled sleep on the mattress on the floor.

The morning report was good. Thầy had less pain, slept for five hours and wanted to train that day.

On the third day, we sat as usual, I on his left and Phap Linh on his right. Thầy put his gentle hand on my cheek.

"Oh, thank you, Thầy. I really needed that." His condition improved every day, and he could train a minute longer each time. He knew when it was enough. I sat with my teacher and sat through my fear every session, "You know, Thầy, you are a rock star with this training." I think he smiled, but it was a little hard to tell.

I came in on day five, and Thầy had decided to go to the beach, which delighted everyone. He hadn't been getting out. On day 6, Thầy pointed to C3. Dr. Quoc, his osteopathic physician, had shown me the fMRI from July, and the hemorrhage had claimed the left frontal quadrant. "This should have killed him," he said. "It may have been white matter that saved him. It is exceptional. Probably from his practice." When he pointed to his left hemisphere, Thầy was deciding his protocol. "You're right, Thầy, but the problem is that training there will increase the arousal of your nervous system and that won't feel so good." He insisted, and he possesses Siddhic consciousness.

Sur Co greeted me in the kitchen the next morning, "You were right, Thầy had a hard night. We are so glad you're here so that you can lower the arousal."

"You know," I said, "you understand more about how this all works than 98% of the psychologists and doctors in the world."

It would be our last session. Thầy trained with unwavering attention on the feedback. When he was finished, Phap Linh told him that he had been training too. Thầy pointed to his head.

"Yes, Thầy. For me, it has made it easier to enter the stream."

Thầy nodded, encouraging him to go on, "Thầy, do you think that neurofeedback is a new dharma door?"

I could have swallowed my heart. I had no idea that Phap Linh would ask such a question. Thầy nodded his head enthusiastically, "Yes."

I could hardly stand up. I could hardly hold back an explosion of tears. Phap Linh had to remind me to say goodbye to Thầy. I went to his room and bowed to him, tears streaming silently down my face, before I pulled my way up along the stair rail and collapsed in the upstairs room where we'd been meeting every day. I couldn't stop sobbing. The day in the monastery went on, while I just sat and cried, the stress of this suddenly over, Thầy was much better for the training, and the years of invalidation swept away with a deep nod of Thầy's head.

John came to take me back to our apartment. He insisted that we stop for dinner at a nice restaurant he'd scouted on the way. We were in San Francisco, and I had no skull. My neurons were firework displays. I needed to cover more than dinner. He'd found that you could climb the hill using the escalators in Target, and he guided me through. I was nearly blinded. He wanted me to get a book for the six-hour flight home, and it seemed to be the first time the woman at the check-out had ever been asked where to find books. It was a small collection, and I needed to get out of there. I handed John the first possible book, *Whiskey and Charlie*, a book, as it turned out, about twin brothers, one of whom had had a stroke.

I emailed Arles: "Every once in a while, and tonight is one of them, I become aware that I am riding a very big horse. It is no longer the trauma mount; it is the new paradigm mount. The fears and hopes of so many people with this book. I don't regret writing it, but it comes with an oddly unimagined and immense responsibility."

He wrote back: "Let me suggest this view is still part of the trauma thinking, the big horse pressure of mastery and responsibility. These are projections onto you and, worth considering, yours onto them. Think, instead, as a thought experiment, that you are riding a wind horse. Ride the wind, and there is no ego, and if ego comes, let it flow through you. Become a wind horse, that is the new paradigm."

I still wonder about the nature of the energetic gales that swept through me for days after Thầy nodded his endorsement of neurofeedback. I have described it as my whole field buckling at the knees. The heavy bones of self.

I had my third neurofeedback session since returning on Friday. After the first, I felt brighter and noticed that my sacrum felt steady and strong, as if, for the first time in my life, it actually held me up. I had no pain, and I felt energy in the sacred space. It is the root chakra, the site of sexual assault, the kick, chronic pain, three-way blowouts and the strong sense only six weeks ago that my sacrum held all of my illness. It was the point of collapse. I asked Lee today if she would stay just there, and it released and released and released again; there was no pain. Then I was opening to Thầy, to ask him if he had ever cried in the midst of the horror, the blood, the gas, the napalm, the bombs, the bodies, the grief, the strewn wreckage of his birthplace. I saw the image of the crying Buddha, which I so wish I could draw. I felt this coming together, the interbeing of trauma and release of trauma, of transformation, of the impossibility of transformation, of the complete oneness of it all.

Phap Linh called shortly after I returned home with a small boxwood Christmas tree and a pumpkin pie. I'd been losing a little of my oneness with Thầy each night. I told him about it, listening to see if he understood. He did. I will see him again when Christmas has passed and before the year turns. I will live in the same house as Thich Nhat Hanh for eight days.

Chapter 22

Thầy did not greet me, but after Chan Khong insisted, he passively allowed the neurofeedback. In my absence and on my recommendation, Thầy had been trained by a practitioner with a different approach to brain training. It hadn't helped him. He seemed shut down, almost depressed, and he was refusing most treatments. Ram Das had sent one of his healers. Thầy dismissed this poor fellow after only a couple of minutes. After two neurofeedback sessions, he began to sleep again. By the third, he was animated. He started to move his leg up and down, to lift his foot and to move it back and forth on the bed. Nerves were regenerating in the sole of his right foot. Dr. Quoc was there with me at Thầy's bedside, and he said, "This must be the neurofeedback because I can't get near these areas."

It was the end of the six months that Thầy had decided to be in the United States. He wanted to go home to Plum Village. Everybody was worried about this. His niece arrived, sick with bronchitis, to ask him to stay. He lit up when she came into his bedroom, but he did not reconsider. She came to say her goodbyes to those of us she found sitting and talking in Phap Linh's office, before she left to catch her plane back East. When she came to me, she said, "I really don't know what to say to you. 'Thank you' doesn't even begin. You have helped Thầy so deeply, and I feel such deep gratitude... It's beyond words." Chan Khong said, "Thank you for coming to heal Thầy." These feelings and expressions were important. I felt invisible to Thầy.

A woman introduced herself as Brigitte as she took the cushion next to mine. There were many visitors this morning gathering to sit in meditation with Thầy before he left. I welcomed her with a bow, and we talked. She asked how it was that I was here, in this privileged moment of farewell. I shared a brief version.

"You must feel so proud." I shook my head and began to weep. I couldn't stop.

"It is so deep, it is so deep." She and her husband cradled me. They were my container.

Many came to say goodbye. Allan Badiner was "floored," he said, by the changes in Thầy, many of which I knew had only come or come back in the last few days with neurofeedback. As a result of medical tests and the endless stream of visitors, I didn't end up seeing Thầy in the last three days. I had no blessing. No moment with him. After he left and the crowd of teary well-wishers dispersed, I wandered to Pete's Coffee, just a place to go. In the kids' clothing store next to Pete's, there was a T-shirt with an Obama logo saying, LOVE. I bought it for my own supreme being back home. I fought off my dejection. We had lentil stew and King's cake at Thầy's acupuncturist's house that night to celebrate Phap Linh's 36th birthday, and he rose yet again to the occasion. I didn't learn until the drive to the airport how much that took.

There, the waitress at Napa Farms brought me an espresso. "Did I order this?"

"Yes, and I was surprised. That's my drink."

"Here, this must be for you," I handed him the cup. "I don't drink espresso."

When I'd gone with him on his run to Walgreens for Thầy's new prescription, I'd tried but failed to get him an espresso because of the late afternoon lines at Starbucks. I joined him in the pharmacy, we waited for the prescription, and we returned to the car with the keys still in it. I hadn't noticed that he'd left them for me. He said, "You left the keys in the car!" I braced slightly for the reprimand—what else comes in that script—, and he said, "I like your style!"

I flew home still in a pall of confusion, and I was lonely. John fetched me.

On April 20, I got an email from Tom Lesser, our lawyer, that began, *It's a beautiful day indeed. Kinder Morgan withdrew the pipeline!* I couldn't believe it, could not quite grasp the truth of it; we'd won the unwinnable battle, all 700 Davids of us. I'd worked with my group, and as I did, I became increasingly certain. When one would say, "*If* we stop this," I would correct them and say it is not "*if,*" it is absolutely "*when.*" But 'when' came much more quickly than we would have dared to think. Hundreds were being trained in civil disobedience. Hundreds more were ready to stand up at the DPU hearings that kept commissioners in school auditoriums without air conditioning until midnight. One person testifying said he was going to commit civil disobedience and asked how many in the room of 450 or more would also be willing. Everyone stood up. When I got the news, I couldn't hold it in. I got Blake, who said, "I knew you'd stop it, Mom." And then Emily, who said, "We did it!" She asked if we made history, "We did, you and Emily helped." She'd taken the information cards to school to help raise consciousness, her first political victory in many actions she'll be called upon to take. And finally, after five calls, I got a hold of John, who hadn't heard. John has been a guardian angel, a legal foot soldier and a rock star at every meeting. Many were testifying. He'd entered our energy bill as evidence in our senator's hearing. It was $5.78. Solar power. There was, in a way, no meeting this moment. We talked about what it had meant that we stood together every Sunday for a one-hour vigil on the small rise at the edge of 116, our little group, on the site planned for pipeline construction materials to be stored in Plainfield. It mattered; I just can't possibly imagine how.

During our interviews for the book, Roger Lewin, Marsha's ghostwriter, asked, "I've heard what you did for Marsha, but it's not clear to me what she did for you?" This question had occurred to me and to her and I can't answer it except to say that this is not the currency of our enduring friendship. She was telling me about her fears of betrayal by her senior students. At the same time, she talked about her will and giving Geraldine and her sister her fortune. I asked her, momentarily hurt, if she was leaving me anything, and her answer was brief and informational: "No." I wasn't surprised. It is the answer to Roger's question. She loves me dearly, knows of my financial situation and can't seem to provide. (She did send me a money tree plant.) She isn't curious about me. She doesn't ask questions, and every conversation turns back to her within a few sentences. She did want to explore writing a book together, one about our recoveries.

"When did you recover?" I asked her. "It took me until neurofeedback."

"We aren't telling them it will be 35 years!" The toll of her life, of her mother's hunger, and her devotion to all the suffering women is manifest. Her memory is going, she is in chronic pain, she is accident-prone and at some level still deeply lonely. I've helped as much as she will allow around the book, and she is resigned to its fate and hers as it configures around its publication. She is fierce in protecting her mother and suspicious, truly, of the almost singular focus on parents in dynamic therapies. She did say about terrorists that most of them would do anything just not to be forgotten. She is definite when she said that Putin is not a sociopath and that professional organizations cannot come out about Trump.

I have thought, and still think, that my sense of self depended on memories that I did not have. But even as that scaffolding slips away, she stays herself. So, as she has done, she forgets me, all the time loving me, grateful, willing to do anything for me and never doing it.

Arles listened and said, "Your sense of self was not established through memory, Sebern. It was established through me."

This morning, after many nights of segmented sleep and vivid, meaningless dreams, I grabbed a sour cappuccino that I didn't like and some eggs at the Green Bean and drove to Hanover to see Eva. It's been a long time. My brain kept slipping off center, wobbling, at times scarily, on the road. I assessed my competence the whole trip. Was this the coffee?

The sleep? the drug still afloat. The me? The sugar fast? Maybe I need sugar? It took me almost half an hour to find parking, and I was still unsure, watching myself make turns, cautious in the rain and with the distracted parade of students and self-important professional men, very rapidly interpreting and double-checking my understanding of traffic lights. I jumped when Eva called. She wouldn't have known because it smooths out so quickly. It wasn't until I was walking up to the Hanover Inn that I recognized it was Charlie. I was fully aware that I was going to the place where I had last seen him, and fully unaware until that moment that something of this was kicking my brain around. It is nothing like dissociation anymore, but it shares a birth story. I'm not at all clear why this would create this neuronal storm that puts me at risk driving, or why, once I see it, once I have insight, that the storm subsides and driving is again reliable.

I showed Eva the picture of Thầy and me at his hermitage. I am, in fact, radiant in this photo. I'd told him that more cells were stunned by stroke than were killed. He did a double-take. He'd never heard this. "The job of neurofeedback and you with neurofeedback is to wake them up." This is his language, the language he still teaches. I asked him if I could show him a photo of my granddaughter. He wasn't enthused. I laughed, "I know you must have had thousands of people wanting you to see pictures of their grandchildren, but I promise you, you'll like this one." When it came up on my phone—Emily in her light blue shorts and T in standing meditation—he turned toward it, touched my cheek with his palm and then touched the photo with the side of his hand. He blessed her. "For all you know," Peggy said, "he ordained her".

Part Three

Chapter 23

It was at the Nugget Point in Queenstown, New Zealand, overlooking the stream and the mountains, that we learned that democracy had voted itself out and certified the oligarchy in America. I felt wave after wave of visceral terror. I felt I might throw up. Blake called. I was confused because it was just happening, and it was a day after it had happened, and she was crying, and Emily was crying, both in shock. Blake understood the real meaning of this; Emily was just stunned. Obama to this. The cruelty and ravages of our democracy. I moved out of my own descent into bleakness, the sense that there was no way out of this, that Emily would live with the terrible consequences of this terrible election for her whole life, to take the call, to confirm the reality of the horror of this, but to offer hope. I had to offer hope I had not attained. Emily's sobbing quieted. I reminded her that we defeated the pipeline. There would be fights ahead, but we would win them. Love and light always ultimately win. I ask her not to take part in the violence, that violent language is violence, and it always lacks imagination.

John and I have each other to share our loneliness and being away from our country. I looked around the hotel lobby and the restaurant to see if this news was registering. Life, it seems, just goes on. But the Kiwis felt their own shock. The headline in the paper the next morning was in a font that almost filled the front page: WTF.

We met Bessel and Licia a day later in Sydney. Being together brought us all some comfort. Back home, we had dinner with them. Bessel was down with a cold. "It was always America that was safe," he said. "I know that because I grew up in postwar Europe, and now it's not. This is the truth of it. Now it's not."

People asked me if there would be a civil war in the US. "No," I said. "There is a major divide, but there are no sides to go to war." But I do ask that question myself, to myself, "Could there be?"

I'd written to Arles from Sydney. "*Yes, of course I will see you. Be in touch when you get back.*"

"What I most need is the solace of your presence," I said as I sat down on the long black couch in his sunny office. He assured me of this when, as I was leaving, he laid his cheek on the top of my head.

By the time we got back, Blake and Emily had righted themselves and were ready for resistance. Molly was taking a gun safety course, and classes are apparently filling up fast. Who am I to judge this? It scares me how scared she is, but hate is let loose over the land, pumped up by Trump, sanctioned if not yet sanctified. Hillary won by 2.7 million votes, but we elected a sociopathic reality TV host to lead our nation.

As we walked down the stairs to the T station at Alewife, a cheer went up. The T had opened its turnstiles. There would be no charge. People were riding out to this furthest stop just to be able to get on the subway into Boston. Peggy, John and I were there to join the Women's March. The train stopped at every station. Every platform was filled to overflowing. Above ground, rivers of people were walking. There are millions of us just in the US. Nothing is secure.

❧

It was terrible; it wasn't the same, it was not explosive. I didn't have the buffer of dissociation. I wasn't blown apart. Memory was forcibly yielded into his hands at my throat. It was slow-moving, and my tears spilled over his hands. I heard him reminding me to open my eyes, and I looked at the ceiling. I see the ceiling, I was in the time of this ceiling, on this table, in these hands. That was good, but it didn't alter the course. I couldn't stop it.

"They don't know how close they came to killing me." I looked up at him, "It wasn't sadistic." This feels strange to say, but it seems correct. The attic was revenge. My death would have been incidental. Bob couldn't move it any further. I felt like a child in a quake, but I wasn't a child. I wasn't reduced. I was cared for. I was not humiliated. This too is just. I wanted to write, "Even as it obliterates me," but that's what was different. I was not there; I could not be obliterated. And, yet, here I am claimed by it yet again.

"This was not about my patients or me; it was the suffering of every child, and it went out horizontally forever. One vibrating field up against another and another, and they bang and set up new vibrations in the other, endlessly out into time. It is vibration within vibration."

"Yes, I understand this. Let yourself expand with it. You won't lose yourself." Arles knows these fields.

"I won't lose my mind?"

"No," he said, with a trace of impatience, as if this were a silly question. I knew when I said it that there were stakes, but that's not it. I'm still in the aftershock, and the inner formations organize and disperse and tell their versions.

"Are you ready to grab my wrists if you need to so I can speak?"

"Yes, I am", he said as if he already felt my body organizing to spring.

"Do you know that I am not quite as competent as I sound?"

"Yes, I do," he answered. "And you aren't as non-competent as you fear." It was as if my consciousness was blinking, like eyes adjusting to a brighter light than expected, and I could get where I was and breathe again.

"It wasn't aftershocks," I wrote Arles, "it is 'afterpools.'" I wasn't a child on Bob's table. It wasn't a reenactment. I guess there is no other word than flashback, but it didn't have the twist and jolt of a flashback. I was a large wave crashing over a smaller wave. The sense of being spent is different, too. It is much closer to the feeling I had after coming home from Thầy the first time in September two years ago. This really surprises me. It isn't as thoroughgoing as that or as multiply enriched as that collapse was, but it was of that nature.

I am attending the death of a young woman who is no doubt me. The cause of the death was unclear. In the dream, I saw her the whole time, but I was in a different room, and I couldn't see her. I would think "go attend to her," but I believed that she was already dead or unconscious, so I didn't have to go. Finally, I decided I needed to get up and go into the room where she was and be with her. She was lying in a bed in an alcove with a shaded window. I saw someone else was also there making a meal. The dying youth greeted me by name and without resentment at my neglect. She seemed actually quite robust. I thought maybe she's not dying at all, maybe not even sick.

When conditions are right. Pattern match. Amplitude. The reality of states in the brain. I teach these things. I tempt these states of terror with a slight shift up in arousal. My state can go from solid feet in the present, to wilding, to active need to protect myself, to temptation to harm, to silent fits of rage, to "fuck you" aimed at whoever I imagine will contain this. It is as if the only way to recruit containment is to be in opposition to it.

The flame comes close.

"Would you still interpret an accident? Would you notice one?" "What do you think?!" I summoned him to my mind and fought him there. These states of mounting terror take me to the brink of dissolution. The lick of the flame quiets it. Amplitude rises, adrenaline, pattern activation. This is memory itself, and it has within it its own forgetting. A lethal confusion. I am a baby rocked in the arms of my killer.

Arles will step up to this. He will find a way to shut this down. I will say fuck you.

He did what he needed to do to assure me that he was there, a presence greater than the force of dissolution, obliteration, murder in my heart, in Moses' heart. The bomb in North Korea and the bomber in the White House are part of the conditions, but I hardly hear them over the din of war in my brain.

Coffee amps me up. I tinker with amplitude, looking for new information. It is so aversive, I get so scared and rearranged, and I am in a state of active threat. I hate it, it is not real, it turns on the strobes.

"Stop drinking coffee," he says to me in my voice.

"Fuck you." I say to him in my voice.

I felt almost liquid driving in. My mind was clear, my memory was excellent, and my thinking was fluid. Then I felt it slowly begin to build again. Bob said he was surprised I wasn't feeling more. "It's like the Aurora Borealis, energy moving everywhere, in your vena cava to your pelvis, to your sacrum, to your neck, to your head, your face, your heart, your kidneys, your adrenals."

This is exactly true to my experience, and when I'm in it, I make mistakes, and my knees get weak. I was looking for Emily in the schoolyard, and she arrived behind me.

This morning, when I was getting coffee, an awareness began to arise. I was outside the attic. For years, I couldn't leave my office during the day. If I had a cancellation, I couldn't walk into town or go to the market. I wasn't a free agent. I was held there, hostage. There is a cost to being obedient.

I turn away from Arles.

On Sunday, I drove in and trained. It was almost night and day. It was more bearable. When I wrote him that I had done this, he agreed with the decision. Both of us wanted to change this through and within our relationship. It couldn't be done. John remarked on the difference. Who is it really who suffers all this?

"In, in, in and it will get better." I heard him.

"Sensation is not just sensation; it is meaning. The splintering of the root chakra that had never organized to begin with." I cried, and I felt rage at all the White men, the rapists, the wife beaters, the pedophiles, the petty molesters, and I couldn't stop. My colleague Clair said she didn't know how to explain it, but last Thursday when we met, my state felt "neurological" to her. Something in the way I moved. I don't know what she saw, but she's right, this is neurological.

I wrote Arles, "I know why I am doing this. I am coming to know her. She will not be buried in an unmarked grave."

Sam held my forehead, and my brainstem unwound and unwound, and I cried, moving very little, gasping at what I could not see. The unwinding continued, and he sat with me. I am not dissociated or in another time. I am, I think, not in time at all. I said to Sam, "You've seen this in other people, too, right?"

At first, he didn't respond, but then he smiled slightly, tears in his eyes, "No, Sebern, not like this". I was finally able to get up off the table, and I hugged him. I held onto him. This is where we are after 30 years of work together.

"I think the most real you ever felt was with Moses," Arles said with a note of despair. He has been dealing with everything that I have been dealing with, all the multiple states and state shifting, the discovery of the reptile, which I called the iguana, and he calls the snake.

Bob said I was "a living still point" when I couldn't turn over to my stomach. I learned later that if you turn a lizard on its back she will go still and could die. They don't have diaphragms, so they can't breathe on their backs. After 10 minutes of intense will and mental focus, I finally turned over and immediately began to belly off the table; lizard flight. This happened three times. The second was the Wednesday before I was to travel to London for the interview with Ruth and her graduate students. I'd phoned her to warn her that I was not the person who had agreed to come.

"I don't know, Ruth, how competent I'll be."

"Have no worries, Sebern, I can take care of you if it gets hard." After that session with Bob, I felt cleared and grounded.

"Burning off the shells of multiple traumas," Arles said.

Everything, including these blowouts, has been recapitulated. I think his metaphor is layers, the one most used in therapy, but my experience within is now horizontal. I can feel my brain shift into some pre-existing patterns and my eyes, my shoulders, the tilt of my chin, follow it. To him it's 'snake; to me it is inevitability. Certain patterns arise in my brain when conditions are right – the content, his nearness or distance, his anticipation of the exhausting, even hated, sociopath and circuits rearrange. He has said about Trump (his election was the beginning of this, then Weinstein, Epstein and Kavanaugh) that it is reptilian; it cannot be treated. I think that it is exactly what he has been treating, what we have been treating, even before it was identified to me in the wilding moment. It has arisen, in the connective tissue, in my walk, in my eyes. I can't always hear it in my voice, but he does. He contains the wild child; he hates the sociopath.

"I am not a sociopath, Arles." He hesitates to agree. "You know that. You wouldn't have continued working with a sociopath." I am a little worried about his hesitation, not for me, but for him.

"Yes, ok," he conceded. "But you do have a soft spot for the sociopath."

This is true.

I watched my mind churning in old familiar ways. He and I have to change this, to evolve this. I also, quite suddenly, felt a physical sensation that I was releasing him from my body. I'd felt this once before. Years ago, I was sitting in meditation when suddenly, physically, Thầy left me, and there, in his absence, was Buddhism. He had said, "Meditating for me is like counting someone else's money." This was Thầy's warning about transference. It was a clear and certain shift today with Arles. I have yet to know if it's enduring or if it sets a clear course for us.

When I wake up, I am breathless. There is a weight on my lungs. Trump unleashed a slow-building terror in me that I reasoned with and meditated on and prayed for. I returned to therapy, upped my bodywork, discovered my reptilian centers and the terrible flight path that whatever I do, other than neurofeedback, remains activated. It overtakes my working memory, my agency, my proprioception, my appetite, my coordination, my mood, the alignment of my muscles, my balance, my mind. I told Bob last night that I have a silent film running in the back of my head that has no pictures.

I'd asked Arles about hypnosis.

"You get hypnosis in the body work every week, and I trust this process more." I think that might be true, but I am trying to discover the yield. There is discharge. There is validation. There is the truth of it, some specifics. "My body does yield memory..."

"This is the first time you've said 'penis in my mouth', that you used those words and with some ease actually". I was unquiet, "Fucking Trump!"

"He is not the first president to be a sociopath," Arles said, and I cut him off.

"The others were the living room, Trump is the attic!" and a lizard turns over in my brain, gasping for air, near death. Is it the PAG fighting for its life? On my stomach, those three times I could have belly-crawled right off the table. But I have a mind, and not even a terrified iguana would have flown off the ledge. How do I make it from the attic to the second floor? How do I orient my body? What is the blessing of waking up already scared?

Arles reminded me of the nature of memory, particularly in early childhood. "It is an atmosphere."

He was upset with me and even seemed to hold me responsible for having the colonoscopy that bruised the wall of my colon.

"Every decision you make right now takes place in this context." He pointed to the rough floor plan I drew of the house in Bronxville. I thought of pushing back on him for making me responsible for the injury, but I really can't. I think he's right.

"You are being very tough on me."

"I am, it's too important. This state of being is endangering you." He focused on the likely rage Moses had at my mother, that he raped me as a proxy for raping or killing her. He said he had no doubt that this happened, and much as I reported. We are now talking about how I got down the stairs, and then, whether I ever went back up. What the transition was, what the mind was. Maddy, giving me a bath.

"You make a mistake to think this is repetitious," he said, responding to my earlier complaint. "It is not. These are new cycles, new levels, new understanding, new experience, and they all deepen you."

He chided me for going to present at the Networker Conference. I think he expected me to be defensive.

"I go where there are therapists, and there are very few of them that get any of this. This isn't a collective of deep consciousness. I don't go to any gathering of therapists and find that it's any different. They don't get it. And you, Arles, don't get it totally either. And where is your rarified company? Who do you talk to?" He didn't push back because I think, for the most part, he couldn't argue. I'd brought Kleenex. I slid the eco sandpaper box under his chair. "That is the Psychotherapy Networker of Kleenex!" and he laughed.

I realized in the midst of talking with him that I had become my age. I still have the pulls away or inward, the twisting of neuronal linkages, but I recognized there is no refuge to take in all the other age positions that I have inhabited since Trump. These twists don't become a child or a teenager. I remain my age.

"You aged suddenly. What's it like to be a woman in her 70's?"

"It's quite a shock, actually. It is as if I have awoken from a coma. It's like the landing. I don't know how I got here. I feel an unexpected dimensionality."

I took a swallow of my tea, "My childhood is becoming more real, not more known but more real. These representations, these 'others,' were preservative in a way. They kept me young."

Who am I? Where am I? I can address these questions, and yet I have no trace of my past at all, of the life lived. It isn't adequate to call this dissociation; it doesn't provide the scope.

"I have two primary positions related to this therapy: 'Yes' or 'No'. Reading the journals and coming to therapy and bodywork was 'Yes', but approaching therapy, both kinds, I also felt a clear 'No.'"

"Maybe," he said, "when you came through the door, you inhabited both positions simultaneously, 'Yes' and 'No.'" The twins, "Yes and No."

"How do I say yes to this? When you say yes, it's consent." He got quiet. This is a very real dilemma. It accounts for the jerk of my head away and the re-formulations and the discharges in my brain. "People lapse back into comas, Arles, and this is why."

We shared our silence before he said, "Sebern, you have to be real about this. No one can recover from what happened to you; it's just not possible."

"Then we need to shoot every trauma survivor before they reach age 20 because this is an epidemic. There has to be a 'cure.'"

"This is another realm; really, it is all ephemeral."

"Penicillin mattered, Arles. Training matters."

"Yes," he said, as if poised to disagree, "penicillin mattered." But for 24 hours, his hopeless churn was lodged in my chest—not quite in my heart—and it's become my practice to quiet it. To separate. To find my compassion for him, to reinstate it. As it returns, or more precisely as it reorganizes, we are OK. His gift, his curse, his rage; his heart.

He acknowledged it when I asked him directly. The therapy wasn't easy in those months that I was fragmenting and shifting, not the butterfly in Thailand, the tornado on the plains. I told him that I knew it, that I might have been able to shut it down—other than the terror—but that this was the therapy. I wanted, we both wanted, to quiet this through our relationship, but I couldn't. It had to be calmed in my brain. He spoke about the failure of meditation and gamma production to lead to interpersonal transformation, and that neurofeedback and meditation were somehow quite different. Finally, I feel he sees it.

"Yes, very different, and one of these gamma llamas exploited his female students." He was making sense of all this and then something that I said pierced his heart, and we are again caught in my history, recently recycled and his arousal and his almost religious devotion to psychoanalytic teachings. It is my unconscious. It is my aggression. I am always at the short end of these interpretations, devoured by them. I hate this fundamentalism. It's what drove people to develop CBT. Finally, I get quiet with him.

"I get that you may just not be able to do this, Arles." I try to make peace with this that he will never understand. And this is a loop too, and he can't get me out of this one: the loop that is him and me. He can help me out of the others. I did draw that drawing. I did fall hard at the gym. He is both right and wrong in his insistence that there are no accidents. I get caught. And we get caught, well, mostly he gets caught, and instead of looking for the door, I look now for a momentary break in the loop, for a new space of possibility, and I try to take us there. I still hold all the ways he sees this, weighing it like dough, deciding whether or not to bake it.

I have signed up for a 10-day retreat at the Forest Refuge.

"We are loyal to our suffering," Jack said at the Networker conference. I repeated this to Arles.

"We are not only loyal to it, but it is luscious." He's right, there is that element of lusciousness. I saw green marsh grass and the clear water that sits on top of the fetid decay that gives off life. But suffering is only luscious in anticipation that it will, somehow, be met. Decay becomes fecund. The only comfort of this lusciousness is its knowingness. Desecration is not luscious. Desecration only seems to be used about buildings and artifacts, not children, but we are talking about the desecration of children. Next week, we will engage with the drawing of my brain I made during the worst of this last eight months, a drawing that was luscious, not extraordinary like van Gogh, but luscious like van Gogh, before you see the registry of his face.

I wrestled with this angel on the mount. He couldn't do better, or he would; he knows what neurofeedback can do, and he has access. He could ease his suffering that kindles and loops and threatens the integrity of the universe. It is up to him. It is not something I have to offer. We are in this relationship with his exquisite sensitivity, sharpened jewel-like by suffering. His suffering and what he brings to the world are measured in karats.

I was looping in this, and then I set it down. I realized on Friday that I was filled up, that every cell knew the love, care, the intentionality, the touch, the devotion of my therapists, that they were in residence and settled in me. When I described this stateless spaciousness, this no-self, to Arles, he told me that he'd sent me a transmission. I asked him shyly, as if this were his business, not mine, what it was, and he said, "May you be free of hypnotic memory," and he sent it about the time all of this settled. "Perhaps you sent this transmission as a demand loud enough for its vibrations to reach me."

"Given where you are, do you still need to write the book?"

"The book is not about me. It is a neurofeedback memoir told within the context of you and me. The 'you and me' is not replicable. Within the constraints of the millions of therapeutic dyads, the contribution of neurofeedback is replicable. I am, when captured by this history, living in an animal brain. I am a mangy wild horse, but unlike this prey animal, I can't throw off the wild cat that has its teeth in my neck. It's not even mammalian. There is no evolution possible in this brain. It is survival alone with thoughts and perceptions, and, if you're lucky, a metaphor, surrounding it. If you survive, you use the same strategy again, influenced but not changed by the relationship that is therapy. One of the necessities of this latest round was to see that I could only quiet this reptile, this wild horse, with neurofeedback. This is the reason to write the book. No one knows this. And in the field of neurofeedback, they don't understand the relationship, that the capacity for relationship is the measure of neurofeedback, nothing less. Neurofeedback is a new dharma door. Thầy said this. I know this. Many will come to see it. Neurofeedback is another route out of suffering to awakening. I hope this book will be a light on that path."

He still sits in the chair between me and the door. He leans back, and his long legs almost meet my bare feet. There is no self-consciousness. We are just in this conversation.

He is tired of hearing about body work. He thinks it is "iatrogenic."

"I wasn't looking for the lizard, Arles, nor was Bob. I was animated by it, and the body work gave it form, and it asserted the truth of this in my body. It's just what happens. You would know that if you'd experienced it or even could see one of these sessions."

We ranged over the distances between us and around us, from Trump and Bolton, their individual horrors and visitations, briefly into physics, the Market, then to Jesus Christ Superstar. He really wanted to linger here, but I exerted my patient privilege, and we used it only as a touchstone.

"Christ did not say 'who is my mother, where is my mother?' or if he did, it is not recorded in the Gospels so that we won't know."

"But it was the piece of the lyric that I found so validating, that Christ on the cross would cry out for his mother."

"For you," he said, "the cross is motherlessness. This opera is written from the point of view of Judas. Without his betrayal, Jesus would not have become Christ. He must be betrayed by Judas and forsaken to achieve oneness with the light."

I could feel the moment, a ping, a green flash of neuronal knowing. It was returning to the second floor, to my mother, to my mother's lack of recognition of my broken body that set me on the path of madness. There was no choice. I kept hurling myself down stairs until I was finally gathered up, tightly, unrelentingly held, wounds attended, wounds healed, self-organized, self-regulated, affect quieted, eruption eased, self and other realized. And now... whatever else happens, this is the legacy of Arles in me.

"If the cross is motherlessness, who is my Judas?"

"Moses."

This is because that is. My path to the realization of the Buddha within, to the divine, was this. These were for me the absolute, necessary conditions. They don't in themselves ensure transformation; it just is. It became the path because it became the path. I found myself without myself at all, in a vibrating field, vibrations of nuclear explosion to vibrations of Bach, with all that is left of me slightly at the edge of it, speechless. At one moment, all I saw was the beauty of his head, it may have been haloed, in my love and gratitude and in a certain amazement. In the waiting room, I'd thought of him as my therapist, my teacher, my advisor, and my practice. I've been listening to Jack. He talked about the difference between awakening and transformation. Mindfulness is duality. What training has brought me is a deepening experience of non-duality. To become mindful, we need to be free of threat from our own CNS and to achieve non-duality and no-self, we must step through the portal of mindfulness.

"Quite a chat," he said as he walked me to the door.

"I don't," I said, "even have an ego that can enjoy this." He smiled, and I found myself wishing for his pride in me. That is gem-rare. I'm a little confused about wanting it, even embarrassed by the contradiction.

"I have the sensation that there will be no one there to gather up at the end of my 10 days at the Forest Refuge (which I tend to call the Forage Refuge)."

"What's wrong with that?" He asked. "You will inhabit new possibilities. You will not oscillate between 'here' and 'there', you will experience here from there."

❧

"You know, Lee, with all this, I don't think that body work dispels body memory. It's all still there, but it is less dense, and it is different by the very nature of having been touched and of having yielded. Memory is memory. It is reactivity to memory in the body or in the brain/body that matters."

Lee feels this absence of breath as absence itself. To her, it represents being alone when it happened. The reactivity in my body, however, seems to be about physical harm done. The holographic bruise is memory. In my trajectory of "mental illness," it comes down to one moment. They don't recognize what happened to me. Life went on even as I fell down the stairwell through space and time.

"You kids think money grows on trees," I remember this not by remembering her but by remembering the tree with money as leaves, not fruit, and leaves falling to the ground, leaving it as bare as a mother's skeleton.

"I've never felt this before," Sam said.

"In me?" I asked.

"No, in anyone. You are releasing slowly and thoroughly, but there are no layers. It's usually a more recent layer that is distinct and yields to the early stuff. It's like it's all mixed together, not layered. Very different. Fine, all fine. You are releasing, it's just slow and thorough and different."

I talked with Marsha early in the morning of her 75th birthday, and she told me she's not got Alzheimer's. "It's what football players get." And I could hear several times when she slipped away from the moorings of daily memory, of calendar, of time. And then she was back, but so scared and lonely and alone. She could never enter the stream. She walked and created the "as if" path, and I fear that now she may know the limits of her massive contribution. She couldn't make herself whole —better, but not whole—with all she did because of all she didn't do. She had no willingness or capacity to care for herself. She has always dropped away from herself, and now this final, fatal fall into tau dementia.

The distance between us is the length of his legs stretched out, his feet at the base of the couch. He wants to chat, but gathers himself. He begins an inquiry, then stops and says,

"It's begun, hasn't it?"

"No, not quite."

"You're at the edge of it."

"Can you see it?"

"Oh yes, your eyes first, and there's a change in the energy."

I feel slippery, my mind like Dali's clock flattened and slipping over a curb into traffic, always ready to materialize and run me over. My voice changes, I can't stop it.

"This change is the only way to be faithful to her. It is a true path back, but as twisted as my body and my voice." It's a brief incursion, but it's real. "I want only what is true," a plea, against theory, for a new mind, for curiosity, openness, newness, even as we once again uncover the mossy lock.

At lunch during the Trauma Conference, I had reason—I don't remember what—to tell my friends briefly about the attic. Melanie leaned into me, horrified, with a disbelief that is the most profound belief, and Lori was empathic, the way therapists are. Our reserves for the personal horrors of the world are not endless. Lori was there with me; Melanie validated me. Another stitch in the garment. Matt Sanford's experiences of his paralyzed body are impenetrable to me. At dinner, he said to me, "Everyone sees their story in my story."

"Oh," I said, "I don't at all. It's almost inconceivable to me what you have endured." And right there is the line we can't quite cross. My experience is also inconceivable to him, but he doesn't know it.

"I learn so much," Ruth said to me. Imagine this. It is unheard of. The leading neuroscience researcher in trauma and dissociation wants to hear from those who have experienced it! She doesn't quite understand how significant this would be to the former patient, to the one who can belly off the table. She used a description I'd given her in her keynote, and later I confirmed it with her: a little shiver went through the audience when they heard it.

May 29th was the 10th anniversary of Johnny's death. It didn't register with me until John mentioned it. He said it had slowly gained in him over the day.

My fear circuits were aflame. Arles worried that I could be re-traumatized by the brain drawing I'd given him and that I'd asked to see. He was concerned about my eyes, my antisocial position when I came in, and we made progress, both of us in understanding that he was getting set up by this and that he could take a different, even empathic position. I think he got there; these eyes, too, are of fear. When these circuits fire, my 'identity' becomes fluid, shifting fields of color. I can't look right, swallow predictably or hear.

"It's not a defense," I pleaded with him to understand. "It's not personalities, it is not failed neurofeedback or failed treatment," I was crying. "This is the 'Isness' of this level of trauma; this is my meditation." He slowly but then deeply came to understand what I am trying to say and to feel the ground of time we inhabited together. "It frames up as I prepare to come in, and it only happens here. Well, only here so completely. You're part of it. Our relationship sets a certain rectangle of time that I enter and, to a greater or lesser degree, exit, as I leave to enter another geometry of time. Could you be empathic with the 'snake eyes'? It's the only way I will become empathic with all that I have been through, with this very person I've become."

"I appreciate what you're telling me." He paused before he asked. "Knowing all this, do you think you might reorient before coming into the room?"

"I really don't know how to do that, honestly, since my brain can be so locked by state, and it is exactly this that we have to treat. I think this means that we set aside the understanding or misunderstanding of 'defenses' that has governed our whole world and become empathic with what happens for our patients that recruits this circuitry and its somewhat predictable manifestations. And then learn how we can enter there and keep them company in the vast emptiness between their spines and their skin. And all of this without an invitation."

This is my plea to Arles, "Come in that close and at those moments do whatever you can do to stay there, to lean into the bare bone of my back away from the flashy pretense." I looked more squarely at him.

"It doesn't matter if I dissociate when I look at the drawing," well, it could, "it is you keeping me company."

"Company at the rim of the black hole."

I had a flash of recognition.

"This isn't black; it's bright white light." We were both surprised.

"Tell me about this."

"It is the light," it had sent a jolt to my brain, "that I can't hide from... on the landing. Oh god, I see this white light." I was a little gone with this, and I ignored the light of the attic that had seeped into the back of my eyes, that is gray or not light at all.

She tells me of her father laying out the newspaper and lining up the shoes, the precision of oils, polish and brushes. The way mink oil rendered the leather. The immigrant family's pride in footwear. I remembered my father shining our shoes with Kiwi polishes, taking the cloths and the single brush, the sweetish smell, the darkness. As she talked, I felt the longing to be somewhere else, in a world where the language is not English, where they use mink oil to restore their shoes, where the walls are plaster, not plasterboard; church bells and open-air markets that are every day, not precious like our farmer's markets. It is mostly the cool, smooth plaster wall and someone else's art I am feeling hungry for. It isn't about accumulating experiences, as Arles had once impatiently suggested. It is about immersion into the space made by someone else's wall, falling sweetly into those aromas, finding newness. It is why I love therapy with Arles and why it scares me. His walls are different, his art, his language, and it invites me still into the newness of my own psyche as I explore even more deeply its own recesses. It is the other walls I crave—not the cave or the ocean—the unexpected smells, the welcomed surprise.

"Is all of this," I asked him after yet another convulsive episode, "Is all of this just to have it over?" He didn't answer. It is a deep meditation, this question, not a provocation. There is no answer but silence, silence that acknowledges the vastness of the endeavor, the honesty and the endless existential sadness of the question. "Overness" is to Bessel the promise of treatment with MDMA. I have held "overness" like a fine cut emerald, but that isn't it at all.

"'Overness.' Is that all?"

I went to the session expecting to look at the drawing of the brain I'd done in a six-hour frenzy in October. He had it out. I wanted to begin by showing him the house on Google Earth, where you can't see the third floor from the front.

"This is the outside, though, not the inside," he said, and he asked to look at the floor plans I'd drawn from memory. I had the pad with the drawing next to me. I ignored it. I put it in different places on the couch. We focused on the landing, on the white light that obliterates all detail, that is the nuclear flash where the convulsion begins. He sits deeply, he surrounds me. He is no longer the idle bystander, the school teacher who must have known something was wrong, the gardener.

He remembers that I repeated kindergarten. He asks me if I was given a reason for this. I wasn't humiliated. I may have even been relieved. I probably felt both.

"It's amazing I went to kindergarten at all."

"Yes," he said softly, "it's amazing you went to kindergarten at all."

I did not completely regain the present. It is that a predictable present time, that I want more than it is "overness."

I looked at the drawing. It's difficult at first to find the baby with the wings or my discrete four-year-old body. The sulci outline a pile of dead or almost dead bodies, some of them bewildered, some of them copulating like the baboons on the beach, a holocaust scene.

"Are you repulsed?"

"No, not at all!"

"No one wants to see this, Arles."

"Because no one wants to see what this actually does. This is the truth of it." He took it back gently, and I did not protest.

"I don't draw this well," I said, and, some sadness in his eyes, he smiled warmly, broadly. I looked again at what he was holding. "It is like I've given birth to a deformed baby, beautiful in its wretchedness, but it cannot live; it will be humiliated, misunderstood, tormented. What is my responsibility to this being?"

He gave me a rare bit of praise. He said how well I'd done this therapy. "You didn't lose your mind" was the nub of it.

"Your presence," I said to him, "has endured this last experience of landing. These forces push you to the furthest perimeter. You can't get too close, or you die, but you still disappear at the edges of the shimmering desert sky, at the rim of the black hole." He follows this like someone who knows the native language that is about to go extinct. What a miracle it was that this time he didn't just blow to pieces like every other time, or drift away like smoke. "And the reason for that, Arles, is because I know that you will only let the explosion travel so far; your body contains it, it will not reach the door or break out the window. I know this because of what you did for me, that you contained me, that you would." I reached the newly felt perimeter of him and me and began there to assemble a nervous system along the midline, to use all that energy that intends to explode, to bind. He has made this possible with his hands, with his body, with his voice.

At the tea shop, I mentioned that Tulsi was a medicinal plant for stress. Emily almost did a double-take, looked around at me, clouded and asked, "Stressed?" As if to say, "You?" As if to say, "you just rearranged my universe or at least the clear blue sky."

Kennedy resigned. Today may be the end of the world as we have fought to make it. I can imagine a civil war. What the fuck was that old White man thinking to hand over this country to mad men, thugs, liars, thieves and rapists? The glaciers are melting for Christ's sake. What is he thinking?!

I look for a harbor; I need somehow to provide a harbor. My rocky brain is holding its own, but my psyche wants to find even the thinnest, fragile thread that could lead me out of me to safety.

In response to the catastrophe, I sat. I quieted everything related to Justice Kennedy. I chose meditation over my skull blowing off, and it was the far better choice, now possible.

Tomorrow, John leaves for Pakistan to introduce neurofeedback at Lady Reading Hospital in Peshawar... Peshawar!

Emily keeps introducing herself to me in our shared time as we both arrive almost magically but without question, suddenly, in the present. There we are face to face, literally, as she has grown tall. I talked to her about being unpopular in my public school in Bronxville and deciding, as I prepared to go to my new school in my new town, to make myself popular. I studied the popular kids, and I learned how to be like them. She looked interested, and then her face clouded over, and she asked, "But what happened to 'You?'" The question stopped me, and I smiled. All I could say is "That is a profound question, that 11-year-olds don't ask, that no one really knows to ask, and that I don't really know how to answer." She described them as skills I had, and this comforted her, and I agreed. I did not want her to confront the reality of 'no me' when she's barely past grieving Santa.

Chapter 24

I am trying to recall my last session with Arles. I had trained at PZ 1-20 Hz down. I could feel that certain inflammatory currents were out of play until the moment when he insisted on something, when he became the boss, and then I felt my eyes flit to the side, barely, but to him noticeably. I pointed it out.

"Yes," he said, clearly tired of this, "I saw this." But for me, it was different. I'd never felt the crawl up my neck like lightning, in immediate opposition to his insistence on our relationship. I noticed it happening too when I saw he had the drawing pad out. He remembered me, and I, as if on cue, turned away as he turned toward.

"Why is the pad turned over?" he asks, and it begins. To say it is visceral would be wrong. The energy takes me over at the back of my neck, "It's like," I told him, "when you turn your computer over to an engineer somewhere who you've never seen, whose location you don't know, and he turns your head at the neck." My cheekbones burn, then my skin, my eyes skitter away to the left. Once it begins, it's hard to shut down. He starts there. It is why I am there. The drawing. He is holding the drawing of my brain that arose in a propulsion of discovery. "I will burn it; I would never burn it." He punctuates my desperate longing, the despair, the vitality, the exposure, the uselessness, the beauty, the shame, the disgrace, the truth, this illumination and my impulses to destroy it, "It is staying here." I expect to protest, but it's not there. "This is not a drawing. It is not art. Art is looked at from the outside. The light shed on it is external. An icon is illuminated from within. This is an icon. Even if you tear it up or burn it, it would not be destroyed. It can't be." He brings the metaphor of the monstrously beautiful child to a close. He talks about the sacred, the ethereal sacred and the sacred in the body, which includes the violence and the degradation.

I dreamt *I gave back an adopted baby. She is so beautiful, they say. They will have no trouble finding another owner family. They can't quite understand why I am turning in such a perfect baby, but for me, it's just too late to raise her.* I have dreamt several times, deeply felt, believable dreams *that my eyes are stuck closed, that nothing I can do will open them, and nothing anyone else can do will open them either. I feel panicky* and wake up believing this. The eyes of my unconscious are sealed with epoxy. It doesn't seem, though, like there is anything left that I don't want to see.

Arles responds to my thought of ending, "That won't happen." When I think about it, the thought comes that I don't share, "I could make it so you would surrender me." This goes on like some vital, habitual, endless "Hold me, fuck you, don't touch me, I'll kill you, don't let me go, ever." The volume on this is low, but its gravity is escapable, and it persists—life and death, creation and extinction. What was it like to be delivered by Moses? It was white light oblivion. It makes me breathless.

I realized the obvious that the story is about being a hostage, but not only when I was held there and done to, but every day that Moses lived there, every day I heard their footsteps overhead and every day since. I obeyed the rules of not leaving, even when I was working on my own schedule in my own office in Northampton, Massachusetts, over 65 years later.

"Did this happen only once?" Bob had asked, and my body, ambushed, froze. I felt pressure inside my head. Was the answer "Yes" or was I beginning to register that it actually happened every day?

I asked Arles when we'd be done looking at the drawing.

"Done? What do you mean, 'done?'" And automatically, suddenly but necessarily, my eyes narrowed, leveling on him. He went on, "When you no longer look like that, like you want to kill." I shake my head and smile an equally true smile.

"It's unbelievable that I still do that." He's going to be away. I asked him to think of me.

"Yes," and then he adds, "Every day." I opened the door and turned back.

"I love you, Arles. Thank you."

Bob put his hands on the back of my head, and he described his experience later. "Is she not feeling this energy bouncing every possible way around her skull?" I lay still, unprovoked and largely unaware. But I'd gone quiet when he touched the center of my right cheek, and I pulled away from him, and it began: the tears, the "No," the opening, the attempt at refusal, the utter surrender. He said it felt at first that my brainstem was splitting, but it stayed connected and kept opening, and then, when he put his hands around the pons, it yielded too. I was still. Then it felt like the cerebellum untethered and opened down the center, and I said something like "Wow," and he stopped himself from laughing. He went back to my cheek, first the right, then both, and I spilled out, "No," and tears and "No." I clasped my hands over his that held my face, and the tears slid over our knuckles, and everything kept unwinding in my lumbar spine, in my face, in my brainstem. He sat with me, still unwinding, and he said, "I've never had an experience like this, the nature and quality of the opening."

On Friday, I will fly to Seattle to spend the weekend with Marsha, who is stumbling her way through her latest misery. I'm going in part to see if I can guide her toward Vielight gamma stim, the best option out there to help reverse or contain dementia and then, because I won't be successful, to hug her and say goodbye for the last time.

It might qualify as the worst and, still to be known, one of the most important trips I've taken. Marsha reintroduced me to the mind of my mother. They had liked each other. Before I went, I had the broad outline of a biography ending in madness. I had not inquired into what happened between my birth and Moses. I had the photos. Being with Marsha sucked me into a familiar universe of negation, of self-satisfaction, of a stingy generosity, of no self and no other. Marsha said that she had a good brain and a bad memory. In a way, this has always been true. She could never hold the reality of the other, even their actual existence. I wonder about what it was like for her patients, all of whom, like her, suffered this as their original condition. If she hadn't offered them skills and flashes of brilliance and irony and care enough, she would have made them crazy. And now she is becoming demented. When I think of her, I don't know what tense to put her in. She recognized me at the airport, and she was warm. She climbed into the backseat with me. This would be the only time. The rest of the 2 ½ days felt like a groove on a chipped LP, like being in the vast, uninhabited universe of my mother.

I asked her if she missed her patients, and she said, brusquely, No. I doubt she could remember them now, even if she could have kept them in her mind. She never could, so she focused on stopping behaviors, never deeply understanding the reasons for them. They were, after all, her behaviors and mine. Her memoir will come out soon, and thankfully, she will not know its reception, although of course it could be well received. Her therapy has been, even in its emptiness, very useful for a lot of people, both therapists and patients. She was, in that sense, not alone. When I asked her if she was lonely, she said "Yes," without hesitation, almost emphatically, "But what is there to do about it? You cope." These could be words swabbed from my mother's mouth. Her first moment of waking, she turned on CNN in her bedroom, then switched on the theater-size screen in the den before getting her bowl of Raisin Bran to bring in to sit down to watch, and it stayed on until she went back upstairs for bed in the early evening. She is proud of her method for falling asleep. She counts until she falls off and advises me, "Don't quit counting or you're done for!" I asked, as apparently others had too, "You mean like counting sheep?" and she answered a bit sternly, "No, just counting, no sheep." I've tried this, and she's right, no sheep.

John McCain died that weekend, and 90% of the coverage was of him, stories on loop that were merited, I suppose, for the occasion, like those remembrances at a funeral that are far from the whole story and never wholly true.

She was mad at me for not coming up to bed at 7:30 when she went up to sleep. I pleaded email, but it was the spaciousness and the quiet of the living room without CNN or Toby, "Baby Boy," the gnarly little terrier saved from the "quick kill" shelter, who is wary of her and at times nips her. That's the thanks she gets. She's been mother to this unlovable dog, and the only breaks we got from CNN were brief excursions to MSNBC and taking "Baby Boy" out for walks in the neighborhood. Fire surrounded Seattle, and the many paths of smoke converged there and sank into the persistent drizzle. When I didn't follow her up to bed, she stomped down the stairs, insisting. I think she glowered silently, almost like a kid holding her breath, because she couldn't think of any reason to be so mad at me for not doing as she was doing. When I remembered why I had come, I followed her up and gave her a hug goodnight.

She is thinking of writing another book to be called *Losing My Mind Twice.*

"You know, Marsha, losing your mind is also losing your memory. You might want to take notes."

"No, I can't do that now, I am writing this other book on DBT with cancer patients, and I know what's important to say: 'You must acknowledge what is wrong and face it.'" Marsha will not allow the use of the words Alzheimer's or dementia. This is all so her, even as we lose or have lost her.

Marsha will forget me. She may have already. But I will never forget her. I loved her. She has left her mark.

It was extraordinary. I walked away from my office and out of my house when I was supposed to stay there, strolled down the street in full view, went into Nourish, the new little veggie restaurant, ordered a smoothie, waited, took it outdoors and stretched out on the skeletal chair, in the warm sun. My first patient had canceled. I pulled the drink up through the straw, which they would compost later. I felt it; I'd broken through a hard, invisible shell, and there I am sitting here, outside it. Long after the threat is over, hostages comply. I leaned over, my elbows propped on the little table and settled myself into the sun. Like a rabbit out of the hat, the thought, "I have led a moral life."

It is true. It is factual. So are the antisocial, the feral, even the sociopath. They are approximations, characters, stories riding the frequencies of my nervous system, playing to an empty house.

Two days later, with a trill of trepidation, I told Arles my revelation that morning in the sun.

"Oh yes, Sebern," he said, "you have led a highly moral life."

I am writing this at Forest Refuge at the end of my first full day. I spoke with Caroline, the teacher here, about my exhaustion and my brain/mind/trauma confusion and the deep questions I have that give rise to others about treatment and meditation. Rest first; questions, as they arise. We both agreed.

Once during my meditation, I began to order treatments, perhaps erroneously, but definitely too literally and the systems they address. Neurofeedback is a first-order treatment; you can't be better than your brain. Bodywork that encounters trauma is also a first-order treatment, but it can be overwhelming to meet what your body has kept without at least a semblance of a regulated brain. Memories are held more literally, more concretely, more stubbornly in the body. EFT, EMDR, etc., are second order and meditation and therapy are third, higher order. I can feel this slip away even as I write it. There is no schematic or order or model except that neurofeedback comes first and never, in trauma, by itself alone.

People come and go in the meditation hall. They arrive and arrange themselves and then fall into silence, and I fall into it with them. We go down the chute of silence, we disappear into our own heads, but here we do that together. We create a field that amplifies, deepens and quiets.

When I decided to apply, I was just beginning to recover from the terrible fall I took after Trump, Epstein and Weinstein into the lizard reality of survival. I knew I had to deepen my practice. I had a mind then, and I had suffering; it was the purchase for the deep dive. Even then, as engaging as it all was, as believable, it never coalesced into a personality. If there was anything like a core self, it did not invest, it absconded, it leveraged states with coffee or sugar. I was fascinated by how labile and deeply conditioned this was. I couldn't eat; I couldn't think. Only action, often just discharge, made me coherent to myself. But somehow, at least as I remember it, I never lost "non-self" during it. I formed in awkward clumps around terror, and this arrangement was propelled through time and space, from appointment to appointment. It was the deepest engagement yet with the reality of what this has done to me, without me, as me, there at all. In her talk, Caroline quoted Larry Rosenberg, saying that meditation is understanding that fear is workable. I said to her in our interview that the definition of trauma is that fear is not workable. It has you, you don't have it. So here I am, in the midst of this great privilege, the sanctuary and kindness of Forest Refuge, and I don't quite know what to do. I listen to Joseph's teaching on CDs in the library, and almost at the beginning, he says, "Be mindful about good periods too. Let them be, submit to your happiness, don't over-inquire, this is a happiness practice. Submit. Rest."

When I wake up here—I slept hours during the day both yesterday and today (I don't do that) and last night I slept from 10 to 5 straight through—I realize first thing that there is no demand, no one requires anything of me, every minute of the day and night is without obligation. I wash windows and will go for my interviews, but that's it. The rest is the gift of time to reach Anatta, and there's nothing there to solidify. It's airy. Empty. Thoughts pass through like the turkeys I heard tonight or the bells from IMS calling the kids into talks. I don't want to waste this time, but I don't think that's possible. I am wrapped in it. Tonight, sitting, I realized that I may be further along in this practice than I think.

I have been thinking of Marsha a lot today and the deep sadness of her life. Her therapy failed her, and she failed her therapy. Her therapist,

Dick, I think, was quite devoted to her, but she couldn't find her way to abide with him, in part because it was not DBT. She has suffered exactly what I have. It's not rare. When I told a friend recently that she has dementia, he put his hands to his face and said, "It seems even worse when it takes such an intellect," and I agree with him.

At one point during our last weekend, she said to me, "You don't seem like someone who likes to talk," and I thought, how do I talk with someone who has no memory. Memories were really what sustained us, and they are gone, except for the times I blew cigarette smoke in her mouth as she stood at the edge of the seclusion room, because then, due to the burns on her arms, she was forbidden to smoke. I showed her pictures of Thầy and reminded her that she'd gotten permission to use the practices from his book Miracle of Mindfulness without mentioning Buddhism. I'm sure if Thầy were ever consulted, he would have been delighted to permit this.

"He could have taken them from me!"

"No, honey, you got them from him." She turned back to CNN. At our last dinner, she told the story of how Geraldine became her daughter, and it still made Geri cry. All of this experience, which I had had at all, was only certified back home when I heard a report on NPR that the worst air in any city in the world that weekend was in Seattle.

In meditation last night, I tried to influence the flow of blood from my left hemisphere to my right hemisphere as a way to shift from aimless thoughts to awareness. What is the nature of this mind, the most precious gem in the universe? There is no weight to this. It is as if I need gravity boots and a weight belt to help me sink into this inquiry.

Last night, peeing, I felt a wasp crawling up my upper arm, and I swept it away with the back of my hand. It landed on the baseboard and crawled away, limping a little. It was suddenly an elderly man, very clearly looking over his shoulder at me, sad, saying, "And what did I do to you?" I rescued it in a cup provided, apologizing to it, now again a hornet, and whispered, "Don't be afraid." I stepped out into the rainy night and set it free. This morning, I couldn't find my peanut butter-soiled napkin and thought someone may have mistaken it for theirs. I'd put my toast in and came back to a woman grasping it with wooden tongs. She looked at me, and I registered that it was mine and gave it to her. She was beautiful in this exchange and in an acknowledgment tonight in the Yogi kitchen. I had touched her back, and tonight she touched her heart. I put in another piece of toast and went to prepare my egg. Once again, a Yogi took my toast, but he was unaware. Someone must've taken his. I got my toast on the third try. As I was walking to my room, I found the soiled napkin in my pocket. The thief was me.

A pin dropping in that hall would be startling. I've never experienced this quality of stillness. The space has formed by the practice within it, now 13 years of continuous meditation. I am held in it; everyone is. It is a stillness that creates reverence for itself.

Wild turkeys flock at the feet of the Buddha, whose back is to us, who looks out on the forest. I am struggling to understand basic concepts fundamental to my training here and my training as a therapist. In those who have suffered early neglect and abuse, I do not think that it is their minds that create suffering; I think it is their brains. Stopping your prescribed psychotropics is grounds for dismissal from retreat. Isn't this an acknowledgment of this? It is not the mind that gives rise to the erupting nervous system. It is the earthquake at the brainstem that gives rise to this wild mind.

The practice here is deep. It's what's invited. I don't want to make trouble as I look deeply into my mind and find my brain.

Western psychology - What is all this planning?

Eastern psychology - Who is planning?

Caroline completely supports my finding my right hemisphere and the importance of rhythm.

I woke up this morning in a dream. *John and I were in a new city, and I was being swarmed by bees. I said to him, "No, they aren't stinging me, I just can't get free of them."*

Tonight, the thought comes of Brett Kavanaugh and all the rapists, molesters, wife beaters, pedophiles and petty abusers who violate everything that is human and decent. I feel the energy shift in my body to gray and cold, almost white, and I noticed that I was annoyed that there was only one other person in the meditation hall. I am becoming aware of an awkward ambivalence in me about being free, of letting the tether to all of this go. How is it possible that the Buddha was ever human? It is no wonder to me that this gets confusing for people, this line drawn in water. And then there's how trauma throws a wrench into all of this and the question Caroline struggled to address with such kindness. "Fear keeps coming, and it's so big I can't stay with it. What is the next best thing?" She answered with a quote from another Buddhist teacher, "When you feel afraid, be fear." Of course, this neat linguistic solution is not a solution at all. The person who asked the question is already fear itself.

I dreamt in a semi-lucid way of a man lying on his side who was dreaming also in a semi-lucid way of a woman who was dreaming, lying on her right side.

I lift the coffee pot and note, as I always do, its reassuring weight. At some metric of registration, I decide there will be enough. I am reassured, "I made this coffee; there is more, almost freshly ground, in the refrigerator. I am not hungry or thirsty." I've just gotten up from an hour of meditation. I have patients who could have starved as children, the frozen parrot; milk toast for dinner; another scolded for using too much peanut butter at the shelter after the flood that washed away the trailer park. I have always had enough to eat. I have usually eaten too much. I have not been deprived of even a morsel. My mother's milk did not come in. I didn't know this, but there may have been rumors. It's not that. Her appendix burst, and she was in the hospital for two weeks. These were the first weeks of Mary, who was 18, an orphan and hungry, stepping in. It could be that my bicep is weighing. How did the viscera absorb this burden of absence and develop its own metaphor? How do I follow this thin fascial thread to its source? How is this history still represented here when I am about to turn 77 in the beautiful little house that I share with my beautiful husband in this beautiful, clear landscape? It's not that it's too old a trail, it is that, without a body, it has always been too faint.

I have been pitching a book to John for him to write. We are drowning in dystopia. It is the fashion. It is what we all believe. It is hip and impossible. It predicts its own inevitability, making it seem inevitable. I want a utopian novel about the meaning and ascendancy of self-regulation. What would that look like? How would that come about? Who would lobby against us?

The troops in the forward operating base in Afghanistan expressed their wariness of brainwave training. They asked questions. "Will this make me like Obama?" "Will this make me gay?" "Will this make me a Democrat?" When they were reassured, they settled into training. Records were kept. A regional commander flew in to find out what was happening. There were no suicides; few sleeping pills were dispensed; there were fewer injuries. The army major who told this story told another. These boys wanted to do Alpha-Theta training. As one did, he went into his office next door and leafed through a sailing magazine. He went back at the end of the session, and the young soldier said, "I feel great. I don't know why, but I kept seeing all these boats."

Emily was worried when I told her I had to go feed the meter while she waited for the pita with cinnamon and the tea. I could hardly bear how fearful she could get, "You are so precious to all of us, Emily, that we get worried that we will lose you. That worry gets mixed up with a 24-hour news cycle. There is no perfect safety, and where you live is the safest place in the world. You are competent, strong and mature. You can take care of yourself." She was still reluctant to let me go, but she did.

Later, just in the course of the conversation, I said something about being ordinary, and she said, "No, Grammy, you're not ordinary." I repeated myself because being ordinary was so hard won. "No. You are," and she searched for the words she wanted, "'one above.'"

In a sense, it has only been in the last month that I realized the swath or the scope of my treatment, the arc of it; perhaps that it was treatment at all. I lived my internal life in his office, a thread pulled out of ongoing time and lived mostly there with him. He can't quite bring himself to endorse the reality of neurofeedback. He has turned his waiting room into a spare anteroom.

"It's about as comfortable as a museum, and museums at least have benches."

He went off on the "6000 neurofeedback sessions" I'd had.

"Yes, exactly and if you'd had 6000 neurofeedback sessions, you would never have designed it this way". He laughed. It does, though, display some quality of his mind—this spareness. He also hung a thangka of the Wrathful Deity.

"That," he said, "represents the energy in me that healed you." I can see this actually, but I turn away from iconography; it is to me a representation not just of belief but of a kind of fanaticism. He stays just this side of that, but it does mean something that he ended up in the Tibetan Buddhist tradition, and I with Thầy.

At the end, he said,

"Don't wait too long to write. You have a story to tell."

"No mud and perhaps no lotus either."

This was how I started my talk on meditating on my brain at the weekend forum on Buddhism and the Brain at Plum Village. My chair happened to be placed at the spot where I sat on the last night of my first retreat. There were only a few of us left that night, Anne, Allan, Marion and Shantum. It was that night, sitting on my brown cushion, that I fell in love with the wall.

My focus on the brain and on neurofeedback was well received. Phap Linh and I caught up in the music yurt.

"You know this is all happening mostly because of you." When I demurred, he said, "Oh come on, Sebern, take this in!"

"It's not that I don't recognize the facts of what you're saying," I said. "It's that I don't know what to do with the 'you.'"

"Oh yes," he said, recognizing this, "I have that problem too." Phap Huu, now the Abbot of the Upper Hamlet, had been away in Luxembourg accepting a peace prize for Thầy. He found me to say hello, and he said, "You know you planted the seed for this." Same problem. In truth, it was Thầy who opened this door.

Michel and I reasoned our way through making our French press coffee. We both like it strong. He made me scrambled eggs as we got to know each other in the stone-walled kitchen with the long wooden table that had accumulated the effluvia of food—bags of chocolate, almonds, granola without gluten, raisins... Lionel, who lives in the other half of this house, tidied up for us. Peter Levine wandered in on his way elsewhere, said good morning and then lost track. Mirjana finds us an exquisite cappuccino in the café at the outer edge of Eymet's plaza. She proved, as she'd said, she has a nose for good coffee.

"Train your mind," Phap Lu'u said, "or someone else will train it for you."

I hadn't regained my sleep after France, waking at 2:30 and, at best, only slightly dozing until 4:30. After the last training, I shifted. Sam found all systems organized and quiet, and I described my statelessness that has no words. Arles seemed muted, and I am not able to respond to that as neutral. He is gone. I had no spontaneous thoughts. They only arise with his engagement, so I was stranded there. Somewhere within this profound statelessness, there is a harmonic, a familiar yearning for connection to him, and he pretty much disappears when he is so... stationary. Who have I come home to? My slight but rising panic betrays the truth of statelessness. I feel his resistance to it as well. It was a cloud meeting in that room. He did form up at the end when he commented on Michel and the French phenomenologists, and he said, "I ended up giving you an object."

"Yes, and thank you. It's like small weights on my ankles." He smiled.

We had dinner with Bessel and Licia, and I trained them both at the Inion like I had done to recover what I could of my sleep. Bessel has been dealing with insomnia. Licia reported that it felt like mushrooms. Bessel texted the next morning that he'd slept from 10:45 to 8:20 straight through, and adds with a wink, "But this couldn't have anything to do with neurofeedback."

He was first a wild, terrorized adult screaming uncontrollably at Molly's. I could hear him over the phone. She was calling to ask me to take him. I was going to be having surgery and just couldn't, or couldn't bear the destruction of equanimity. Molly would just go silent, and I would hear him, and I just couldn't take him. I didn't. I woke up distressed, and it took me some minutes to realize that Johnny wasn't here, that this wasn't happening, that he would never come, that he was OK, that he was dead. I fell back to sleep enough to dream, and *he was back now as a little boy who was terrified and could not be soothed. We were trapped in a car in a pileup accident, and it helped him to bring me things from the car. Then, in a house, I was trying to find him a place where he felt safe enough to sleep, but where I could sleep too. The upper bunk of my bunk bed? No. I couldn't sleep with him so close and so perilous. He couldn't sleep. He arrived at the door of Bessel's living room, my tiny supplicant in his pajamas. Bessel was empathic with this little boy and made him a bed across the top of mine, over my head. In the morning, we hadn't slept much, all in this big living room. There was a note of resentment as I looked at the clock and realized how little sleep we'd gotten, but it passed quickly,* and I woke up.

"The antisocial is a condition of your existence." He quickly moved to cut me off. "No, not everyone's, yours!"

"Why are you sitting in that chair? Wouldn't you be more comfortable in yours?"

"I sit here to contain you."

"What are you containing?"

"The part of you that doesn't think I exist."

"So, you know that still happens?"

"Yes, I do."

"Are you discouraged?"

"No. Are you discouraged?"

I talked with him about how this organizes in me, that it is a hole, like the ozone hole, torn and ragged around the edges, non-conforming. When he said "existence," I thought he'd said "resistance."

"That," he said, "would also be true."

"It is feral and sometimes caged, sometimes not, but it is a molecular hijack that by its nature has neither you nor me in it, and I can't quite grip the edge of my adulthood. This element is young and has no sense of mortality. It is lively."

"Of course," he said. He wanted me to cut back on travel, which I have said I will do, but don't. "What do you think you're getting away with?"

"Getting away with? I don't think..." He cut in.

"You are stealing time, relationship, nature, and the opportunity for spontaneous insight by doing all this travel."

I have a deep problem because in this configuration, I can't hear him. I said, "Your imprint is your hands, nothing else has left a trace." He nodded. "How do I write about the truth of this? I am below the tear in the fabric of my being, and I look up at it like a hopeless ecologist." He didn't respond. I stood up to go.

"Sit!" I did, faster than this "me" would have.

"Look at me." My chin popped up, and my eyes followed. "Are you hearing me?" I hesitated, making sure, "Do I need to get louder?"

I shook my head. "No, I am hearing you."

"When you leave here, you are to leave knowing that both of us were here. Take that with you."

"I don't know quite how to explore this territory without you, but by its nature, I have no choice."

"That's a hat trick," he said, as he turned away.

There was a mix-up in time. I'd been very careful to arrive on the dot of one and prepared myself to wait the typical 10 minutes. His door opened. Then the waiting room door. He looked angry and said, "It's 1:30 today!"

"It would have been helpful to have been informed," and with a snarl, he snapped,

"You were!"

I left, heart pounding, and looked at my email thread with him. The message was weeks before and he had changed the time. I sent an apology for interrupting his session, which I repeated when I entered his office. He was angry but, I think, frightened at what he was about to say.

"Do you know that you slammed the door?"

"No," I didn't.

"This was dissociative then, because you did." I think you can not notice these things when you're upset, and it's not necessarily dissociative, but it was not a time for debate. His chin trembled ever so slightly.

"There has to be a consequence to this. You won't like it." This was going to be a warning. "If this happens again, the therapy is over." I felt no protest at all. I was not quite shocked at this, and I noticed. I agreed. I understood there were ample grounds for protest or for my ending it, or for tears, or forming up the feral position, but none of this was happening. That was over. I saw, really for the first time, how my behavior affected him, that of course he was pretty hopeless about me, and I knew from his chin that he would suffer ending too.

"I can't guarantee that the Tony Soprano element won't form up if the conditions are right, but I can guarantee I won't act on it. There is a well of sadness beneath it all."

"Yes," he said, "A well we will visit."

A workman hit a live wire in the wall of our cabin across the driveway. The power surge traveled backward into our house, burned out the surge protector and took out our furnace, the garage doors, and half of our lights. It didn't affect the cabin.

"Does this happen?" I asked John.

"Ah, no, this violates the laws of electricity."

I wrote Arles. He responded, *"There are dark energies in the air. Be careful."*

"The backward power surge is an expression of the unconscious, Sebern. What other explanation could there be?"

I watched as the conversation happened to see if any part of me was getting away with something. That, astonishingly, did not occur, and I was using a precision instrument to measure it. I understood that Arles could not know or believe that this antisocial takeover was gone. He had despaired of it ever ending since year two, when he talked about even the futility of exorcism. The sociopath is untouchable. This element was inevitable, but it had remained untouched. I described it as where the breath is. There is some brain truth to this, too. Ruth will not endorse my use of "sociopath"—"That's a very strong word, Sebern"—but she too sees the antisocial in developmental trauma and acknowledges that this is rarely talked about. We discussed shoplifting and the brain dynamics rather than the psychodynamics of it.

"I would steal at great risk to myself. Looking back, I think that the risk was the thing. I didn't want to get caught. I didn't want the items. There was, though I think, a heightened sense of aliveness in the terror of getting caught, and the rapidly dulling thrill of getting away with it. It may reduce to adrenaline and a momentary firing of the default mode network. It would establish me in me. I would steal from a five n' dime on Broadway and take the toys down the street to the fire station, Toys for Tots."

"We are discovering your mind, your unconscious. There will be no talk allowed here about neurofeedback."

"No! Arles! You will not 'X' me out. Neurofeedback is a vital part of all of this!"

He seemed surprised and delighted.

"Differentiation! Good! Do you think my intervention about ending the therapy was like a neurofeedback moment?"

"Yes. Sudden, electric, surprising, and organizing."

In two weeks, I will be back at the Forest Refuge. Every corner I turn, I realize "It is enough, everything is perfect. I am perfectly cared for, I need nothing."

My mind, in its low amplitude, wandering on the cushion, encounters the image of a white shirt front and a red tie. It took up a lot of the screen and then dissolved. The next morning, I had the image again, but smaller this time, maybe half the screen and quickly gone. This afternoon, it was there again, but almost like a miniature or at a great distance, and it was also discharging from my body. My second night here, my mind was held securely by all the minds together in the room. I was taken by the power of it. There had been others in the hall when I entered. When I opened my eyes, I was alone. It is the nature of this place. The teaching today: the deep dive of the electron microscope into the human body ultimately reveals two things, emptiness and rhythm.

The low-level hectoring, nattering in the background, a low rumble of effluvia, slowly slips away into acceptance, then compassion and then the crust breaks, and my mind cracks open. I open my eyes, stretch out my arms on the floor and then I sit again. The bells sound. Getting to the dining hall takes my complete presence to stay organized enough to walk. Each step, I name, "Here," then "Now," then "Here" again. I named them to believe them. I could smell lunch, and the smell was there. My feet were here. Can I eat? Should I walk to get my glass? It felt as if I needed the force of attention and the grace of intention to walk at all. The reality of the molecular dissolution tingled through my whole body down into the marrow in the bones of my feet. My head is not mine. I sat down next to the young man who seemed to have the deepest practice, and I kept my eyes on his hand every time he set it down between bites. I asked myself, "Do I need protection?" No. I had protection, of the place, of its walls, of the intention of everyone. I went, painstakingly, back to the cushion. "It will move through," I said to myself, "or it won't. It will do what it does." I got up after an hour and a half because I was afraid of breakthrough vocalizing, but this process is roaring through me, and it sends all the molecules vibrating, reorganizing, looking for a new way to arrange me as not me. I had to grip the handrails and stick close to the wall. The tackiness of my socks on the carpet helped orient me. Every step, "Here" or "Now." Another 70 minutes of sitting, then a light meal, another hour and a half. This is not over. I didn't know how to get up, so I decided that I would leave when the next person entered. It was hard to keep that vow, but I did.

Was this a neurological event?

"Only in this state of not having to react can the self 'begin to be.'"—Winnicott

In my interview with her, I asked Caroline if she had ever been to jail. She looked bemused or perhaps a little taken aback. She hadn't. I shared the image with her that had occurred several times in my meditation, of the door. One side is the holding pen. It smells terrible, a gray metal degradation and fear and then they take you through the door, and there you are in a courtroom of polished wood, perfumes and a sense of decorum, if not dignity. Just one door, two completely different worlds and yet in neither are you free.

I lowered the glass bell over my head and struck it so I was inside the vibration, surrounded by it. I was only the wave form, abating, flowing, swelling, dying away, rising again. This was the image that kept coming. I tried several times to penetrate the meaning of this molecular rearrangement, and it didn't yield to any question I could ask.

Walking down the hall, I said almost out loud, "I am free." The intensity of the revelation didn't outlast the declaration; it closed quickly, but I remember it. From then, I started a practice of mind clarity. Clarity of mind that has nothing to do, I learned, with clarity of thought. On Sunday morning, entering the meditation hall, I remembered Larry saying, "This isn't Buddhism." It may have been a foreshadowing of the vast incomprehensible opening that I rolled around in for three days. Caroline said, "Remember, Sebern, you have everything you need to weather this, and we are also here." She followed this with a scrap-paper note on the board: *Protection of the Buddha, the Sangha and the Dharma.* In trying one more time to penetrate this experience, I saw a disc, gray and unyielding, that then became a full eclipse—a totality.

When I focused instead on the ring of light, I felt overpowered by this rare privilege of being.

I asked Emily why she was in here alone. She was 2. She looked at me, clear-eyed and said with a note of protest, "No one was paying attention to me."

"So why are you in here, by yourself?"

"Because I wanted someone to come and find me." This child, the most well-attended of any possible child, felt bereft and upset when not attended to. This scene came to me on the cushion and then with the clarity of the glass bell: "It is all infantile, as in infant, as in before 3." The question is, "What do we do about it?" Back then, I sat down on the carpet next to her.

My mother did not hate us. Her field alternated between shaming and vacuity. I could feel the streams of her consciousness in my own critical mind as I looked for her and for my dad. They are both known to me, and I can't find them anywhere. To be out of your mother's mind is to be out of your own. To be hated by one's mother is annihilation.

I had my brain map on the day I left the retreat. I could not discern any change in my brain and said, "But, Bob, there is a very big change in my mind." Will any of this show up in the material infrastructure, in the generator of rhythm and emptiness?

Shortly after coming off retreat, I dreamt that *John and I had been asked to adopt a baby younger than one who needed to be held. We took care of her lovingly. We learned that she could not just talk but spoke meaningful, thoughtful sentences. Somehow, even though she could not yet walk, she seemed to leave to attend to important matters and then return. How do we take care of this baby who can so clearly take care of herself?*

I don't know when this happened, but it was as if I were pierced by some tiny speck of gravel at high speed at the breast bone, and the body cast shattered and fell off in a discernible piece to the ground in front of me.

I hit a buzz saw. John told me how disappointed Blake had been in my response to her new VW bug. He was talking about the social lie that smooths the seams. "But they were willing to contribute to the destruction of the earth! How could you buy from them! How could you in any way condone or look away from this lie, this greed?!" John and I are on different planes, and I began a descent. In my vivid post-retreat awareness of the effects of Trump's lies and the men and women who believe them, I felt overwhelmed by what he was saying. There in our bedroom, I felt it all, and I cried out, "I can't lie, I can't lie", over and over in wild desperation. I was devolving, opening and descending at the same moment of absolute truth. "It would kill me to participate in this lie." This had its own integrity, but it felt like madness. It had that power and that tone. I felt alone and inconsolable. It came to a natural end. John came to the couch to hold me. Later, I asked what it was like for him and whether he understood.

"I didn't understand how deep it goes for you." The descriptors he used were "intense" and "violent." He said he would help Blake understand. As I began my ascent, I was crying, "I'll never have her. I lost them all, and I will never have my daughter." I was agonized. And then I remembered meditation. This is exactly what meditation is for, and I looked forward to sitting with it all, with her and trying to find my mind. Her accusation, "It's all about you," was on repeat in my head. Suddenly, I realized that she was right. It had been all about me. To see this clearly, I had to set aside the inevitability of this, the necessity of it. I'd been dreading Christmas, trying my hardest, walking the line between authenticity and "as if" as best I could. After sitting the second day, I texted her that I now saw it had, in fact, always been 'all about me'. She thanked me, also by text.

At Christmas, she embraced me easily, and we were just there, happy with the Christmas tree, the dogs and each other. 'This is a happiness practice.' Everything before that realization was lived out in the haunt of double meanings, of asking myself 'what did she mean by that' or, at moments, ascribing the worst possible meaning. I remembered that 90% of the judgments I made at the retreat were wrong. I fell into a well of peace.

Chapter 25

Marsha is in assisted living, but she is spending most of her time in the memory care unit because she worries that people in assisted living don't like her. I have often wondered how she has lived such an important life so friendless. I don't think she could ever block out how lonely she was. Geraldine did her best to fill in that daily emptiness. There's a unit in her skills book on making friends. This is such an essential skill that she could not know how to teach. She'd been mad at me when I was there and called her caretakers many times to vent her anger and disappointment in the two hours that I spent trying to steady my brain with my mind. When I returned downstairs, I described the hypoglycemic episode I'd just been through. She said, "I'm glad that doesn't happen to me." I'd come to understand long ago that this was Marsha's empathy. I laughed and said, "I am too." But Marsha's is a cautionary tale. Loneliness got her. No one but Geri, her sister and me to build memories with. No mother and now no mind.

BRONXVILLE

I drank the last of my weak tea and settled into a meditation I can't remember. Maybe breakfast would help, just the eating, the demand to digest, to move this malaise through and out of my body. I got some way into the PowerPoint, but I couldn't even cut and paste. Exhaustion gathered at my sternum. As I started to do it again, I became aware that I'd been rapping my fist there for a couple of weeks, ever since I heard back from the people in Bronxville. I'd been surprised to get his email, almost forgetting what I'd set in motion. A month before, I wrote to *THOSE OF YOU LIVING at 40 STEWART AVE., BRONXVILLE, NY.* It was a note in a bottle, and they responded. I slept fitfully, finally fully awake at 4. I was not sick from lack of sleep, strangely, I thought. I saw Bob first. At moments, I shook his hands off the way I used to. The way his fingers were on my forehead or up under my skull in the back provoked it. He felt whatever it is he feels and said it was "reactive," as of old, but not "weighty." It's primarily vagal, he says, but it pools at my sternum and at my sacrum. I haven't had these responses since the Trump-Weinstein-Epstein predator era. My bowel kept up, and with it my hope that it would just move out of me. At road construction on King Street, I made the absolute and clearly wrong decision about which lane to inhabit. The cop showed me his exasperation, moved a cone to free me, and I felt stupid, momentarily. Later, I saw Sam. He held the back of my head on the tips of his curled fingers as heat poured out from deep in my nervous system, up, it seemed to me, from my sacrum. He had to breathe so that it didn't take residence in him. His breathing felt like empathy.

Early that morning, when I sat, I thought "this is body memory," an occult kind of memory, specialized, opening only to touch, not really to inquiry. That awareness could have been enough. Body memory. This must, though, I thought, also have some kind of psychic representation. I imagined going into the attic on Friday, which is likely no longer thought of as an attic, and finding... What is this in my body that pours out into their hands?

I have made a vow of care. I will step mindfully. I will not fall or get hurt. The threat is in the field that is propagating within me. That's the nature of it, and it's a field I must find a way to bind. If it isn't bound, it is madness. This is what I talked about with Arles. I try to see through to an image, and what I see disturbs me. He asks me what I'm feeling when I see this. Dizzy at the very top of my head—oh right, I realize now—at the crown chakra. It's like a tight swirl there and then, in response to being asked, nausea and the sickening, hopeless bowel. When Sam was holding my head, my left foot, ankle and calf went numb. My feet were cold, and both he and Bob moved energy down to my feet, particularly to my abandoned soles. I had nothing to stand on, no way to climb the stairs in the Bronxville house. I was caved in, collapsed and a light, ready as tinder.

I propped myself up in my bed with my phone as always at my left ear. Since the pandemic was declared, we have only met by phone.

"What do you see?" he asked. "What is there in the attic?" I don't see or expect Moses. He has been expunged somehow from this field. He's gone.

"I'm afraid I'll find myself there. I see a small child, flattened into the wall, a presence in the wall mostly in outline, but I see her eyes most clearly, large and smudged with dark circles, like a charcoal drawing. I saw this first this morning in meditation." As I write this, circuits change in my brain. I can feel it mostly focused in the left temporal lobe, a similar swirl, a vortex there, while the rest of my brain is swampy, and my chest and my stomach, in turn, collapsed and sickened. "My head is hot."

I could hear Arles finding his own mind, giving it time to align. He has faith in this, and so do I. I told him that I was endangered by the field that was propagating in my brain, not by an unconscious wish and that I am being careful. It is a very powerful field. It attracts injury or assault, and my cooperation with it. He understood this.

"It's very important to bring this heat to your feet. Remember my hands. Let them cradle your brainstem and quiet it." I lay my head on the firm edge of a pillow right there at the junction of these consciousnesses, the brain, the body. This was the memory of his hands. There were his hands. I focused inner attention on my brainstem and let his lullaby of tones quiet the mute, dumb terror. I couldn't really retain the words. I'd tried to remind myself that this was over long ago, but it was futile because it wasn't true. It is never true except in fact and time. All that happened there 70 years ago is coded outside time and fact. It was never real. What from the brainstem is real? What can be believed? All of that is in the realm of thought. There is nothing here like thought, nothing as hard as thought. But of course this is very real, this sacrum, this sternum, this stomach, this sweep of nausea and dizziness, this bowel that tries, repeatedly, to expel.

"If you were with me, I would know what to ask. I would ask, as I have before, for you to pick her up—even if she is as thin as the second dimension—carry her down the stairs, almost weightless and out of this house."

"Yes," he said, "that is what I would do."

"I just don't know what I must do. I guess I can't know yet. Do I bring her home; do I leave her there?"

"Bring back what you must bring back; leave there what you must leave there."

The pill drifted back up my throat like a thought, as if there were no gravity, no peristalsis. I was surprised to find it there again in my mouth. I need to take caution too in swallowing. It's not something that I can take for granted. Forgetting is a property of this field.

I drugged myself that night. The dreams that fill the spaces between wakings are vivid and important. The next days, Tuesday and Wednesday, were easier. These therapists really helped me. Today, the day before I return, I'm on edge. All of that is back, but at a lower amplitude.

Body memory, what is it?

Sarah was on the broad front porch when we arrived, but retreated back into her house. A few moments later, she greeted us at the door and explained that she thought it might be important for me to approach the house on my own. She was warm and offered us coffee and water. The house was small—this mansion of my childhood—teeming with children but cleaned and tidied as if they did not live there, as if her mother were coming, not these strangers she was welcoming in. All the surfaces were clear. Will came down from his office on the third floor. Everything was where I remembered it, just smaller. My parents' room, the alcove for my mother's makeup table with the mirrored top and flowered cover. Did I remember the fireplace? How could I forget the fireplace? I don't think I remembered it, but it was covered by their bed. [Even as I write this, I am rearranging furniture in the architecture of my brain. I don't know how to trust this process, but I don't distrust it either. It's like playing with a doll's house under my skull.] They were painting, and there was no sign of that either, just apologies. I almost imagined them in there, my mother in her costume as a Bloody Mary, "Come as your favorite drink." They had twin four-poster beds, my father's nearest the bathroom. Hugh's bedroom was next off the hall. My bedroom was in the corner, connected to Kevy's by our playroom, where Raggedy Ann and the others came alive at night. Before we moved, we got walkie-talkies for Christmas.

"Do you remember the bathroom here?" Sarah asked. And it was, except for the wall at the end of the tub, as I remembered it. There used to be back stairs from the kitchen to the second floor, but I couldn't see where they would have been. Maybe there never were. I remember seeing Moses go up the stairs, the stairs I was now going to take.

"I think it's best if I do this part alone." They were gracious and went down to the kitchen to give us the most privacy the house could allow. Will apologized for the mess in his office—he works, at least now, mostly from home. He'd been a district attorney who prosecuted crimes against children. His office is in the room where it happened. I stood at the door briefly but never entered the room. It was his office, filled with his work. I didn't want to intrude further on his privacy and his generosity. I wonder now about that. I did step over the threshold of his son's room with a large poster of Steph Curry dribbling out from the wall. This is where Moses rocked me, his tears rolling off my cheeks. I was disoriented in space. The attic part, now wrapped in heat foil, was it over my parents' room? John had to assure me, taking my shoulders to orient me. My room was under this bedroom where Moses and Maddy slept. I heard their feet. I pointed to the banister. "That's the banister he held me over." I didn't look over it. I didn't touch it. Perhaps I didn't need to —the space felt cleansed of all that had happened here—but I wonder about this too. It wasn't exactly a decision or an avoidance or a refusal. I just didn't go there. I was not drawn. The field was not propagating; there was a new information field here. It didn't bury the old; it replaced it.

We sat together in their TV room downstairs.

Will spoke about being a DA. "It was easier actually," he said, "selfishly," and he put his fingers on his heart, "to prosecute a child's murder than their abuse." His face darkened. "I was usually the third, no, the fourth person they'd have to tell their story to, and when I looked into their eyes, they weren't there. Psychologists told us not to get attached; not to allow them to become attached because it would have to end, and they would lose me. But I was with these kids typically two or more years... and most of them didn't do well, whether or not there was a conviction."

When it came time, Will clasped my hand with both of his broad firefighter hands, hands that could rescue. We asked Sarah where to get some lunch, and she recommended turning left at the end of Stewart and going to the first intersection. We turned right and headed out of town.

I told him first about Bronxville.

"Moses was not there, Arles. The energy was clear."

"But didn't you just say that you didn't go into Will's office?"

"Right, I didn't. It was his workspace."

"Hadn't he said you were free to go in there?" He had. "And you didn't go into the bathroom either?"

"The door was open, and the toilet seat was up. That's all I saw".

"I think you protected yourself, Sebern." Everything went quiet on the phone, and then I broke the weighty silence.

"I think you're right, Arles. I think either way. If I'd gone in and there was his energy, well, there's that and if I went in and there was no energy... I couldn't do it. After all that, I couldn't do what I went there to do."

❧

I told him about Hannah and David Bohm—they were lovers briefly—and that I was thinking of him as I watched Infinite Potential, the film about Bohm on YouTube. Some of this was what I had begun to see at the Refuge, the constraint on us of the repetitious infantile patterns and even the possibility of infinite potential.

"What coalesces there for you?"

"I think it is the opposite of coalescing, it is—there is no less violent way I can think to say this—the blowing apart of molecules." He murmured his understanding. "I was constantly constructing you, Arles, and the construction would fade or fall apart or be under attack. You kept coming through. I'm not terminating. The only other place that 'termination' is used is around abortion. And I don't think we have ever been in 'treatment'. We have been in the making of a self. I rode this unicycle of biology and cognition, only the slimmest of structures beneath me, and it wasn't enough." I stopped to listen for him. I heard the quiet "Yes."

"When I look in the mirror, I see I am old. I've only been old for three years, Arles."

"I'm glad it didn't happen any sooner." It sounded like he smiled.

"Trump's election threatened to vaporize me. It took me back to the brink of the black hole. But if it hadn't happened, I would never have had the certification, yours, that it happened exactly as I thought. I would not have understood the descent from the attic into the madness of no one seeing what had happened just above me." Whenever we talked about the landing, I was standing right beneath where he hung me. "I would not have had to contend with my own antisocial leanings. It was brilliant, it was compassionate, it was daring."

I asked him again today about the toll on him of this relationship. "I just need to know if there have been any enduring costs, Arles."

"Absolutely not. Be assured." It took neurofeedback before I could look at him, and this would be a time when I would have to make sure.

When I told Peggy that I felt cudgeled with each new murder, each lynching, she wasn't quite where I was. She understood, she felt something too, but there was a sliver of separation between our experiences that usually isn't there.

I spent last night trying to walk away from my dream, but I couldn't. The dream content, whatever it was, called me back into it. I woke several times; it was a thin and haunting sleep. I woke up, beginning to know that this reality is inescapable.

"The image that keeps coming," I told him, "is of my being in a cell, the lights fully on, sitting on the floor with my back against the bars. I can't see my face. I don't turn away, I don't avert. I know it's me, but there's more to it; more, I guess, than skin and trauma." I asked Arles if we could change the frame, and he is open, completely open to wherever I am.

"I am having a hard time," and then the torrent of discovery began. "I am feeling all of this chaotic pandemic threat, but mostly I'm being taken down by the murder of Black people, in their beds, walking home from the store. It's almost like I can't get up."

"Like there's a knee on your neck?"

"Yes." I wouldn't, I couldn't watch the video of George Floyd.

"You are not as separated from this as you 'should be', are you?"

"No, not nearly as much as my living here in these hills in this white skin, this age and this privilege should allow." I pushed back against where I was going.

"I have never hated him or turned on him, Arles."

"No, Sebern, you haven't."

"Every other memory I have, every other possible sensation is absorbed by the last moment of his rocking, his tears. I feel this almost entirely on the left side of my head that lies against his body. It is as if the portal is there, but there is no leaving this behind me, no detaching from this 'identity'. I am not a Southern belle who walked away and said, 'they are not me'. They are me, all of them, Mary, Maddie, Evaline, Alma, Moses. They are more in me than my mother or father."

"Yes, I think that is true," he said. "You were tender when you talked of Moses." I couldn't recognize this, but he said it again, and I had no rebuttal or need for it. I have no words. I'd begun by telling him that I woke up with a pulse rate in the high 80s that came down only to 75 when I sat.

"This is not identification with the aggressor." He already knew this.

"Your willingness to know this, to live within this reality that is outside of any cultural frame is likely to help, in a minuscule way, to affect 'the conversation', the field of race in the US."

"Thank you, Arles." I lingered there in the field of gratitude. "But in fields there are no minuscule effects, a butterfly wing or no butterfly at all."

"Right. That's so, isn't it?"

This is affecting me.

"My brain is a bruise—it's a bruise—black and blue and pulpy. I can't quite see how the trees glisten in this clear Covid air. I can't see the beauty of where I live. I know it's there, but I am numb and clenched."

"Lying in Moses' lap, cradled there, you had such a terrible hunger..." I stopped him.

"I did have a terrible hunger, even worse, probably, after Moses, but it wasn't the hunger that made this transfer happen. I was four, alone, often naked, brutalized, raped, exhausted, abandoned. Before and after, I had no language. I had no way to, to interfere with or to intercept or to fail the download. You and I have dealt with the hunger throughout this therapy. This I've known. I'll have Moses within me forever, and I didn't know that. I don't know Moses, but I am joined with his consciousness at the far left of my own, and when I am, I feel the rapid, loud beating of his heart. But when this joining happens, it feels like lightning."

"Thank you for telling me this, Sebern," and then we were both silent at each end of the phone. It was five minutes before four.

"This could just be piling on, but there's something else too that's here in this field." I stopped to listen for him, and then went on, "I hear the boots."

"Yes," he said, quietly, "I thought you might be experiencing that too." He paused as if there was advice that had disappeared. "You are very open."

Our therapy began on the charnel grounds, dark, cold, windswept; demons and maggots, the naked heart. It has been a Tantric practice. I have intonations, when I am still, I feel my way toward the depth of this human experience, the infinite unfolding.

I am trying to get home and walking through Harlem. A Black man approached me. He had an aqua tattoo on his right temple. He asked, "Where?" He was soliciting me. I said "No," and he left. I became afraid, thinking I'd taken the dangerous route and looked for escape. I saw a street uphill alongside a church or a monastery, a brown stone wall. Maybe the remnants of a fortress. I got to the top, and there was a courtyard and a fire going in a fireplace. It is a beautiful place, safe and warm. Allison (friend and neurologist), Charlie (friend and DBT expert), and another unknown man are playing cards at a table. I stood over them, greeted them and then asked if I could join the game. I thought it was a high-level card game and that there was a place at the table. It turned out to be poker. They wouldn't seat me. I was shunned and had to leave the safe enclosure.

COFFEE

When he was sick, Arles found the residue in him. He raged at me about my refusal to face my aggression. I hear it as a kind of analytic sloganeering. It is as if aggression forms outside of a relationship, a freewheeling, unconscious psychic force. The baby's aggression makes the mother turn away. I was refusing this again as I began my meditation, but very quickly, I came up against what I came to describe as "the hard problem of the horse."

Coffee was the beginner's horse. I'd ridden harder horses. As soon as I settled in the saddle, he threw me off. We were still in the stable yard, I was in the dirt, and he reared again. I scrambled under the bottom of the ring to escape the battering of his hooves. He may have caught the back of my leg. What explains such bizarre behavior? A horse does that when a panther lands on its back. I didn't want to kill the horse; I was afraid of him, but it became irrefutable in this blockchain in meditation that I wanted to kill someone. They had to capture and calm Coffee. This led to the moment that I'd had with Blake, where I knew she was right about my withdrawn mothering. My psyche reorganized and opened a wide door to her. Then to Arles. I kept turning away, and it hurt and exhausted him. How could any of that not be true? It was a reckoning, an understanding that I thought would free me, but it dropped me into despair. I'd felt a quantum shift toward forgiveness and acceptance, but it ended abruptly, and there I was in that gray, damp atmosphere, stuck. This is what Bob found.

"There are adhesions and constrictions on the right down from your head to your sacrum. They are either new or very old, even original contractions pulling in and away." He opened where I pulled away. "I knew in a way this was there, but it was never available to me, never close enough to hand."

Later, I described the wave forms to Sam. One was massive and dark and kept getting stuck in a web of myself in history, in the Supreme Court, in Roe v. Wade, in George Floyd. But there was also a bright, clear wave for moments that would extinguish itself before it could develop. I asked Sam if he would move the dark wave through and out. It took a lot from him as it had from Bob and all along from Arles. It is a terrible energy.

Karlen Lyons-Ruth spoke on Ruth's webinar about her longitudinal study. "There are two predictable factors that lead to 'borderline traits' and suicidality in adolescence. The first is the mother who withdraws, and the second is the baby who keeps trying. Abuse, although always clinically significant, washes out as a predictor." I had pushed Arles into his tendency to withdraw—the soft-spoken analyst far away—and when he did, the primal terror and rage worked itself into the fuck-you-swagger that he feels cannot be analyzed, so he never sees it as anger and beneath that fear and sorrow. Instead, there is something in me that is "untreatable," that he hates, that he turns away.

I had a shocking realization. I would call out, begging desperately, "Don't leave me," usually with Lee or Sam or Bob. Who was I asking not to leave? It was, of course, them so that they didn't leave me dumped in the attic with him. It was also him. What is the word for this? He cried for me or for us or for him. He rocked me and rocked himself. His sweat and mine sucked our naked chests into each other. I am left there, and they are left there, and my mother withdraws further from my raw state, and I protest, cry and collapse, headfirst in a screaming, mute heap. This was the terrible dance of the transference.

I'd told him about losing it with John when he turned away from the hot bath I'd drawn for him. It was my empathy for him working outdoors in the cold rain. "I got it, this is my mother. This was why I was scared of being 'caught' doing something to help her. She never received this. There was no acknowledgment." Arles told me about Harold Searles, who wrote about the mother's disdain for the child's care of her. "Searles said that 'madness was the defense' against this." I got riled.

"It is not a defense! It is the only possible, primary response."

"Yes," he said, "That's true. It's primary."

"You couldn't accept my gratitude before I recognized this aggression, could you?" He answered quickly but not too quickly, "No, I couldn't, Sebern."

Last week, I don't remember before or after his explosion and our evolving reconciliation, *I dreamt of a mental hospital with bright lemon-yellow walls. No one, I think, knew why I was there or still there, and I had the run of the place. I was outside and had a key to get into my room. It wasn't clear, maybe not even a question until I woke up, whether I could use the key to get out. The room has no furniture, like a seclusion room, I think, with an indoor/outdoor rug. There were two other women, both walking, aimless in their disordered minds, back-and-forth. I went to sit in the corner. Kinnery from the Institute came and said about one of the other women and me, "I am disappointed in you for being back." She exempted the pacer. She was not back; she never left.*

I asked him.

"Yes, when I read the dream, I thought, 'Oh, she's back there'. I was disappointed."

"Would you be disappointed if I were a Holocaust survivor and dreamt of the camp in lemon-yellow?" We are on the phone. "You've said several different times that no one recovers from the things that happened to me. I can live with this. I have the key, and the walls are lemon-yellow."

"Right, that's right."

I weave my way into a dream about *being at a conference in Iceland, trying to meet some demand for writing an academic paper on something akin to personality or borderline disorder, and not getting it right or not being able to conform to the expectations. I was watching a man surfing in the night. He was with his baby son, who also surfed. At one point, it was body surfing, and I could see the boy in the curl of the wave, fully illuminated by the light generated within it. When I asked the father how old he was—he seemed many ages—he told me nine. I wanted to learn how to surf, and he wanted to teach me. I looked back at the restaurant that housed the conference, and it looked dark, as if nothing were going on.*

Bessel was at a table there. He was writing a response paper that I couldn't write, and Ruth was there too, to tell me what the woman who wanted the paper would accept. It would mean rewriting my section entirely. Instead, I asked this man to teach me to surf. The surf was high, and the board was a two-foot plank. When we got to Wales, an announcement came through that the next outing into the night surf would come on September 8. I realized with grief and disappointment and some new awareness that life goes on, it just goes on.

"You are learning now in this late stage of life to surf the Living Water, the vast, infinite expanse of Being. It is a choice between an enduring, awakening self and the illusions of Mara. Don't fall asleep."

Deep Brain Reorienting

Ruth invited me to London to meet the author of a new therapy that had "brain" in the title. She wanted me to try it. I demurred, thinking to myself, "There is no way other than neurofeedback to reach the brain. It's a day to get to London. It can't be what the title claims it to be, and on like this until Deep Brain Reorienting faded from my awareness."

"I've been doing this new thing, and I'm seeing results that seem pretty close to those you see with neurofeedback," Peggy told me three years later. "It's called DBR, and it's about the brainstem. I can't keep up with the neuroscience, but it works. I've stopped using EMDR. We do this instead." She told me about some of her cases and this strange approach, and I remembered Ruth's invitation to meet Frank Corrigan, the author. I helped Peggy pass the test with what little I knew of the brainstem. "You know, Sebern," she said, "it would be a shame for you to write this book on trauma without having tried this. You might even be able to work with Frank."

In mid-September, I began Deep Brain Reorienting with Frank. On November 1st, I went on retreat at the Forest Refuge.

"Dear Arles,

"I am trying to find a pad of paper here and an envelope to write to you. It's very important. I think I am beginning to see, hear, feel, and taste, at least the beginnings of what you've been wanting me to get, but my revelation has to come through you. I have come down to my car, and the signal here is ok. I dialed my recording, and I could hear it. If you can talk with me on Monday, I will come here to do it. Anytime in the afternoon. I will look for your response."

I smiled at the bumper sticker on the car from Louisiana, parked next to me: "Humidity."

"This is a moment of awakening. You know what they're like. I need you to be closer to open further to this mystery. No theory, not even Buddhist ones. Moment to moment, you and me. Absence is a powerful field. You can get lost in it too, particularly on the phone in a car in a parking lot." He let me know he was there and listening.

"I woke up happy and knew immediately that I was in your care. You'd found me. I was secure. My mind went to Butch Cassidy and the Sundance Kid, charming thieves, and they were in custody, I guess in your custody. So maybe somewhere between care and custody," I paused and shifted on the cold seat. "You would materialize, then I would and then the events of my life. My pale heart will fill up with blood."

After realizing that I was feeling secure and happy, I remembered a fragment of a dream. *I was in some kind of written interaction with a bank in London that was laundering terrorist money.* Fuck. It's still fucking there.

"I am trusting you with my mind. My heart, too, but my mind. Hold me to it."

He wrote back, "I will."

There are two kinds of suffering. There is suffering that leads to more suffering, and there is suffering that leads to less suffering. Last night in meditation, I saw it again, that I have suffered the first way most of my life, and that somewhere, ambivalently at first, it changed to the second. It was when I began my deep work with Arles, and then with neurofeedback and the body work and now also with DBR. It was always my instinct, but I was caught in the deepest condition of trauma, well, that, yes, but even more the condition of absence.

I wrote to ask Arles if I was the most unmothered of his patients, and he answered immediately, "Yes." In a second email a few hours later, I asked, "Am I one of the most brutalized patients you have treated?" and he wrote back simply, "Yes." I read each mail several times, as if they were long, complicated paragraphs that I had to unravel. The two arise together, the possibility and the refusal of possibility. I turned my mind to it, like a fair and honest lawyer or perhaps a DA, and I assembled the facts, mostly from body work. I don't, haven't, couldn't be making that up. Or the times with Arles, with the footfalls or the bruises that would just appear. The narrative is untrustable, it is so far away. Once any of this is spoken, it disappears from the page. I don't believe what I have just said.

Something surfaces in a dark pool. I am spilling over with tears, fumbling with the key code to my room, and then, once inside, I begin to sob.

"I made a vow. No one would ever know what happened to me."

When I put this into words, it is like disappearing ink, but the feeling, the rush of empathy and grief for the little child that made this vow, that cannot be denied. I cannot deny it. I shared this with Arles in an email so I wouldn't lose it entirely. I sent it and just watched as I turned against it.

"There was a part of me that has always been in opposition to you."

"Yes, always."

Ruth's slide of the absent Default Mode is the expert testimony. Arles is the witness. When I began this therapy, my brain had no default mode network. Now I do, and I must be responsible for it, not to, as the Buddhists call it, habit energy. There is a "him" and a "me." My opposition is like a small boulder, or a period at the end of a sentence. I made a new vow to dissolve this habit, to begin a new practice of turning toward. I woke up Tuesday morning, secure and happy. Happy has seemed like such a limp word, like floppy, but this happiness felt robust.

There he was, his face formed as a face, a little in the darkness, but discernible, not quite his face, but like in a dream, I knew it was his face. I wrote to him, "I am in your care. Or somewhere between care and custody." He wrote back, "Yes, you are in my care." By Saturday, it was eroding, and I felt desolate. I caught it, my muscles tensing up to once again turn away.

That night in the hall, I took this on. I arranged the cushions to help my back sit meditation into the night. I settled in. An exchange came from years ago, "Nothing will happen in this therapy that you don't want to happen, but that does not mean that you are in control here. You are not." His voice, his clarity, his hands set up a corral around the herd of wild horses that are my habits. I bit his hand; he smacked mine. It got me back to him. Turning against "You are in my care," this is just conditioning, this is just ego, this is just habit. I dissolved it again and again until my back said, "No more tonight. Time for bed." This came in his voice through my voice in my ears. I slept until 5 and woke up happy, although a little tremulous at this, "in his care."

There are different kinds of trauma memory. There is trauma you remember, and there's trauma you don't. And when it is remembered, when it surfaces slowly from the bottom, like a dead body without enough stones in the pockets, it is believed. There is an 'aha' moment or many, and they can be shocking. This person needs a lot of help, but they believe what has surfaced. They just see it, the corpse of it. And then there is trauma memory that surfaces, without narrative, without a self to validate it, no self there to have experienced it to begin with. Frank had said to me, "You will believe it because you will feel it." I responded from years of progress, "Feeling it makes it, at best, more proximate to real." I'd said to Arles on the phone in the car, "For this to become real to me first requires that you become real to me." I began to get a headache.

"Is there a 'No' in the headache?"

"No, Arles, there is no 'No.'" Even in all the tidal ebbs and flows of this in the last few days, the tide of him comes in. I can use the contact point, the memory of his hands when I felt contacted for the first time by another body, his hands that left an imprint and slowly, meaning. And then the tide goes out, and I am stranded in the effluvia of habit, but there isn't a 'No.'

Trying to experience who that baby is, the baby in the photo, is like trying to tie a dinghy to a fog. Without intervention, she is one month away from an inescapable psychiatric illness.

Caroline asked me how I used retreats, and I answered partially, predictably and Buddhistly. We have been out of sync, and I put it together last night, sitting with my chamomile tea with honey. I came on Tuesday, she gave the dharma talk, I saw there was an opening on the interview sheet and delighted, I took it. I went in for the community sit the next morning expecting her, and there was a total stranger, the other teacher. She was attending a memorial service. I did register the slight shock at seeing him and then let it subside. But I did count the days. He told me she would be back Sunday night, but off on Monday. After the interview with him, my light, spacious mind with its high, thin clouds collapsed. At some level, I was frantic. It may have been then that I doubled down on making access to Arles, knowing Arles, getting the reality of him, the focus of my meditation for the rest of the retreat. It's what I have to do.

I don't know, really, what to say to Caroline, but it started there. My meditation has been focused on discerning the qualities of this infant's mind, and, for seconds, that she is me. This mind formed in absence, not neglect. I want to know the texture of that reality, the nature of this mind that cannot certify its own reality, the reality of her, of being at all. I put my hands around that small head and gently extracted that mind from the true mind of emptiness and luminosity. I want to do this for me, I want to do this for everyone who suffers like this, and I want to do this for those who treat, and those who teach those who treat. It is my calling. It is my bodhisattva incarnation. I want to discern the truth that obscures the truth.

I sat down that night to experience luminosity the way Anne and some of her students have described it, lights dancing at the crown. I closed my eyes. I sat for almost an hour and a half, opening my mind. I feel this in the center of my brain. My mind, dark sepia tones, came up against the edge of space and fused with it. It was absorbed. I whispered to myself, "This isn't so hard!" and smiled. Soon after, almost as an instruction, the thought arose, "Bring the baby here." The photograph that Arles had protected from me, that baby arose in a circular cradle of light. The space that opened in the midst of my brain was not luminous, but it was lit up, like the full moon behind cumulus clouds, enough to see the baby in the bassinet in the bottom half of the space. Her expression didn't change, but I was able to hold both images, one within the other.

I sat in the airless phone room with the white noise machine outside the door. I had begun to mourn the end of all the work we had planned.

"Let's see how this unfolds," he said, his voice threaded across endless miles of phone line. "You are in my care."

More muscles let go in my shoulder. I had just gotten him. This can't be over.

I opened my eyes after meditation, sought out the shivering young beech tree in its orange leaves, and it came, "I am alone." It wasn't, I told Caroline later, ever as cold as "a fact of life"; it was simply "Isness." She nodded and smiled. I closed my eyes again, and after a while, I felt an energy, like a warm coin in my palm. Someone had left it there for whoever might pick it up. Energy entered the tip of my middle finger and up into the cocoon of my head. The second round was all energy, running through me, and surrounding me almost like one would swaddle a baby.

I stayed in my PJ bottoms, John's undershirt, soft with his smell, and my sweater that I wore often during my meditations on retreat. John couldn't be home, but he anticipated what I needed. He had made the meals. I folded into time. I just lived in time. When I went to meditate on Wednesday, I realized I was worried about the stress on my brain. It felt like my personality was melting off me. I said to myself sweetly, simply, "Just meet life where it is."

As the sky darkened, the woods outside my large window, he told me of his state shift when I said, "I rely on you." His voice broke.

"This is the first time you have allowed me into the inner sanctum of you." And still, even with all this deep attention, I was surprised. He told me later that after that session, he went to his bookcase, wall-length and height, and his hand landed on a book of commentary on the poems of a Holocaust poet. He opened to a poem, Black Milk, and there was a card I'd sent him years ago. It was a picture of a little girl, sucking her thumb with a tiger cub's alert face poised on her neck as she slept. It was, he said, a kind of reverie.

"This card was both a presentation of you, but also a revealing of you."

"It is a miracle, Arles, a miracle of us."

"I don't want to go back to the attic, Arles."

"I hope we won't need to."

Toward the end, I asked him, "What would the signal be that we might have to?" He took a long time to answer.

"Our experience will let us know, but why are you asking that now in the flow of this? It casts a shadow."

Slowly, realizing it, I answered. "It is about you saying that I am in your care. You just got here. I am just now, newly in your care, and I don't want to lose this. Not yet. I want to sleep in a hammock of light, but you have to be there, Arles. You have to be there."

His voice is soft, and he fades away from me on the phone. He wants the solitude of the pandemic; he has this final opportunity for the monastic life. He will not say that I will never see him again, but I know I won't.

Somehow, even on the phone, I know when I have his complete attention. We were talking about our excursion into the underworld.

"I think you're right. I don't want to go further in this direction," I said. "I'm willing to bear my unconscious. I am just trying to make sense of what you called 'Hell.'" I looked out the window and turned back to the phone. "The depths of the unconscious are endless and unknowable.

My mother's mind and your mother's mind, it's a field that is beyond psychology, philosophy, meditation, even the deepest, most devoted conversation." He waited for me. "Maybe it is that I'm too old, Arles. Maybe it is that I have finally made peace with myself. Maybe it is that I lack courage, vision or commitment. Maybe it's that I am tired. All of that could be true. But I think, more simply, that I treasure this peace and want to engage in practices that deepen it. And, you know, it just may be time for a pause and a new direction either for us together or for me on my own. Wherever we go, it has to be different than this."

He joined me, right there. He began softly.

"I have been thinking about this, too, Sebern. The thought that arose was 'the unconscious is an infinite set' and that it cares only about its own self-replication. It does this automatically once it is given any sustained attention. I think the unconscious is agnostic with respect to peace. Spirit, though, is eternal. It has always been with you, with us. In contrast to the infinite unconscious, it is gentle and spacious. Its fabric is peace, a very different kind of mother, present from before the beginning." My cell phone went off, and he waited until I had buried it under pillows. "We have related from this space many times. I think now it is calling us forth with a new gentle imperative." My cough interrupted him. "When you get back, I will welcome you into our spiritual home, and we will celebrate all the richness you have accomplished in your precious life."

We observed a mutual silence, and then he added, "And, Sebern, be careful on this trip. You are facing considerable demand from a starting point of depletion."

"Thank you. Thank you, I will." I paused to swallow and then added, "Wherever we go, Arles, I will never leave you, and you will never leave me."

"Yes, Sebern, I know this is true."

Tomorrow, I am leaving for the UK in great part to meet Frank Corrigan, to learn more about Deep Brain Reorienting and to introduce him to neurofeedback. There is more for each of us to learn from the practice of the other. The absence of my parents and all that happened as a consequence became my life. It becomes everyone's life who survives the many deaths of absence and assault. I live now in the abundance of presence, and I am safe. It is still my life. As I am writing, an image emerges: the dream boulder filling the gap in the mountains just under the sea. And then the question, "How do we dislodge this from the DNA?"

www.ingramcontent.com/pod-product-compliance
Lightning Source LLC
LaVergne TN
LVHW011533200926
848484LV00001B/258